Cardiovascular Pharmacology
Volume 1

Karen Petty Marzlin DNP, CNS, CNP
Cynthia Webner DNP, CNS, CNP
Carol Jacobson MN

Published by:
Cardiovascular Nursing Education Associates (CNEA)
3324 SW 172nd St.
Burien, WA 98166

ISBN print version: 978-1-7335811-4-1
ISBN ebook version: 978-1-7335811-6-5
ISBN pdf version: 978-1-7335811-8-9

Notice:

Every effort has been made to assure the accuracy of information presented and to describe accepted and current practice. Health care is a rapidly changing field, and new research and clinical experience may prompt changes in practice, including drug and device therapy, that are different from what is presented in this text. Care has been taken to confirm the accuracy of drug information presented, including indications, dosage, and side effects. Readers are advised to check the package insert and the most current information available for each drug to verify correct dosage and for added warnings and precautions. Neither the publisher nor the authors assume any liability for injury and/or damage to persons or property due to application of the information presented in this book.

Purchasing Options

This book is available both in a print edition and as an EPUB.
Go to **www.learn-cardionursing.com** for pricing information and to order.

Cover design by Gina O'Daniel, O'Danieldesigns.com

About Cardiovascular Nursing Education Associates

Carol, Karen, and Cindy are passionate about nursing practice and nursing education. CNEA was established in 2005, when the three of us joined together to offer continuing education and certification review courses for nurses, who were engaged in advancing their knowledge of cardiovascular and critical care nursing practice. We quickly discovered that we had synergy in teaching and helping the learner to really understand and apply information rather than just memorizing facts. We teach and design products to help nurses in every role excel. Our mission through CNEA is to empower nurses to link knowledge to clinical practice for the purpose of improving patient outcomes. We believe that Exceptional Nurses = Exceptional Patient Care.

Go to **www.learn-cardionursing.com** for all of our online classes and educational products.

Acknowledgments

Thank you to Ron Gangnes at Angle Lake Printing in Seattle for helping us with printing.

Thank you to Gina O'Daniel at O'Danieldesigns.com in Seattle for the cover design.

Thank you to Thad McIlroy at The Future of Publishing for his help getting this book into electronic format.

Dedication

This book is dedicated to all our exceptional nurse colleagues who are committed to practicing with excellence and who bring healing to patients and families in the work they do.

Objectives

1. Compare the similarities and differences between ACE inhibitors (ACEIs) and angiotensin receptor blockers (ARBs) for indications, monitoring, and adverse effects.
2. Differentiate between changes in renal function where ACEIs and ARBs must be held and when they are safe to be continued.
3. Describe the differences and similarities between the dihydropyridine and the non-dihydropyridine calcium channel blockers (CCBS).
4. Explain the rationale for using beta blockers to reduce mortality post myocardial infarction (MI) and in patients with heart failure with reduced ejection fraction (HFrEF).
5. Discuss how the hold criteria for beta blockers is different in the setting of an acute MI compared to in the treatment of HFrEF.
6. List the cardiovascular indications for sodium-glucose cotransporter 2 inhibitors (SGLT2Is).
7. Recognize risk factors for the development of euglycemic diabetic ketoacidosis (DKA) in a patient taking an SGLT2I.
8. Define dose equivalents between the loop diuretics furosemide, torsemide, and bumetanide.
9. Clarify how to transition between oral and IV and between IV and oral dosing of loop diuretics.
10. Review the clinical indications in which mineralocorticoid receptor antagonists have demonstrated improved clinical outcomes.
11. Contrast 0.9% normal saline (NS) and balanced crystalloids in terms of potential risk for the development of hyperchloremic metabolic acidosis.
12. Name potential adverse effects with the use of hypertonic and hypotonic IV fluids.
13. Analyze the impact of each sympathomimetic drug on beta1, beta2, and alpha1 receptors.
14. Initiate appropriate interventions in the management of extravasation of a vasoactive medication.
15. Summarize the differences between indications for IV dobutamine and IV dopamine.
16. Evaluate similarities and differences between milrinone and dobutamine.
17. Assess the similarities and differences between norepinephrine and vasopressin.
18. Paraphrase the rationale for the use of vasopressin in septic shock.
19. Distinguish the reasons why hydralazine and minoxidil are not first line agents in the treatment of hypertension.
20. Determine the appropriate process for weaning a patient on clonidine.
21. Create patient education key points when instructing a patient on how to use nitrates and maintain the recommended nitrate free period.
22. Develop a monitoring plan for recognizing potential cyanide toxicity in a patient receiving nitroprusside.
23. Select 3 important aspects of safe medication prescribing or administration that you have learned and are committed to implementing into practice.
24. Commit to teaching a colleague one thing you learned in this book that has the potential to change patient outcomes in your area of practice.
25. Decide the next step you will take to expand your knowledge or skill in your area of clinical or educational practice.

CARDIOVASCULAR PHARMACOLOGY VOLUME 1

Table of Contents

CARDIOVASCULAR PHARMACOLOGY: VOLUME 1

INTRODUCTION

Welcome to Volume 1 of this comprehensive and practical resource that will increase your level of wisdom, provide practical strategies for the application of knowledge, and expand your impact on patient outcomes. While reading this book you will be motivated, challenged, and inspired as you learn.

This book is written from a clinician perspective for the purpose of imparting applicable insights. You will learn the physiology of medication actions and their clinical impact, which provides the basis for safe and effective prescribing, administering, and monitoring. You will also gain education and counseling skills to help patients and families become active partners in implementing their pharmacological treatment plan.

Whether you are a seasoned advanced practice registered nurse (APRN) or a novice registered nurse (RN) this book will take your knowledge, skills, and clinical decision making to the next level.

Volume 1 of *Cardiovascular Pharmacology* covers the physiological basis of drug therapy and the following medication categories:

☐ Angiotensin converting enzyme inhibitors	☐ Diuretics
☐ Angiotensin receptor blockers alone and with a neprilysin inhibitor	☐ Additional antihypertensives
	☐ Inotropes
☐ Mineralocorticoid receptor antagonists	☐ Vasopressors
☐ Renin inhibitors	☐ Vasodilators
☐ Beta blockers	☐ Nitrates
☐ Calcium channel blockers	☐ Crystalloids
☐ Sodium glucose co-transporter 2 inhibitors	☐ Colloids

Volume 2 of *Cardiovascular Pharmacology* will include strategies for improving medication reconciliation and patient adherence and will cover the following categories:

☐ Fibrinolytics	☐ Lipid lowering agents
☐ Anticoagulants	☐ Electrolytes
☐ Antiplatelets	☐ Potassium binders
☐ Antiarrhythmics	☐ Iron & erythropoietin stimulating agents
☐ Digoxin	☐ Ivabradine & vericiguat
☐ Pulmonary vasodilators	☐ Tafamidis
☐ Diabetes medications	☐ Mavacamten

In this updated edition of *Cardiovascular Pharmacology*, we have included the following features to engage you and enhance your learning:

- **Tables and Figures** to compare and contrast pharmacological details and provide visual examples.
- **Linking Knowledge to Practice** nuggets that provide specific ways to implement new knowledge.
- **Prescribing Pearls** with additional insights and considerations for APRNs.
- **Advanced Concept Focus** topics that take a deep dive and give clarity around challenging concepts.
- **Content Boxes** containing standalone information on important and interesting aspects of care.
- **Appendices (**drug tables) at the end of the book to provide a concise reference of medication specifics.

Throughout this book we provide information and applications in a way that brings clarity to complex information. However, this book is not intended to be the sole source of information necessary for prescribing or administering medications. We have purposely not included every fact related to each medication to provide a resource that is practical and relevant for RNs and APRNs. A basic level of pharmacological knowledge is assumed and thus, for example, we do not list allergy as a contraindication for each medication since it is a standard of care to assess allergies before prescribing or administering a medication. We also include only select examples of more common potential medication interactions. This book does not provide information about the use and safety of these medications in women who are pregnant or breast feeding. Pediatric indications and dosing are also excluded in this resource. When needed, it is important for the RN and APRN to refer to the manufacturers individual prescribing information, UptoDate®, Lexidrug™, or other pharmaceutical references for more complete information about specific medications.

PHYSIOLOGIC BASIS OF CARDIOVASCULAR DRUG THERAPY

The primary function of the cardiovascular (CV) system is to provide oxygen (O_2) and nutrients to every cell in the body so that each cell and every organ system can optimally perform its own individual function. Basic components of the CV system include:

- The heart which serves as the pump to eject O_2 rich blood into the arteries.
- The arteries that carry oxygenated blood to the tissues.
- The veins that return blood to the heart after the tissues extract O_2.
- The blood volume that fills the vascular space and maintains hemodynamic stability.

While the heart's basic function is to serve as a pump, the pumping effectiveness of the heart is more complex. It is determined by multiple factors including the status of the myocardium, electrical system, cardiac valves, blood volume, and blood vessel tone. Dysfunction of the CV system can lead to hemodynamic instability. Hemodynamic parameters are evaluated by physical exam or hemodynamic monitoring, and these same components can be altered with drug therapy to restore hemodynamic stability. The sympathetic nervous system (SNS), renin-angiotensin-aldosterone system (RAAS), endocrine system, renal system, and endothelium are involved in regulation of CV hemodynamics. CV pharmacology can be used to optimize the physiological response of these systems to enhance CV function.

The physiological concepts below provide a basis for understanding CV drug therapy:

- Determinants of cardiac output (CO).
- Myocardial O_2 supply and demand.
- SNS.
- RAAS.

Determinants of Cardiac Output

CO is the amount of blood pumped by the heart each minute, normally 4 to 8 liters in a normal-sized adult. It is the product of heart rate (HR) times stroke volume (SV). SV is the amount of blood ejected with each heartbeat and varies widely among individuals, normally around 60 to 120 milliliters (mLs) per beat.

Understanding this formula is key to understanding drug therapy aimed at optimizing CO.

Formula for Cardiac Output

$$CO = HR \times SV$$

The two sides of the equation must balance each other. Therefore, if the CO is low, look at the other side of the equation to determine why: it must be either an abnormal HR or a low SV (or both problems). Conversely, if you want to increase CO, you must go to the other side of the equation to do it: improve either HR or SV.

The three major determinants of SV are preload, afterload, and contractility.

Linking Knowledge to Practice

- ✓ *A low SV is the most common reason for low CO. When SV falls, HR will increase to compensate and maintain an adequate CO. In this situation the focus is to improve the SV, not to correct the HR.*
- ✓ *Less commonly low CO is caused by an abnormal HR such as occurs with complete heat block or the development of a tachyarrhythmia. In this case the treatment is to correct the arrhythmia.*

Preload

Preload is ventricular fiber length prior to contraction. The Frank-Starling law of the heart says that up to a certain point the longer the fibers, the better they contract. In the ventricles, blood volume is what stretches the fibers, so we think of preload as volume in the ventricles at the end of diastole. Up to a point, the more volume in the ventricles, the better they contract. However, if the fibers get too long or are overstretched their performance declines and SV is reduced.

Each ventricle has its own preload. When using a pulmonary artery catheter, the right atrial pressure (RAP) is used as the clinical indicator of right ventricular (RV) preload. This is an indirect measurement of RV preload and assumes that increased volume in the RV will generate an increased pressure that will be transmitted back to the right atrium thus generating an elevated RAP. This is true when cardiac function is normal, but RAP is not always an accurate indicator of RV volume. For example: tricuspid valve stenosis will result in an elevation of RAP in the absence of RV volume overload. The central venous pressure (CVP) can also be used as an indirect indicator of RV preload. RV preload can also be evaluated noninvasively. Jugular venous distention or jugular venous pulsation more than 3 cm above the sternal angle when the head of bed is elevated 30 to 45 degrees is an indicator of RV volume overload.

When using a pulmonary artery catheter, the pulmonary artery occlusion pressure (PAOP) is used as the clinical indicator of left ventricular (LV) preload. The PAOP is an indirect measurement of left atrial pressure which is an indirect measurement of LV pressure. As with RAP there are limitations of using the PAOP as an assessment of LV preload. Mitral valve stenosis and diastolic dysfunction are two examples where left atrial pressure and the PAOP can be elevated even in the absence of increased LV volume.

LV preload can also be assessed non-invasively. Orthopnea or bendopnea are two signs of elevated LV preload. The evaluation of a patient's hemodynamic status is discussed in detail in the *Cardiac Essentials* book within this series.

Factors Impacting Preload

- Blood volume: Hypovolemia reduces preload, hypervolemia increases preload.
- Distribution of blood volume: The following factors determine whether blood returns to the ventricles or is distributed away from them.
    - Venous tone: Venous vasodilation causes volume to stay in the dilated venous system rather than being returned to the heart.
    - Body position: Sitting upright with feet on the floor is the best position for a patient in pulmonary edema because it uses gravity to help distribute blood away from the heart into the dependent extremities. Conversely, lying flat with legs elevated is a body position used in hypotension to help redistribute blood from the peripheral circulation back to the heart.
    - Intrathoracic pressure: The heart sits in the thorax, and it is affected by intrathoracic pressure. Normal intrathoracic pressure does not interfere with ventricular filling, but if intrathoracic pressure rises, that pressure is transmitted to the heart and pushes on it from the outside, thus limiting the ability of the ventricles to expand and fill. Examples of high intrathoracic pressure that can lead to preload reduction include pneumothorax and the addition of positive end expiratory pressure (PEEP) to a ventilator.
    - Intrapericardial pressure: The heart is surrounded by a non-distensible fibrous pericardial sac that normally contains between 10 to 30 mL of fluid to lubricate the heart as it moves during contraction and relaxation. If excess fluid accumulates in the pericardial sac, it limits ventricular filling in the same way that a pneumothorax does, by constricting the ventricles and limiting their ability to fill.
- Atrial kick: Atrial kick refers to atrial contribution to ventricular filling. Normally in sinus rhythm, the atria contract just before the ventricles and contribute 20 to 30% more volume (over the volume added during passive filling in early diastole) into the ventricles just before ventricular contraction, thus increasing preload by stretching ventricular fibers a little more, just prior to contraction. Any rhythm that causes a loss of atrial kick, such as atrial fibrillation, atrial flutter, ventricular paced rhythm, or any rhythm that results in atrioventricular (AV) dissociation, can reduce preload.
- LV function: How well the ventricles handle blood volume is determined by LV function. Normal functioning ventricles can handle additional volume by increasing the HR and force of contraction. With LV dysfunction, however, the ventricles are unable to compensate for increased volume and, therefore, ventricular pressures rise, resulting in venous and pulmonary congestion and ultimately heart failure.

Figure 1 summarizes the determinants of preload. Table 1 outlines clinical conditions impacting preload.

Pharmacology and Other Treatments to Alter Preload

- Volume administration with crystalloid, colloid, or blood products will increase preload.
- Stopping diuretics and venous vasodilating medications, or decreasing their doses, is a strategy to increase preload.
- Reestablishing and maintaining sinus rhythm in atrial fibrillation or flutter also increases preload.
- Loop diuretics and venous vasodilators are the two main methods of decreasing preload.

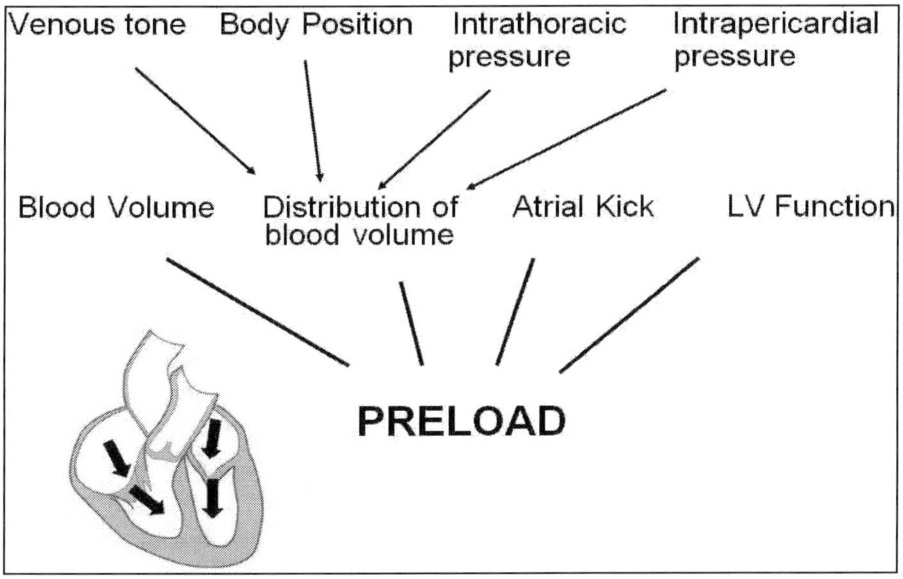

Figure 1: Determinants of Preload

Table 1
Clinical Conditions Influencing Preload

Conditions that Decrease Preload	Conditions that Increase Preload
▪ **Hypovolemia** √ Hemorrhage √ Dehydration / over diuresis √ Burns √ Third Spacing	▪ **Hypervolemia** √ Overhydration / Excess IV fluids √ Heart failure √ Renal disease
▪ **Altered Size of Vascular Space (venous vasodilation)** √ Sepsis √ Spinal or epidural anesthesia √ Anaphylaxis √ Venous vasodilating drugs	▪ **Altered Size of Vascular Space (venous vasoconstriction)** √ Vasopressors. √ Hypothermia.

Linking Knowledge to Practice

- ✓ *Venous vasodilation is one of the strategies available for reducing preload in a patient with symptomatic heart failure. Nitrates (NTG and its relatives) are primarily venous vasodilators. Venous vasodilators redistribute existing volume by dilating veins which results in more volume distributed in the periphery and away from the heart.*
- ✓ *Loop diuretics also reduce preload by reducing total circulating volume.*
- ✓ *Any other pharmacological or non-pharmacological treatments that result in improved SV will improve LV emptying and therefore reduce LV preload.*

Afterload

Afterload is the amount of work a ventricle must do to eject its volume. Clinically we think of resistance to ejection as afterload. Systemic vascular resistance (SVR) is used to assess LV afterload, because the LV ejects into the systemic circulation. Pulmonary vascular resistance (PVR) is used to assess RV afterload because the RV ejects into the pulmonary vasculature.

Noninvasively the pulse pressure is a good indicator of LV afterload. A narrow pulse pressure (< 35 millimeters of mercury [mmHg]) indicates an increase in SVR, and a wide pulse pressure (> 40 mmHg) indicates a decrease in SVR. RV afterload is difficult to evaluate noninvasively.

Factors Impacting Afterload

- SVR is determined primarily by the amount of vasoconstriction or vasodilation of the small peripheral arterioles. PVR is more evenly distributed between the pulmonary arteries, the pulmonary capillaries, and the pulmonary veins. PVR is about $^1/_{10}$ of SVR. Vascular tone in the systemic and pulmonary vasculature is influenced by the SNS activity and by circulating vasoconstrictor or vasodilator substances such as endothelin, angiotensin II, kinins, histamines, and others.
- When a patient is treated with vasopressors for hypotension there will be vasoconstriction of the arterioles and an increase in SVR. This increase in SVR can adversely affect LV function in a patient with systolic dysfunction.
- It is important to remember that the process of compensatory pulmonary vasoconstriction that occurs in the setting of any alveolar hypoxia will increase RV afterload. Placing a patient on positive pressure ventilation or any increase in PEEP will also increase the workload of the RV.
- Vascular compliance refers to the "distensibility" or ability of blood vessels to stretch to accommodate blood volume. A stiff, noncompliant aorta increases LV afterload, and a noncompliant pulmonary artery increases RV afterload.
- Valve stenosis also contributes to the work of ventricular ejection. Pulmonic and aortic stenosis increase afterload for the RV and LV, respectively.
- Outflow tract obstruction from hypertrophic obstructive cardiomyopathy (HOCM) is obstruction of the LV outflow tract due to septal and LV free wall hypertrophy. This contributes to an increased afterload for the LV in the same way as aortic stenosis.

Figure 2 illustrates determinants of LV afterload.

Pharmacology and Other Treatments to Alter Afterload

- Drugs that cause pulmonary or peripheral arterial vasodilation are used to decrease afterload, commonly referred to as afterload reduction therapy.
- The intra-aortic balloon pump is a non-pharmacological strategy that can be used to reduce LV afterload.
- Drugs that cause systemic vasoconstriction increase LV afterload and increase the workload of the LV. Many of the vasopressors used to treat systemic hypotension will also increase PVR.
- Vasoconstrictor drugs (called vasopressors) include norepinephrine, epinephrine, high dose dopamine, phenylephrine, and vasopressin.

Linking Knowledge to Practice

✓ *It is important to remember that while a vasoconstricting medication may increase BP in a patient with hypotension, it will also increase SVR. An increase in SVR will increase the workload of the heart and can adversely impact SV in a patient with poor ventricular function.*

✓ *Vasoconstriction of peripheral vessels also increases resistance to blood flow and therefore an improvement in BP does not always result in an improvement in blood flow. A patient on high doses of vasopressor therapy can develop distal peripheral ischemia of the toes.*

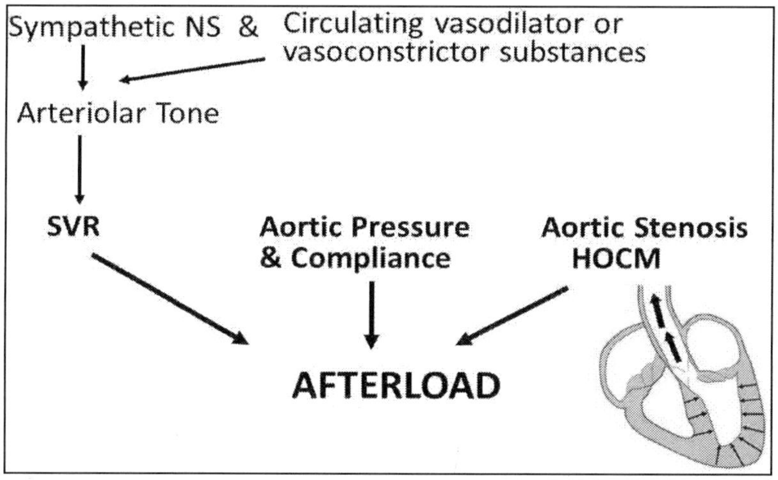

Conditions that Alter Afterload:

Vasodilation
- Sepsis
- Spinal or epidural anesthesia
- Anaphylaxis
- Arterial dilating drugs

Vasoconstriction
- HTN
- Compensatory vasoconstriction
- Arterial vasoconstrictor drugs

Figure 2: Determinants of Afterload

Table 2 lists common afterload reducers.

Table 2

Common Afterload Reducers

Systemic Arterial Vasodilators	Pulmonary Specific Vasodilators
▪ Angiotensin converting enzyme inhibitors (ACEIs) and angiotensin receptor blockers (ARBs) (by preventing arterial vasoconstriction) ▪ Calcium channel blockers (CCBs) (also used for pulmonary vasodilation) ▪ Direct smooth muscle relaxants (e.g., hydralazine) ▪ Selective alpha$_1$ blockers (e.g., doxazosin) ▪ Centrally acting alpha$_2$ agonists (e.g., clonidine) ▪ Nitroprusside (Other medications that contain an arterial vasodilator (e.g., milrinone [used as an inotrope but also causes arterial and venous vasodilation] and labetalol [a beta blocker that also contains an alpha$_1$ blocker])	▪ Prostacyclin Analogs √ Epoprostenol √ Treprostinil √ Iloprost √ Selexipag ▪ Endothelin Receptor Antagonists √ Bosentan √ Ambrisentan √ Macitentan ▪ Phosphodiesterase (PDE)-5 Enzyme Inhibitors √ Sildenafil √ Vardenafil √ Tadalafil √ Avanafil ▪ Soluble Guanylate Cyclase Stimulator √ Riociguat

Contractility

Contractility refers to the ability of cardiac fibers to develop tension and shorten. Shortening of cardiac fibers causes ejection of blood from the chamber. The term "inotropic" refers to the contractile state of the heart. Substances or drugs that increase contractility are positive inotropes, while drugs that decrease contractility are negative inotropes.

Contractility is difficult to measure in the clinical setting. LV ejection fraction (EF) (LVEF) and the assessment of RV function from echocardiography are commonly used to evaluate the contractile state of the ventricles. LV stroke work index (LVSWI) which considers both systolic and diastolic dysfunction can be obtained by a Doppler transthoracic echocardiogram. Low LVSWI is associated with short term and long-term mortality in patients in the cardiac intensive care unit (ICU). The noninvasive assessment of LVSWI may be a tool to guide clinical decision making in the future (Clark & McNamara, 2020; Jentzer et al., 2020).

> ***Linking Knowledge to Practice***
>
> ✓ *Patients with an LVEF ≤ 40% are considered to have impaired inotropic function.*

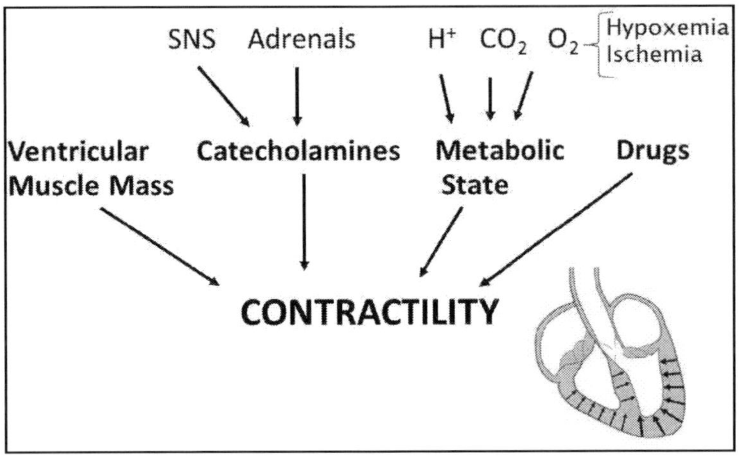

Conditions that Alter Contractility:

Increase

Pheochromocytoma

Hyperthyroidism

Positive inotropic drugs

Decrease

Myocardial infarction

Cardiomyopathy

Ischemia

Hypoxia

Acidosis

Figure 3: Determinants of Contractility

Factors Impacting Contractility

- Adequate ventricular muscle mass (the number of alive and functioning fibers in the ventricle) is necessary for normal contractility. Myocardial infarction (MI) destroys muscle fibers and reduces the number of fibers available to eject blood.
- Catecholamines, circulating substances released by the SNS and the adrenal glands, increase contractility of muscle fibers. Epinephrine, also called adrenaline, is a hormone secreted from the medulla of the adrenal glands. Norepinephrine, also called noradrenaline, is synthesized, and released by both the medulla of the adrenal glands and the neurons of the SNS. Epinephrine and norepinephrine are both released into the blood during the fight or flight response, and both can exert a positive inotropic effect.
- The metabolic state of blood perfusing cardiac fibers is a very important determinant of contractility. Metabolic acidosis and reduced delivery of O_2 to the myocardium (either from hypoxemia or ischemia) cause tissue hypoxia and thus decrease myocardial contractility.

Figure 3 illustrates determinants of contractility.

Pharmacology to Alter Contractility

- Positive inotropic drugs increase contractility and include moderate dose dopamine, dobutamine, milrinone, epinephrine, isoproterenol, and digoxin (considered a weak inotrope).
- Negative inotropic drugs decrease contractility and include beta blockers, CCBs, most antiarrhythmics, many sedatives, anesthetics, and some chemotherapy agents.

Heart Rate

HR is the 4th major determinant of CO. Unless HR is very slow or extremely fast due to a cardiac arrhythmia, it is unlikely to be the cause of a low CO.

Factors Impacting HR

- A slow HR due to a bradyarrhythmia such as complete heart block will reduce CO because CO is determined by SV x HR.

- Mathematically an increase in HR will result in an increase in CO, however, there is a point where an increase in HR will decrease CO. Tachycardia can decrease CO in three ways:
  - Since the ventricles fill with blood during diastole, rapid HR decreases preload and SV by reducing diastolic filling time.
  - The coronary arteries perfuse the myocardium during diastole; therefore, a rapid HR reduces coronary perfusion time.
  - The higher the HR, the more O_2 the myocardium requires. Thus, tachycardia increases myocardial O_2 consumption (MVO_2) and can contribute to angina and heart failure.

Pharmacology and Other Treatments to Alter HR

- Drugs that slow HR include beta blockers, non-dihydropyridine CCBs, digoxin, adenosine, ivabradine, and class IC and class III antiarrhythmics.
- Cardioversion from atrial fibrillation, supraventricular tachycardia (SVT) or ventricular tachycardia (VT) corrects the arrhythmia and thus decreases HR.
- Drugs that increase HR include atropine (parasympatholytic medication that lyses the parasympathetic system), and dopamine and epinephrine (sympathomimetic medications that stimulate beta-1 (ß1) receptors.
- Pacing the heart with an external, temporary transvenous or epicardial pacemaker, or a permanent pacemaker are non-pharmacological strategies to correct an abnormally low HR.

> ***Linking Knowledge to Practice***
>
> ✓ *HR is not the most common reason for a reduced CO. However, HR is almost always abnormal in the setting of a low CO because HR will increase when low SV is the reason for a low CO.*
>
> ✓ *When a patient has a low CO and an abnormal HR it is important to differentiate between an abnormal HR as a cause of the low CO (a primary arrhythmia) or an abnormal HR (typically sinus tachycardia) that is a compensatory response to a low SV.*

Pharmacologic Manipulation of CO

Figure 4 shows drugs commonly used to manipulate the determinants of CO: HR, preload, afterload, and contractility.

Myocardial O_2 Supply and Demand

- A mismatch between myocardial O_2 supply and the heart's demand for O_2 can produce angina. Chest pain can occur with a decrease in O_2 delivery to the myocardium or when there is an increase in myocardial O_2 demand.
- O_2 supply is dependent on open coronary arteries, adequate CO, adequate arterial O_2 content in the blood, and an adequate amount of hemoglobin to carry the O_2. The heart's demand for O_2 is determined by HR, preload, afterload, and contractility.

Figure 5 shows drugs used to manipulate myocardial O_2 supply and demand.

Sympathetic Nervous System

The SNS plays an important role in the CV system in both heart and blood vessels. The SNS works by stimulating either $alpha_1$ ($\alpha 1$) or beta (ß) receptors. $Alpha_1$ receptors are in arteries and veins and when stimulated, they cause vasoconstriction.

Alpha$_2$ ($\alpha 2$) receptors are in the central nervous system (CNS) which includes the brain and spinal cord, and in the periphery. The role of $\alpha 2$ receptors in the periphery is not fully understood. In the CNS $\alpha 2$ receptors, when stimulated, inhibit norepinephrine release and centrally mediate sedation and pain.

There are two types of ß receptors, ß1and ß2. The heart is heavily populated with ß1 receptors, and when they are stimulated, the result is an increase in HR, contractility, automaticity, and conduction velocity through the AV node. In the kidney, ß1 stimulation results in renin release, which activates the RAAS (discussed in more detail below). ß2 stimulation in the peripheral blood vessels causes vasodilation, and in the lungs, it causes bronchodilation.

Drugs that stimulate $\alpha 1$, ß1, or ß2 receptors are called "sympathomimetic" agents because they mimic SNS stimulation.

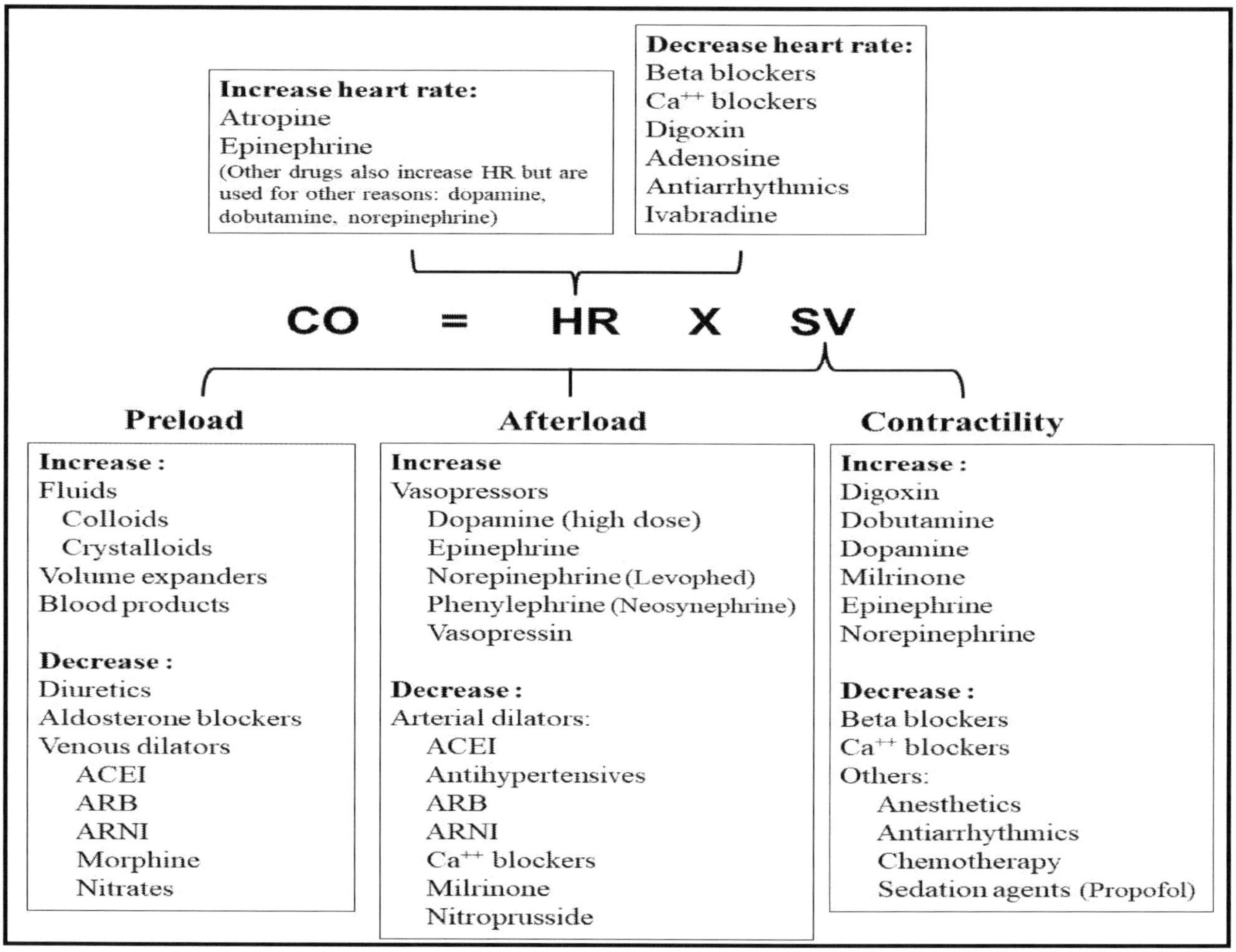

Figure 4: Drugs Commonly Used to Manipulate Cardiac Output

Linking Knowledge to Practice

- ✓ *Both selective alpha$_1$ blockers (e.g., Prazosin) and centrally acting alpha$_2$ agonists (e.g., clonidine) are used in the treatment of HTN.*
- ✓ *Selective alpha$_1$ blockers prevent $\alpha 1$ receptors from causing peripheral vasoconstriction, while centrally acting alpha$_2$ agonists stimulate $\alpha 2$ receptors to inhibit the release of norepinephrine thus preventing vasoconstriction.*
- ✓ *Dexmedetomidine, a sedative used in critical care, is a centrally acting alpha$_2$ agonist that produces non opioid analgesia.*

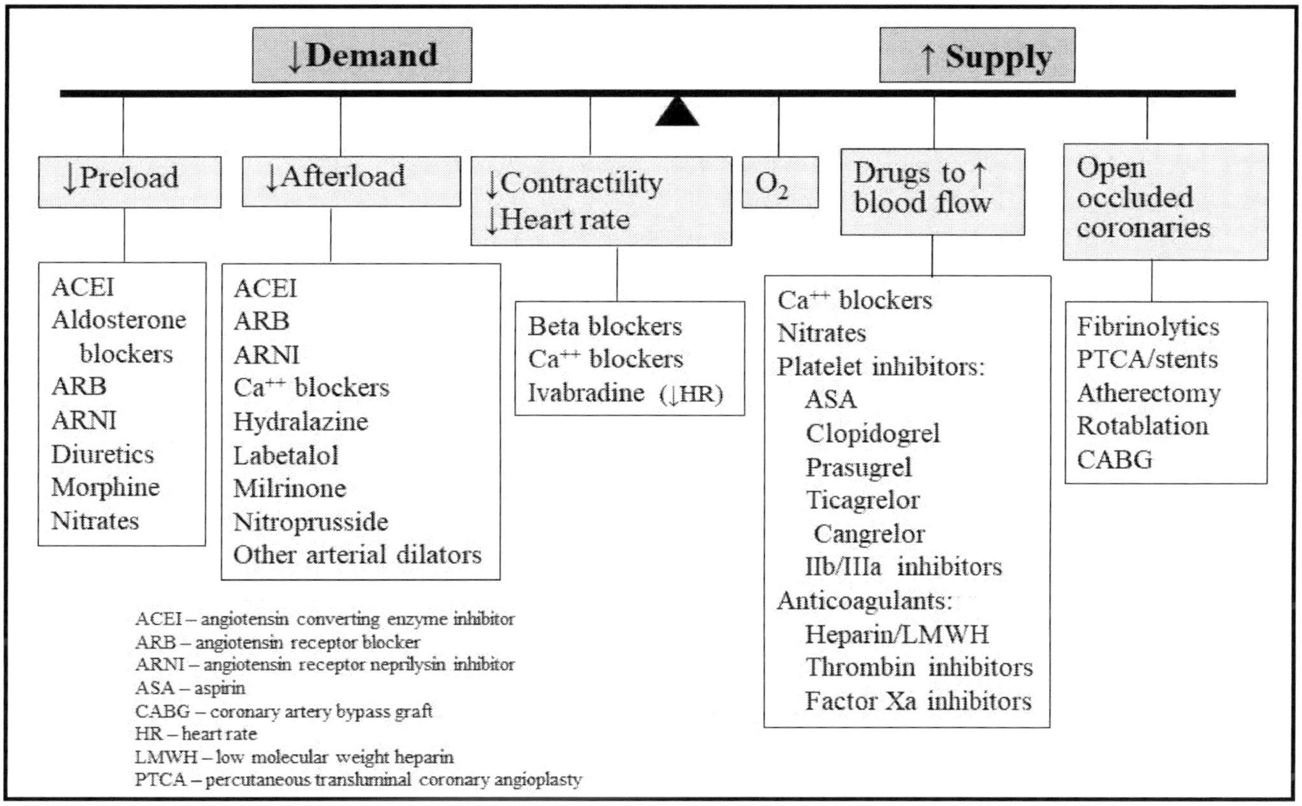

Figure 5: Drugs Used to Manipulate Myocardial O_2 Supply and Demand

Figure 6 summarizes the impact of SNS stimulation.

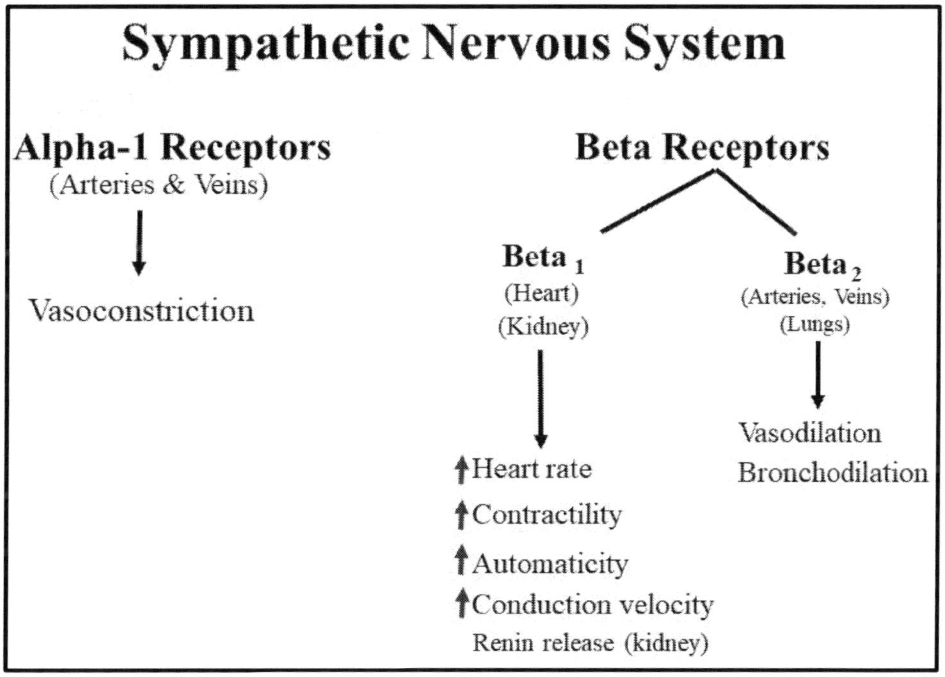

Figure 6: Sympathetic Nervous System Stimulation

Renin-Angiotensin-Aldosterone System

The RAAS plays an important role in CV pathology, especially in hypertension (HTN) and heart failure (HF). The main function of the RAAS is renal protection in the presence of hypotension or decreased renal blood flow, but there are potential negative CV effects when this system is activated.

Renin is released from the juxtaglomerular cells in the kidney in response to decreased renal blood flow (e.g., hypotension, hypovolemia, or sodium depletion), and in response to increased ß1 stimulation. Renin causes the conversion of angiotensinogen (an inactive protein) to angiotensin I. Angiotensin I is converted to angiotensin II by an angiotensin converting enzyme (ACE), found primarily in pulmonary vascular endothelium, but also in other vascular beds. Angiotensin II causes two major effects: peripheral vasoconstriction (arterial and venous) and aldosterone release by the adrenal cortex. Aldosterone causes the renal tubules to reabsorb sodium and water, thus increasing circulating blood volume.

The combined effects of peripheral vasoconstriction and increased blood volume lead to an increase in blood pressure (BP) and increased renal perfusion, which is the main goal of the RAAS. However, when the decrease in renal perfusion is due to a failing LV, the effects of vasoconstriction (higher afterload) and increased blood volume (higher preload) are deleterious to cardiac function and can worsen HF. Activation of the RAAS can also lead to HTN.

In addition to its CV effects, angiotensin II also affects the glomerulus and glomerular filtration rate (GFR) in the kidney. Angiotensin II constricts both afferent and efferent arterioles in the nephron but has a greater effect on efferent constriction. When renal perfusion pressure is reduced (e.g., hypovolemia and diuretic or antihypertensive therapy), the kidney maintains blood flow and glomerular filtration via autoregulation. This autoregulatory response causes afferent arteriolar vasodilation which allows more systemic arterial pressure to transmit to the glomerulus and maintains GFR. With greater reduction of renal perfusion, renin release occurs and results in increased angiotensin II production, which causes preferential constriction of the efferent arteriole. Constriction of the efferent arteriole increases intraglomerular pressure and maintains GFR until these autoregulatory mechanisms are maximized (Hilal-Dandan, 2018; Mann & Hilgers, 2017).

Angiotensin II can also be formed in tissues via non-ACE pathways, including in the heart and kidneys. Whether angiotensin II is formed via ACE or non-ACE pathways, it stimulates angiotensin receptors to exert its effects on the heart and blood vessels.

Six types of drugs can be used to block the RAAS either directly or indirectly. These medications can be used in the treatment of HTN and HF, and for myocardial protection following MI.

- Beta blockers prevent renin release by juxtaglomerular cells in the kidney by preventing ß1 activation.
- ACEIs block the enzyme responsible for converting angiotensin I to angiotensin II and thus only work on ACE pathways.
- ARBs block angiotensin II at its receptor sites, regardless of the pathway used for angiotensin II formation.
- An angiotensin II receptor blocker and neprilysin inhibitor (ARNI) contains both an ARB and a neprilysin inhibitor. They block neprilysin (an enzyme that degrades natriuretic peptides), resulting in increased levels of natriuretic peptides that are beneficial in HF.
- Renin inhibitors decrease plasma renin activity and block the conversion of angiotensinogen to angiotensin I, therefore ultimately decreasing the formation of angiotensin II.
- Mineralocorticoid receptor antagonists (MRAs), also referred to as aldosterone blockers, block aldosterone at its receptor sites.

ANGIOTENSIN CONVERTING ENZYME INHIBITORS

Mechanism of Action of ACEIs

ACEIs block the conversion of angiotensin I to angiotensin II, resulting in arterial and venous vasodilation and reduced sodium and water reabsorption by the kidneys.

They also block the breakdown of bradykinin, increasing bradykinin levels. Bradykinin is a vasodilator itself, but it also causes the release of two vasodilator substances in the vascular endothelium: nitric oxide and vasodilatory prostaglandins (e.g., prostacyclin). The actions of bradykinin are thought to potentiate the beneficial vasodilating effects of ACEIs.

Figure 7 illustrates the components and consequences of the RAAS.

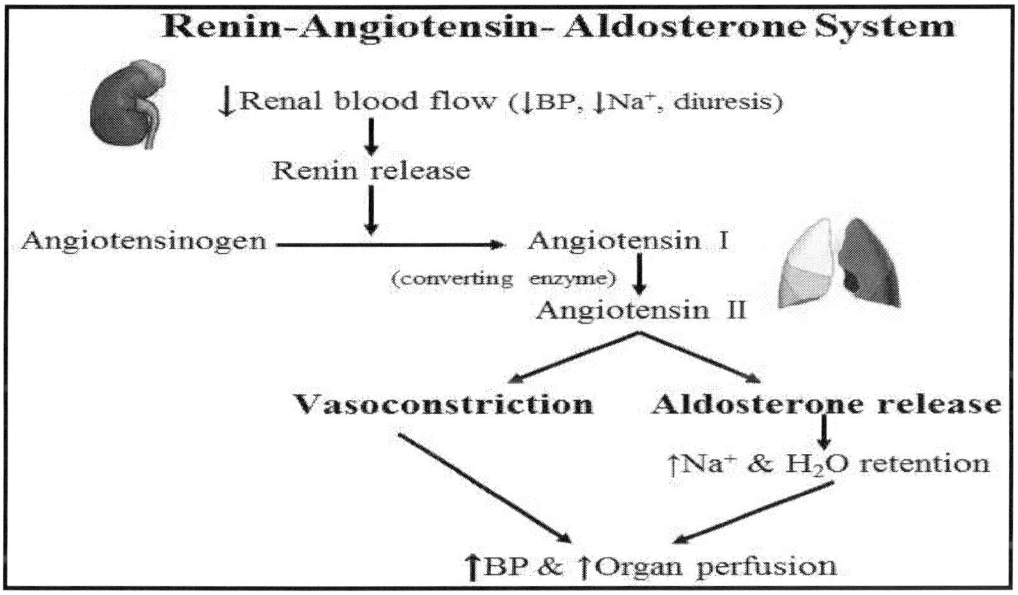

Figure 7: Renin-Angiotensin-Aldosterone System

The net effects of ACEIs include:

- Preload reduction due to venous vasodilation and decreased sodium and water reabsorption.
- Afterload reduction due to arterial vasodilation which leads to improved forward flow in HF.
- Increased levels of bradykinin due to inhibition of the enzyme that breaks down bradykinin, resulting in vasodilation.
- Increased prostacyclin and nitric oxide production in the vascular endothelium, causing vasodilation and endothelial protection.
- Potential raising of serum sodium in patients with HF and hyponatremia by increasing free water excretion when used with a loop diuretic.
- Decreased ventricular remodeling through several mechanisms including reduction of LV preload and afterload (preventing progressive LV dilation) and higher levels of bradykinin, a substance known to have antigrowth effects.
- Renal benefit of promoting efferent arteriole vasodilation and lowering intraglomerular pressure.
- Vascular benefit of preventing platelet aggregation due to increased nitric oxide and prostacyclin.
- Additional beneficial effects on the kidneys and vasculature contributing to the CV mortality benefit.

(Colucci, 2021; Mann, 2019; Mann & Hilgers, 2023; Opie & Pfeffer, 2013)

Indications for ACEIs

Hypertension

- ACEIs lower SVR and both systolic and diastolic BP by preventing systemic arteriolar vasoconstriction and increasing the compliance of larger arteries. ACEIs also reduce preload, which further supports BP control.

- ACEIs alone normalize BP in about 50% of patients with mild to moderate HTN, and 90% are controlled by a combination of an ACEI with either a CCB, beta blocker, or diuretic (Hilal-Dandan, 2018).
- All guidelines for management of HTN include ACEIs among the first-line agents recommended for the treatment of high BP. Other potential first-line agents for the treatment of HTN include ARBs, thiazide and thiazide-like diuretics, and CCBs (James et al., 2014; Jones et al., 2025; Williams et al., 2018).

HTN in Patients with Diabetes

- Major guidelines agree that the amount of BP reduction, not the agent used, is what is important in reducing CV risk.
  - However, in patients with diabetic kidney disease (DKD), ACEIs or ARBs may slow kidney disease progression better than other medications used to treat BP (Bakris, 2021).
  - Guidelines specific to the care of patients with diabetes often make recommendations to use an ACEI or an ARB as a first-line agent in the treatment of HTN, and all guidelines agree with ACEIs or ARBs as the first-line agents in patients with diabetes who have albuminuria.
- In patients with diabetes mellitus type 1 (DMT1) ACEIs or ARBs are the preferred medications to treat HTN if there is comorbid albuminuria.
  - ACE inhibition has been shown to provide renal protection even in the absence of HTN in patients with DMT1 and should be considered as a primary prevention for the microvascular complication of diabetic nephropathy also known as DKD.
  - If albuminuria is persistent in a patient with DMT1, management with an ACEI or an ARB is recommended to help prevent progression to proteinuria

  (Graves & Donaghue, 2019)
- ACEIs and ARBs also slow progression of diabetic nephropathy and retinopathy in patients with diabetes mellitus type 2 (DMT2).
  - ACEIs and ARBs are the preferred agents to treat HTN according to recommendations from the American Association of Clinical Endocrinologists and American College of Endocrinology (Garber et al., 2020).
  - Recommendations from the American Diabetes Association (ADA) include the use of an ACEI or an ARB to treat HTN in diabetes when the patient has albuminuria or coronary artery disease (CAD) (ADA, 2023).

Acute Coronary Syndrome (ACS)

- ACS includes ST segment elevation MI (STEMI) and non-ST segment elevation ACS (NSTE-ACS).
- ACEIs reduce mortality and major adverse CV events in both STEMI and NSTE-ACS. ACEIs are especially effective in patients with HTN or diabetes. ARBs are recommended when there is a contraindication to an ACEI in the setting of STEMI or NSTE-ACS.
- ACEIs are a class I recommendation for all STEMI patients with any one the following criteria (a) an anterior STEMI, (b) HF, or (c) EF $<40\%$ (O'Gara et al., 2013).
- ACEIs are a class I recommendation for all NSTE-ACS patients with any of the following criteria (a) EF $\leq 40\%$, (b) HTN, (c) diabetes, or (d) stable chronic kidney disease (CKD) (Amsterdam et al., 2014).

LV Dysfunction and HF with Reduced EF

- ACEIs not only provide preload and afterload reduction for a failing LV but also curb the adverse effects of neurohormonal activation of the RAAS that occurs in HF. Neurohormonal activation of the RAAS has adverse effects on the heart, blood vessels, and kidneys, and blocking these adverse effects contributes to the positive clinical outcomes seen with the use of ACEIs.

- ♦ Multiple trials have shown that ACEIs stabilize ventricular remodeling, improve symptoms, and reduce mortality and hospitalization in patients with HF with reduced EF (HFrEF) (EF $\leq$ 40%).
- ♦ In addition, ACEIs can prevent or delay the progression of HF in patients post-MI, and in those with reduced EF with or without symptoms of overt HF. When used, ACEIs should be continued indefinitely if tolerated (Amsterdam et al., 2014; O'Gara et al., 2013; Maddox et al., 2021).
- ♦ ACEIs have historically been the first-line agents for blocking the RAAS in the prevention and treatment of HFrEF.
  - The American College of Cardiology (ACC) Consensus Decision Pathway for Optimization of HF Treatment (2021) and the most recent ACC / American Heart Association (AHA) / Heart Failure Society of America (HFSA) Guidelines for the Management of HF (2022) recommend either ACEIs, ARBs or an ARNI, with an ARNI now recommended as the preferred agent over ACEIs and ARBs.
  - The 2022 HF Guidelines add the following statement about economic value: "In patients with chronic symptomatic HFrEF, treatment with an ARNI instead of an ACEI provides high economic value." (Heidenreich et al., 2022; Maddox et al., 2021).

Nephropathy / Chronic Kidney Disease

- ♦ ACEIs reduce glomerular injury by decreasing arterial BP and dilating both renal afferent and efferent arterioles with a preferential vasodilation of efferent arterioles. The vasodilation of efferent arterioles greater than afferent arterioles results in "afterload reduction" of the glomerulus.
- ♦ A lower intraglomerular pressure is associated with less proteinuria. When BP control is achieved, ACEIs and ARBs are more effective than other antihypertensive medications in reducing proteinuria and slowing the progression of all forms of CKD associated with proteinuria (Bakris, 2021).
- ♦ In a meta-analysis ACEIs were superior to ARBs and other antihypertensive drugs in providing the benefits of reduction of kidney events, improved CV outcomes, and decreased CV death and all-cause mortality in patients with CKD, stages 3 through 5, who were not on dialysis (Zhang et al., 2020).

> ***Linking Knowledge to Practice***
>
> ✓ *ACEIs (and ARBs) should <u>not</u> be referred to as BP medications.*
> - *While they may be used in the treatment of high BP, they may also be prescribed for other reasons and in patients without HTN.*
> - *For example, ACEIs or ARBs are often used in the setting of systolic HF where BP is often low normal or even low due to low SV.*
>
> ✓ *It is important to clarify the hold criteria for these medications for each patient because the hold criteria may be different based on the indication for the medication.*

Special Dosing Information for ACEIs

Information below is based on enalapril, lisinopril, and ramipril. Consult Appendix 1, manufacturer recommendations or other drug reference for recommendations for each individual ACEI.

- ♦ A small transient increase in creatinine is acceptable after the initiation of an ACEI. If the creatinine increases by 30% or more within the first 2 months of therapy the medication should be stopped.
- ♦ An ACEI should be temporarily held in the setting of any acute kidney injury (AKI) until the AKI is resolved and renal function has returned to baseline.
- ♦ No dose adjustments are recommended when the creatinine clearance (CrCl) is $\geq$ 30 mL/minute (min).

- A lower initial dose and slow titration is recommended when the CrCl is between 10 (or 15) and 29 to 30 mL/min. Alternate therapy should be considered when the CrCl is < 10 (or 15) mL/min because the risk for complications such as hyperkalemia and kidney failure is too high.
- In the setting of very advanced CKD there is emerging evidence that there is no harm in continuing ACEIs and ARBs and there may be potential benefit (Bhandari et al., 2024). More research is needed.
- ACEIs should be taken after hemodialysis if prescribed on dialysis days.
- There are no manufacturer recommendations for dose adjustments with hepatic dysfunction. However, ACEIs should not be used in the setting of ascites secondary to cirrhosis due to the risk of precipitating hepatorenal syndrome.

(Singh et al., 2025; UptoDate®,Lexidrug™, 2026)

Linking Knowledge to Practice

✓ *ACEIs and ARBs are always held.in the setting of AKI regardless of the creatinine. However, it does not mean these medications cannot be resumed after the AKI resolves.*

✓ *ACEIs and ARBs are used in the setting of CKD to slow disease progression. Historically they have been held when the patient begins approaching the need for renal replacement therapy (RRT) to allow for compensatory efferent arteriole vasoconstriction to maintain GFR and delay the initiation of RRT. However, there is new evidence that it may be beneficial to continue an ACEI or an ARB in the setting of advanced CKD regardless of creatinine (Bhandari et al., 2024).*

Select Adverse Effects of ACEIs

Potential adverse effects of ACEIs are due either to inhibition of the RAAS (hypotension, hyperkalemia, and decreased GFR) or due to increased kinin levels (cough, angioedema).

- Side effects related to RAAS inhibition are likely to occur with all drugs that inhibit the RAAS (ARBs, renin blockers).
- Those related to increased kinin levels are less likely to occur with ARBs, since ARBs do not increase kinin levels.
- However, when an ARB is combined with a neprilysin inhibitor (discussed below) there is an increased risk for cough and angioedema.

Cough

- Cough is the most common side effect, occurring in 5 to 20% of patients.
- Cough is thought to be caused by increased bradykinin and prostaglandin levels.
  - ACE is responsible for metabolism of kinins and thus inhibition prevents kinin breakdown. This results in more kinins which cause bronchial irritation by stimulating production of prostaglandins.
  - ACE inhibition can also result in increased levels of thromboxane. Both prostaglandins and thromboxane can stimulate the cough reflex.
- The cough is a dry tickle-like cough that usually begins within 1 to 2 weeks of therapy but can be delayed for months to a year.
- Women are affected more often than men, and in Chinese patients the incidence is as high as 50%.
- Cough usually resolves within a few days of discontinuing therapy but sometimes lasts up to 4 weeks.
- Treatment includes discontinuing the ACEI and switching to an ARB, which typically does not cause a cough.

(Hilal-Dandan, 2018; Opie & Pfeffer, 2013; Townsend, 2022)

> ***Linking Knowledge to Practice***
>
> ✓ *Cough is a potential side effect of an ACEI, but it can also be a sign of worsening HF. Verify that HF is not worsening before assuming the cough is a side effect of ACEI therapy.*

Angioedema

- Angioedema (swelling of lips, tongue, mouth, face, larynx, and rarely intestine) is a rare but potentially fatal allergic reaction that occurs in 0.1 to 0.7% of patients. However, due to the number of patients taking ACEIs, ACEI induced angioedema is responsible for 20 to 40% of emergency department visits for angioedema in the United States. African Americans have up to a five times greater risk of developing angioedema than Caucasians (Guyer & Banerji, 2020; Hilal-Dandan, 2018).
- ACEIs inhibit the breakdown of bradykinin, resulting in increased bradykinin levels that are thought to cause angioedema by causing vasodilation and increasing capillary permeability.
- About half of the cases of angioedema occur within a week of initiation of therapy, but it may not occur for months to years after starting ACEI therapy.
- There is no quick diagnostic test to determine if a patient's angioedema is bradykinin mediated, or mast cell/histamine mediated. Any patient who is taking an ACEI at the time they develop angioedema should be diagnosed as having ACEI induced angioedema. However, if the patient's medical history and medication list are not readily available some patients with ACEI induced angioedema will be treated with antihistamines and corticosteroids as if the angioedema was mast cell/histamine mediated.
- Treatment for ACEI induced angioedema usually involves stopping the medication and observing for resolution. Individual episodes typically resolve within 24 to 72 hours, but complete resolution can take days. In severe cases, airway protection with intubation or tracheostomy may be necessary.
- Hereditary angioedema is a bradykinin mediated angioedema.
  - There are several therapies used in the treatment of hereditary angioedema including C1 inhibitor concentrate, Ecallantide, Icatibant, and possibly fresh frozen plasma. There have been mixed results in research studies on the benefits of using these treatments in ACEI induced angioedema.
  - Patients with hereditary angioedema have repeated episodes and learn to recognize prodromal signs and symptoms (S&S) and self-medicate or seek treatment early. Patients with ACEI angioedema have typically not had angioedema before and usually present later.
  - If a patient with presumed ACEI angioedema presents early with severe and worsening angioedema, it is recommended they receive one of the therapies for hereditary angioedema if the treatment can be given within the first few hours of symptom onset (Guyer & Banerji, 2020).
- Patients who experience angioedema on an ACEI cannot take any ACEI for the rest of their lives. There is an increased rate of angioedema occurrence if the ACEI is not stopped, and subsequent episodes of angioedema can be more severe and even life threatening.
- Theoretically, ARBs should not cause angioedema since they do not increase bradykinin levels, however there are cases of angioedema occurring in patients taking ARBs.
  - In a meta-analysis of 3 studies the incidence of confirmed recurrent angioedema in patients with ACEI induced angioedema who were subsequently prescribed an ARB was approximately 3.5% (Haymore et al.,2008).
  - However, in one nationwide registry, ARBs did not increase the risk of angioedema compared to other antihypertensives in patients who had previously experienced angioedema while taking an ACEI (Rasmussen et al., 2019).
- HF guidelines recommend the use of an ARB in patients with HFrEF who have developed angioedema with an ACEI or ARNI (Heidenreich et al., 2022).

- After angioedema associated with an ACEI, a 6 week wait time is recommended before starting the ARB (Jones et al., 2025).

(Opie & Pfeffer, 2013; Zuraw, 2022)

> ***Linking Knowledge to Practice***
>
> ✓ *Airway assessment is a key nursing intervention in a patient with suspected ACEI induced angioedema who has swelling of the mouth or throat. The patient may need intubation and mechanical ventilation.*
>
> ✓ *Patients who experience ACEI induced angioedema need to be instructed to list all ACEIs on their allergy list. They need to recognize ACEIs as ending in "pril" and know that they cannot ever take these medications in the future.*

Hypotension

- Hypotension following the first dose of an ACEI can occur, especially in hypovolemic patients with high levels of renin.
- There is a higher risk of hypotension in the setting of hyponatremia, <130 milliequivalent (mEq) per liter (L) [mEq/L], concurrent diuretic therapy, or volume depletion.
- To avoid hypotension, a low initial dose is recommended when initiating therapy. It is also recommended that diuretic therapy be discontinued for 1 to 2 days upon initiation of therapy with an ACEI.
- In HF patients, systolic BP in the 80s or 90s can be well tolerated if symptoms or postural hypotension do not occur.

(Opie & Pfeffer, 2013; Townsend, 2022)

Hyperkalemia

- Hyperkalemia can occur because lower aldosterone levels caused by an ACEI result in potassium retention by renal tubules.
- ACEIs usually raise serum potassium (K^+) concentration by < 0.5 mEq/L in patients with normal renal function. However, ACEIs may cause hyperkalemia in patients with renal insufficiency or diabetes, or when taken with potassium sparing diuretics (aldosterone antagonists), potassium supplements, NSAIDS, or potassium-containing salt substitutes.
- A potassium level should be checked within the first week of ACEI therapy.

(Colucci, 2021; Hilal-Dandan, 2018; Opie & Pfeffer, 2013; Townsend, 2022)

> ***Linking Knowledge to Practice***
>
> ✓ *Patients on ACEI or ARB therapy probably do not need potassium supplements because these drugs cause potassium reabsorption. Hold potassium supplements on initiation of therapy and check with the provider about discontinuing supplements if potassium level rises on drug therapy.*
>
> ✓ *Patients with HTN or HF who may be prescribed an ACEI may also be asked to adhere to a sodium restricted diet. It is important for patients to know they should not use potassium-based salt substitutes due to the risk of hyperkalemia while on an ACEI or ARB.*

Kidney Injury / Failure

- Kidney injury can be precipitated by excessive hypotension, severe HF, or renal artery stenosis.
- A reduction of GFR without any true kidney injury may occur with ACEI therapy and it is thought to be due to vasodilation of the efferent arteriole, which reduces intraglomerular filtration pressure.

Advanced Concept Focus:

ACEIs (ARBs) and Renal Function General Principles

- The renal effects of ARBs are largely like the renal effects of ACEIs so the following information can generally be applied to both ACEIs and ARBs.
- Renal blood flow is autoregulated. When there is decreased renal perfusion, the following occurs:
    - There is a decrease in arterial tone that permits more systemic pressure to be transmitted to the glomerulus.
    - The RAAS is activated resulting in a preferential increase in the resistance of the efferent arterioles (through vasoconstriction) that supports maintenance of the GFR.
- The impact of ACEIs on renal function differs depending on the indication for the ACEI. There are differences in the renal impact of ACEIs between the setting of HTN and the setting of HF.
- The reduction in GFR that can occur with the initiation of ACEIs is related in part to the impact of ACEIs on preventing both afferent and efferent arteriole vasoconstriction at the level of glomerulus. Afferent arteriole constriction results in a reduction of GFR while efferent arteriole constriction results in the maintenance or increase in GFR.
- Angiotensin II constricts both the afferent and efferent arterioles but acts preferentially on efferent arterioles to increase efferent resistance.
    - Efferent arterioles are smaller in diameter than afferent arterioles and constrict more easily.
    - Angiotensin II promotes the release of nitric oxide from the afferent arteriole which opposes its vasoconstrictive effects.
- Angiotensin II also constricts the mesangial cells in the glomerulus resulting in some reduction of GFR by reducing the surface area available for filtration.
- A reduction in efferent arteriole constriction by an ACEI or an ARB results in a lower intraglomerular pressure and reduced GFR.

(Kobori et al., 2013)

Linking Knowledge to Practice

✓ *The impact of ACEIs on renal function is complex and critical thinking is required to know when to hold these medications.*
- *In certain settings ACEIs are considered renal protective and prevent the progression of CKD and are thus given to patients with an abnormal creatinine.*
- *In other settings such as AKI, ACEIs are held to allow the kidneys to improve GFR through the compensatory mechanism of efferent arteriole vasoconstriction.*

✓ *The Advanced Concept Focus section above on ACEIs and ARBs and renal function equips you to make decisions regarding these medications based on the patient's kidney function.*

Advanced Concept Focus:

ACEIs (ARBs) and Heart Failure

- ACEIs (and ARBs) reduce afterload, increase CO, and increase renal blood flow. This increase in renal blood flow, however, does not necessarily translate into an increase in GFR.
- A mean increase in creatinine of 0.1 to 0.2 milligrams (mg)/deciliter (dL) with a small decrease in GFR is a common finding within the first week after the initiation of an ACEI (ARB).
- After this initial change the creatinine, GFR, and renal function typically stabilize unless there are complicating factors such as deterioration of cardiac status.

- ♦ Because of the potential of lowering GFR, ACEIs and ARBs are often underutilized in patients with CKD despite evidence of mortality benefit when used in patients with CKD and renal impairment.
- ♦ Patients are at highest risk for a decrease in GFR in situations where the GFR is dependent on high angiotensin II levels.
- ♦ The following conditions require higher angiotensin II levels to maintain an adequate GFR.
  - The use of high dose diuretics resulting in relative hypovolemia.
  - Relative hypotension (mean arterial pressure [MAP] < 75 mmHg) after ACEI (ARB) administration, indicating a low CO and resulting in low renal blood flow.
  - Baseline serum sodium < 137 mEq/L which is an indicator for neurohormonal activation.
  - The presence of significant renovascular disease which is not an uncommon finding in older adults with HF.
- ♦ There are several strategies to minimize or avoid the ACEI (ARB) induced decline in GFR.
  - Initiating therapy with a low dose of an ACEI.
  - Temporarily reducing the diuretic dose.
  - Avoiding nonsteroidal anti-inflammatory drugs (NSAIDs).
- ♦ An ACEI, ARB, or ARNI should be held temporarily in the setting of AKI until the acute injury is resolved. Holding these medications in the setting of AKI allows for the compensatory vasoconstriction of the efferent arterioles.
- ♦ In the setting of CKD and worsening renal function the following recommendations have been made:
  - The ACEI (ARB) should be stopped, and a specialist consulted for: 1) An increase in creatinine > than 100% above baseline, or 2) An increase in creatinine to > 3.5 mg/dL or if estimated measured GFR (eGFR) drops to < 20 mL/min/1.73 m^2.
  - The ACEI (ARB) dose should be reduced by 50% and the creatinine reassessed in 1 week for 1) an increase in creatinine ranging 50 to 100% of baseline, or 2) an increase in creatinine to between 3.0 and 3.5 mg/dL or if eGFR drops to between 20 and 25 mL/min/1.73 m^2. If there is no improvement in renal function in response to a 50% decrease in the dose, the ACEI (ARB) should be stopped, and a specialist consulted.
- ♦ However, the STOP ACEi clinical trial showed that stopping ACEIs (ARBs) did not cause a clinically significant change in the eGFR or make a difference in its long-term decline. Thus, demonstrating no benefit in stopping an ACEI or an ARB in advanced CKD (Bhandari et al., 2024). More research is needed.
- ♦ Patients with baseline renal dysfunction and those with advanced HF are at high risk for developing hyperkalemia when starting on an ACEI or an ARB.
  - There is decreased sodium and water delivery to the potassium secreting site in the distal tubule and cortical collecting duct in the setting of advanced HF.
  - Adequate potassium secretion is dependent on an increased secretion of aldosterone from the adrenal cortex. Angiotensin II is responsible for the release of aldosterone in the setting of hypoperfusion. Secretion of aldosterone from the adrenal cortex is partially reduced when the production of angiotensin II is blocked by ACEI administration.
  - The risk of hyperkalemia is increased further with the initiation or up titration of spironolactone or eplerenone both of which antagonize aldosterone.
  - ACEIs (ARBs) have been shown to have a variable impact on diuretic responsiveness.
    - ▪ In some cases, ACEIs (ARBs) may increase the natriuretic response.
    - ▪ However, at higher doses due to a reduction in systemic BP and a fall in GFR, there can be a blunted diuretic effect.
- ♦ ACEIs (ARBs) have an advantage over nonselective vasodilators such as hydralazine because they are more selective for renal arteries.

For any given increase in CO there will be an increase in renal blood flow with the use of an ACEI compared to a nonselective vasodilator.

(Colucci, 2024)

Advanced Concept Focus:
ACEIs (ARBs) and HTN

- In the setting of primary HTN there is an increase in renal perfusion pressure and thus the GFR is not as dependent on angiotensin II. This means that the initiation of the ACEI (ARB) will have little impact on GFR in the patient with HTN and normal renal function.
- In very new onset HTN the addition of an ACEI (ARB) may cause an increase in GFR because of blocking the angiotensin II generated constriction of the glomerular mesangial cells.
- An ACEI (ARB) may impact renal function in a patient with HTN who is volume depleted due to diuretic(s). In the setting of volume depletion, the GFR is more dependent on angiotensin II.
- The start of an ACEI (ARB) in patients with more severe renal disease can result in a decline in GFR.
    - Patients with a long-standing history of HTN are at risk for developing renal disease due to hypertensive nephrosclerosis, also called benign nephrosclerosis.
    - In patients with established glomerular disease the afferent arterioles may already be fully dilated to increase glomerular pressure and thus they don't receive any additional benefit of afferent arteriole vasodilation caused by blocking angiotensin II. Also, the addition of an ACEI (ARB) will prevent the compensatory efferent vasoconstriction to maintain the GFR (Kobori et al. 2013).
- An ACEI (ARB) may cause worsening renal function when given to a patient with renal artery stenosis who has baseline reduced blood flow to the glomerulus due to a stenotic lesion in one or both renal arteries. When systemic BP is reduced in the setting of renal artery stenosis intraglomerular pressure is further lowered and an ACEI will block the efforts of autoregulation to improve the GFR through efferent arteriole vasoconstriction.
    - A rise in creatinine is usually acceptable and does not result in having to stop the ACEI (ARB). More than a 30% rise in creatinine or a 30% fall in GFR occurs in less than 10% of patients.
    - An increase in creatinine is more likely to occur in the setting of bilateral renal artery stenosis than in unilateral renal artery stenosis.
        - In unilateral renal artery stenosis, the overall GFR is usually preserved because there is an unaffected kidney.
        - However, there is the potential risk for ischemic atrophy in unilateral renal artery stenosis due to the decrease in perfusion pressure to the affected kidney.
    - In the setting of renal artery stenosis and a rise of 30% or greater in creatinine or a 30% or greater fall in GFR, the patient should be changed from an agent blocking the RAAS to a CCB or other agent. If the patient undergoes a successful procedure to correct the stenosis, then a medication blocking the RAAS can be resumed.
    - In the setting of severe bilateral renal artery stenosis, the kidneys may not tolerate any antihypertensive agent because high systemic pressure may be needed for an adequate intraglomerular pressure.
    - If the degree of stenosis is very severe, renal artery thrombosis can occur if there is an extreme reduction in systemic BP.
    - Any reduction in GFR caused by an ACEI (ARB) in the setting of renal artery stenosis almost always resolves when the ACEI (ARB) is stopped.
- If there is a decline in GFR it will occur in the first few days of drug initiation during which levels of angiotensin II are quickly lowered. Creatinine should be checked within 3 to 5 days of starting therapy if the patient has known renal artery stenosis or has severe HTN and known vascular disease.

(Mann & Hilgers, 2023)

Contraindication Highlights for ACEIs

- Consult manufacturer recommendations for use in children, pregnant women, and nursing women.
- ACEIs should not be used in patients with a history of angioedema while previously taking an ACEI. ACEIs should also not be used in patients with idiopathic or hereditary angioedema.
- ACEIs should not be used simultaneously with ARBs.
- Do not use an ACEI in patients taking direct renin inhibitors who have diabetes or an eGFR < 60 mL/min/1.73 m^2.
- Do not use ACEIs with or within 36 hours of a patient taking a neprilysin inhibitor.

(FDA, 2012, April 20; UptoDate®, Lexidrug™, 2026)

> ***Linking Knowledge to Practice***
>
> ✓ *ACEIs should not be used if the patient is receiving RRT that uses a AN69 filter due to the risk of anaphylactoid reaction (UptoDate®, Lexidrug™, 2026).*

Special Considerations & Monitoring with ACEIs

- Patients with renal impairment are at risk for developing neutropenia on an ACEI although this is rare.
- Patients with collagen vascular disease and renal dysfunction are at high risk for erythropoietin dysfunction. Periodic complete blood count (CBC) with differential is recommended.
- Severe anaphylactoid reactions can be seen during hemodialysis with high flux dialysis membranes.
- See below additional special considerations and monitoring for both ACEIs and ARBs.

(Brown & Vaughan, 1998; Singh et al., 2025; Verresen et al., 1994)

> ***Linking Knowledge to Practice***
>
> ✓ *Patients with long standing HTN can develop renal dysfunction due to benign hypertensive nephrosclerosis. It is called benign because it does not typically result in clinically significant kidney failure in most patients. However, there are three groups of patients who are at high risk for developing progressive renal failure resulting in end stage kidney disease: black patients, patients with severely high BP, & patients with underlying CKD, especially diabetic nephropathy.*
>
> ✓ *Bilateral renal artery stenosis should be considered when there is a creatinine elevation after the administration of an ACEI in a patient who is not volume depleted. Potential differentials for an elevated creatinine after the administration of an ACEI include hypovolemia, renal disease from benign hypertensive nephrosclerosis, and renal artery stenosis.*
>
> *(Mann & Hilgers, 2023; Mann & Hilgers, 2025)*

Key Pharmacokinetic & Pharmacodynamic Information for ACEIs

- Captopril and lisinopril are the only oral ACEIs that are not prodrugs and are preferred in patients with hepatic dysfunction (excluding cirrhosis and ascites). All other ACEIs are prodrugs in which the parent drug is inactive until converted to its active form by hepatic biotransformation. The active form of the drug has "at" on the end (e.g., enalapril is the parent drug; enalaprilat is the active form of the drug).
- Lisinopril is the only ACEI that does not undergo hepatic metabolism.
- Fosinopril is an ACEI with dual excretion including both renal and fecal excretion.
- Captopril has the shortest duration of action and must be administered 2 to 3 times daily. Enalapril achieves a more consistent response when administered twice a day.

Many ACEIs are dosed only once daily.
(Piepho, 2000; Singh et al., 2025)

> ***Linking Knowledge to Practice***
>
> ✓ *In the patient with hepatic ascites the development of hypotension is a concern since lower BP in these patients is associated with poor outcomes. Therefore, ACEIs and ARBs should be avoided in patients with hepatic ascites (Shah, 2025).*
>
> ✓ *Lisinopril and captopril are the preferred ACEIs when needed in patients with advanced chronic liver disease or compensated cirrhosis because they are not prodrugs (Singh et al., 2025).*

Important Medication Interactions with ACEIs

See below the combined section of select medication interactions for both ACEIs and ARBs.

Appendix 1 provides additional details regarding individual ACEIs.

ANGIOTENSIN RECEPTOR BLOCKERS

Mechanism of Action of ARBs

- ◆ ARBs block the effects of angiotensin II at receptor sites, regardless of the pathway by which angiotensin II was formed.
- ◆ This prevents vasoconstriction and thus results in vasodilation and decreased sodium and water retention, just like ACEIs. However, ARBs have no effect on bradykinin.

Indications for ARBs

Hypertension

- ◆ The preload and afterload reduction achieved by blocking of the RAAS results in BP lowering in persons with HTN.
- ◆ All ARBs are approved for treatment of HTN and appear to be equivalent to ACEIs in efficacy in reducing CV events and mortality.
- ◆ ARBs are among the primary drugs recommended for treatment of HTN in all major guidelines for management of HTN

(Hilal-Dandan, 2018; Jones et al., 2025; Williams et al., 2018)

HTN in Patients with Diabetes

The rationale for the use of ARBs for the treatment of HTN in patients with diabetes is the same as for ACEIs and is discussed in the section above on indications for ACEIs.

Nephropathy / CKD

- ◆ ARBs are renoprotective in Type II diabetic and nondiabetic nephropathy, primarily due to their antihypertensive effect.
- ◆ ARBs have the same effects as ACEIs on decreasing arterial BP and dilating renal efferent arterioles, effectively "afterload reducing" the glomerulus.
- ◆ ACEIs and ARBs are the preferred agents for antihypertensive therapy to slow the progression of CKD.

(Mann & Hilgers, 2017)

Heart Failure

- ♦ By inhibiting the RAAS, ARBs provide preload and afterload reduction and modulate the adverse neurohormonal effects on the heart, blood vessels, and kidney that occur in HF.
- ♦ ARBs have been shown to reduce morbidity and mortality in patients with HFrEF and to reduce hospitalizations in patients with HF with preserved EF (HFpEF).
- ♦ Candesartan and valsartan are approved by the Food and Drug Administration (FDA) for treatment of HF, but other ARBs are used off label in HF.
- ♦ The current HF guidelines recommend the use of an ARB in patients with previous or current symptoms of chronic HFrEF and who are intolerant of ACEIs because of cough or angioedema, and when the use of an ARNI is not feasible.

(Heidenreich et al., 2022)

Linking Knowledge to Practice

✓ *African Americans are less responsive to ACEI and ARB therapy than Caucasians.*

✓ *A combination of hydralazine (an arterial dilator) and isosorbide dinitrate (a venous vasodilator) is recommended as part of standard therapy in addition to beta blockers and ACEIs for African Americans with HFrEF.*

(Heidenreich et al., 2022; Saunders & Gavin, 2023)

Acute Coronary Syndrome

- ♦ It is a class I recommendation to start an ACEI or ARB within the first 24 hours in STEMI patients with anterior MI, HF, or LVEF ≤40%.
- ♦ An ACEI or ARB is a class I recommendation for all ACS patients who have high risk features. High risk features include LVEF ≤40%, HTN, or diabetes. ACEIs or ARBs are used in ACS to reduce all-cause mortality and MACE.
- ♦ ARBs should be continued indefinitely if they are tolerated.

(Amsterdam et al., 2014; O'Gara et al., 2013; Rao et al., 2025; Reeder, 2022)

Special Dosing Information for ARBs

The information below is based on candesartan, irbesartan, losartan, and valsartan. Consult Appendix 2, manufacturer recommendations, or other drug reference for recommendations for each individual ARB.

- ♦ Small and transient increases in creatinine may occur within 4 weeks of starting an ARB or increasing the dose. If the creatinine increases by > 30%, other reasons for worsening renal function should be investigated. ARBs are always held temporarily in the setting of AKI.
- ♦ No specific dose adjustment is needed based on renal function. However, ARBs should be used with caution in patients with a CrCl ≤ 30 mL/min. Kidney function and potassium levels should be closely followed. There is a specific recommendation for candesartan to start at a lower dose and to not exceed a specific maximum dose if the CrCl is ≤ 30 mL/min.
- ♦ In the setting of very advanced CKD there is emerging evidence that there is no harm in continuing ACEIs and ARBs and there may be potential benefit (Bhandari et al., 2024). More research is needed.
- ♦ ARBs are not significantly dialyzed.
- ♦ No dose adjustment is needed with mild to moderate hepatic impairment. It is recommended to start losartan at lower dose when there is hepatic impairment. Use with caution in severe hepatic impairment and in patients who have ascites secondary to cirrhosis.

(Rossing et al., 2022b; UptoDate®,Lexidrug™ 2026)

Select Adverse Effects of ARBs

- Potential adverse effects of ARBs are related to the inhibition of the RAAS and include hypotension, hyperkalemia, and decreased GFR. These adverse effects are like the adverse effects seen with ACEIs and are discussed in more detail in the section on adverse effects of ACEIs.
- ARBs, have no effect on bradykinin and therefore are not associated with adverse effects of cough and angioedema that are seen with ACEIs.
- Severe chronic diarrhea and weight loss, symptoms of sprue-like enteropathy, have been reported with Olmesartan (FDA, 2013, July 3). These symptoms can develop from months to years after starting the medication and can require hospitalization. Patients need to know they should report these findings even if they occur after being on the medication for a long period of time. Stopping the medication results in improvement of the symptoms. This adverse effect has not been seen with other ARBs.
- ARBs are much less likely to cause a cough or angioedema than ACEIs.

(UptoDate®,Lexidrug™, 2026)

Contraindication Highlights for ARBs

- Consult manufacturer recommendations for use in children, pregnant women, and nursing women.
- ARBs should not be used concurrently with ACEIs regardless of eGFR and they should not be used with direct renin inhibitors in patients with diabetes or eGFR < 60 mL/min/1.73 m^2.

(National Kidney Foundation, 2026; UptoDate®,Lexidrug™, 2026)

Linking Knowledge to Practice

- ✓ *Patients receiving ACEIs or ARBs for HF are usually also on diuretics and a beta blocker. If the patient is taking an ACEI or an ARB for HTN it is usually in conjunction with a diuretic or a CCB. All these drugs can cause hypotension, especially when used together.*
    - *Check postural pressures the first time a patient gets out of bed to make sure there is no significant orthostatic drop.*
    - *If a significant drop occurs, check postural pressures each time up.*
- ✓ *Teach patients to get out of bed slowly, sitting on side of bed and moving their feet for a minute before standing. This should also be included in the discharge instructions.*
- ✓ *If a patient develops hypotension after taking an ACEI or an ARB, this should not be considered a contraindication to future use. If the patient is taking other medications such as diuretics, nitrates, or CCBs that increase the risk of hypotension these medications may need to be stopped to allow for the use of an ACEI or an ARB when used for mortality reduction.*
- ✓ *The goal of drug therapy with ACEIs and ARBs in HF is to make it easier for the heart to work by reducing both preload and afterload. BP is expected to be somewhat lower when used to treat HF than when used to treat HTN.*
    - *Systolic BPs in the 80s are not uncommon in HF and may be desirable for afterload reduction if the patient is asymptomatic (Masarone et al., 2021).*
    - *Verify with the provider what BP parameters are desired for each individual patient.*

Special Considerations & Monitoring with ARBs and ACEIs

- Potassium should be monitored periodically during therapy due to risk of hyperkalemia. Risk factors for the development of hyperkalemia while taking an ACEI or an ARB include diabetes or taking a potassium sparing diuretic, potassium supplements, or salt substitutes containing potassium.
- Volume depletion should be corrected before initiating an ACEI or an ARB.

- Renal function should be monitored with the frequency determined by the patient's baseline renal status and comorbid conditions.
  - A small transient increase in creatinine is expected after initiation in patients who are dependent on efferent arteriole vasoconstriction to maintain their GFR. This is not a reason to stop the ACEI or the ARB.
  - ACEIs and ARBs are both held in the setting of AKI until the AKI is resolved.
- As with all antihypertensives, ACEIs and ARBs should be used cautiously in patients with significant aortic or mitral valve stenosis because of the fixed obstruction and limited ability to increase CO in the event of hypotension. ACEIs and ARBs can worsen obstruction in HOCM by decreasing preload.

(UptoDate®,Lexidrug™, 2026)

> ***Linking Knowledge to Practice***
>
> ✓ *If BP falls in response to vasodilation (prevention of vasoconstriction) the body's normal response is to increase CO to fill the vessels. Patients with severe stenotic valvular disease have a mechanical limitation to increasing CO to fill the blood vessels and as a result syncope or refractory hypotension can occur.*

Key Pharmacokinetic & Pharmacodynamic Information for ARBs

- ARBs differ in the degree of oral bioavailability, absorption / distribution, lipid solubility, plasma protein binding, metabolism, and route of elimination.
- Candesartan cilexetil (converted completely during GI absorption to candesartan) is a prodrug.
- Losartan has a metabolite that is more active and longer acting than the parent drug.
- The elimination half-life is short for losartan, intermediate for valsartan and eprosartan, and longer for candesartan and irbesartan.
- Dosing needs to be individualized in the presence of hepatic disease for eprosartan, losartan, telmisartan and valsartan.
- Pharmacokinetic drug–drug interactions are not common. However, it is important to know that telmisartan may increase the serum concentration of digoxin.
- Most ARBs are dosed once daily.

(Israili, 2000)

> ***Linking Knowledge to Practice***
>
> ✓ *In general, the more lipophilic a medication the more easily and rapidly absorbed it is and the better able it is to penetrate the lipid bilayer of cell membranes.*

Important Medication Interactions with ACEIs and ARBs

- ACEIs and ARBs should not be used together. The combination of an ACEI and ARB together significantly increases the risk of hypotension, hyperkalemia, and renal dysfunction.
- Renin inhibitors can enhance the hyperkalemic and nephrotoxic effects of ACEIs and ARBs. These medications cannot be used in combination with an ACEI or an ARB in patients with diabetes or an eGFR < GFR < 60 mL/min/1.73 m^2.
- Thiazide and loop diuretics enhance the hypotensive effects of ACEIs and ARBs due to the additive effect of decreasing preload.
  - Diuretic doses should be decreased or potentially discontinued for a period upon initiation of ACEIs or ARBs.

- Diuretics can be reinstituted as needed for BP or volume control in HF.

♦ Nitrates also have an additive effect on preload reduction when used with ACEIs or ARBs and the combination may enhance hypotension.

♦ Beta blockers enhance the hypotensive effects of ACEIs because beta blockers block the release of renin that occurs with SNS activation.

♦ CCBs are often used in combination with ACEIs or ARBs in the treatment of HTN. They have an additive effect on BP. Both classes of medications result in arterial vasodilation.

♦ The risk of hyperkalemia with an ACEI or an ARB increases with the use of the aldosterone antagonists spironolactone and eplerenone.

♦ Captopril can increase digoxin levels by reducing renal clearance, particularly in severe HF (Marte et al., 2024).

♦ NSAIDs decrease the cough side effect, but they also decrease the antihypertensive effects of ACEIs by blocking prostaglandins. They also diminish the therapeutic effect of ARBs. They cause vasoconstriction and can lead to worsening HF; therefore, NSAIDs should be avoided in patients with HF. NSAIDs when used in combination with ACEIs or ARBs can lead to worsening renal function.

♦ ACEIs cannot be combined with sacubitril due to the high risk for the development of angioedema.

(UptoDate®,Lexidrug™, 2026)

Appendix 2 provides additional details regarding ARBs.

ANGIOTENSIN RECEPTOR BLOCKER / NEPRILYSIN INHIBITOR (ARNI)

The newest class of drugs blocking the RAAS and used to treat HF is the ARNI. There is currently one ARNI (sacubitril/valsartan) which is a combination of a neprilysin inhibitor and an ARB. The first ARNI released was under the trade name Entresto. The first patent (a combination patent) for this medication has an expiration date of July 2025. However, there is ongoing legal activity regarding the validity of this patent (Novartis, 2023). Generic alternatives were approved by the FDA in 2024 but the exact timing of the release of these generic medications is not known. Entresto has been identified by the Centers for Medicare & Medicaid Services as one of the costliest medications under Medicare Part D (FDA, 2024, May 31).

Mechanism of Action of ARNI

♦ Neprilysin is an enzyme that breaks down the natriuretic peptides (atrial natriuretic peptide (ANP) and brain natriuretic peptide (BNP), bradykinin, and other vasoactive peptides.

♦ Neprilysin inhibition results in higher levels of natriuretic peptides which are beneficial in HF because they cause diuresis (loss of water), natriuresis (loss of sodium), and vasodilation (both preload and afterload reduction).

♦ The clinical effects of an ARNI are the result of higher levels of natriuretic and other vasoactive peptides and include the following:
  - Decreased sodium retention.
  - Decreased neurohormonal activation.
  - Decreased vascular tone.
  - Decreased hypertrophy and cardiac fibrosis.

Indications for ARNI

♦ HFrEF: In the PARADIGM-HF Trial, sacubitril/valsartan was compared to the ACEI enalapril in more than 8,000 patients with symptomatic HFrEF.

- The results of the trial showed that compared to enalapril, sacubitril/valsartan resulted in a 20% reduction in the rate of death or hospitalization for HF.
- There was also a 16% reduction in the rate of all-cause death compared to enalapril at 3.5 years of follow up

(McMurray et al., 2014)

♦ HF with mildly reduced EF (HFmrEF) and HFpEF: Sacubitril/valsartan might be reasonable in the treatment of HFmrEF and HFpEF although its effectiveness is not well established (Heidenreich et al., 2022).

Special Dosing Information for ARNI

♦ Sacubitril/valsartan comes in 3 strengths:
  - The lowest dose is sacubitril/valsartan 50 mg and contains 24 mg of sacubitril and 26 mg of valsartan. The prescription or order should be written as sacubitril 24 mg/valsartan 26 mg.
  - The medium dose is sacubitril/valsartan 100 mg and contains 49 mg of sacubitril and 51 mg of valsartan. The prescription or order should be written as sacubitril 49 mg/valsartan 51 mg.
  - The highest dose (which is the target dose, if tolerated) is sacubitril/valsartan 200 mg and contains 97 mg of sacubitril and 103 mg of valsartan. The prescription or order should be written as sacubitril 97 mg/valsartan 103 mg.

♦ In HF patients who are at risk for the development of hypotension, ½ of the lowest dose can be considered on initiation with the goal of titrating up the dose as tolerated.

♦ The valsartan in sacubitril/valsartan is dosed differently than valsartan only tablets because of increased bioavailability. Valsartan 26 mg, 51 mg, and 103 mg in sacubitril/valsartan is equivalent to 40 mg, 80 mg, and 160 mg, respectively, in other formulations containing valsartan.

(UptoDate®,Lexidrug™, 2026).

Select Adverse Effects of ARNI

♦ Since sacubitril/valsartan includes the ARB valsartan all adverse effects of ARBs apply with ARNIs.

♦ Potential adverse effects of an ARNI are related to inhibition of the RAAS. These include hypotension, hyperkalemia, and decreased GFR.

♦ There are also the potential adverse effects of cough and angioedema due to the increased levels of kinin produced by the neprilysin inhibitor as discussed in the section on angioedema with ACEIs.

(UptoDate®,Lexidrug™, 2026)

Contraindication Highlights for ARNI

♦ Consult manufacturer recommendations for use in children, pregnant women, and nursing women.

♦ An ARNI should not be used in any patient with a history of angioedema regardless of cause.

♦ The use of sacubitril/valsartan with an ACEI is contraindicated due to the high risk of angioedema.
  - If switching from an ACEI to sacubitril/valsartan, the ACEI must be discontinued 36 hours before starting sacubitril/valsartan.
  - Likewise, sacubitril/valsartan must be stopped 36 hours before switching to an ACEI.

♦ Use with caution and reduce the dose with moderate hepatic dysfunction.

♦ An ARNI is contraindicated in patients with severe hepatic failure and with ascites due to cirrhosis.

(Heidenreich et al., 2022; UptoDate®,Lexidrug™, 2026)

Special Considerations & Monitoring with ARNI

- The special considerations and monitoring as discussed above with ACEIs and ARBs are applicable to an ARNI because it contains an ARB.
- At baseline and within 1 to 2 weeks of starting the medication or increasing the dose, the following needs to be monitored: 1) BP including orthostatic BP, 2) renal function, and 3) potassium.
- Patients with low BP, diabetes, and renal dysfunction need to be monitored closely during therapy.

(Heidenreich et al., 2022; UptoDate®,Lexidrug™, 2026)

> ***Linking Knowledge to Practice***
>
> ✓ *Sacubitril/valsartan, an ARNI, produces a greater BP lowering effect than an ACEI or an ARB. If possible, diuretics should be held the day before and the day of sacubitril/valsartan initiation until the BP effect is known.*
>
> ✓ *Patients should be instructed to stay home and be cautious with activity until after the peak effect of the first dose. If there is a drop in BP, patients and families should be instructed regarding lying down and elevating feet until low BP is resolved. Patients should then notify their provider for instructions regarding the next dose.*
>
> ✓ *In patients with increased risk for developing hypotension, ½ of the smallest dose of sacubitril/valsartan can be considered on initiation.*
>
> ✓ *Kidney function and electrolytes should be evaluated prior to initiation and within 1 to 2 weeks after initiation and they should also be reevaluated with any dose changes (Maddox et al., 2019).*

Key Pharmacokinetic & Pharmacodynamic Information for ARNI

- A steady state of this combination medication is reached in 3 days.
- The valsartan in this combination medication is more bioavailable than in valsartan only tablets.
- Sacubitril/valsartan decreases plasma NT-proBNP because the medication is effective in treating HF. See the ***Linking Knowledge to Practice*** box below for information on the impact of sacubitril/valsartan on BNP results.
- Hemodialysis does not remove key active metabolites of sacubitril/valsartan. However, in patients being treated with sacubitril/valsartan who were receiving hemodialysis the medications stayed in a safe concentration range (Feng et al., 2022).

(Novartis, 2015)

> ***Linking Knowledge to Practice***
>
> ✓ *Because of the mechanism of action of an ARNI, BNP levels may not be accurate.*
>
> ✓ *In the PARADIGM-HF trial 14% of the participants had a doubling of the BNP level with initiation of sacubitril/valsartan. Another 6% had a tripling in the absence of decompensation. The increased levels corrected over time. These increases differed between the type of BNP assays used.*
>
> ✓ *Clinicians who rely on BNP levels (rather than NT pro-BNP levels) are encouraged to utilize patient physical exam to evaluate for sign of volume overload in the early stages of initiation.*
>
> ✓ *Sacubitril/valsartan will not impact the accuracy of NT pro-BNP in the same manner as BNP.*
>
> *(Myhre et al., 2019)*

Important Medication Interactions with ARNI

- Sacubitril cannot be used with an ACEI due to high risk of angioedema.
- See above for select medication interactions for ARBs.

Appendix 3 provides additional information regarding ARNI.

Prescribing Pearls for ACEIs, ARBs, and ARNI

- The initial dose of an ACEI, ARB, or ARNI should be low (e.g., 15 to 25% of the maximal recommended dose) and slowly increased over weeks to attain treatment goals.
- Once the response is known (e.g., BP, creatinine, and potassium level), the dose can be increased if the drug is tolerated.
- Correct volume depletion before initiation to avoid the risk of hypotension and syncope.
- In patients at high risk for ACEI induced reduction in GFR, (as described in the Advanced Concept Focus section above on ACEIs and Renal Function), a temporary reduction in the diuretic dose should be considered and NSAIDs should be avoided.
- Creatinine level and potassium should be checked within 3 to 5 days of ACEI therapy if initiated as an outpatient. Creatinine will be checked more frequently if the patient is in the hospital.
- Titrate ACEIs or ARBs generally every 2 weeks in patients with HFrEF based on tolerance. Start low and titrate to tolerance. Patients need frequent monitoring during titration. Titrate more slowly in frail older adults. Titration may occur more quickly in clinically stable patients.
- ARNIs should be titrated every 2 weeks (or more slowly) because of risk of hypotension. BP monitoring is more important when titrating an ARNI. Loop diuretics may need to be held or decreased when starting or titrating an ARNI.
- When titrating ACEIs, ARBs, or an ARNI renal function and potassium must be considered.
  - Renal function and potassium should be assessed 1 to 2 weeks after titration.
  - A dose reduction is needed for hyperkalemia or an eGFR < 30 L/min/1.73 m2.
- Obtain a periodic CBC with differential. Patients with renal impairment are at risk for developing neutropenia; patients with both renal impairment and collagen vascular disease (e.g. systemic lupus erythematosus [SLE] and rheumatoid arthritis) are at even higher risk of neutropenia.

(Maddox et al., 2021, Mann & Hilgers, 2021)

RENIN INHIBITORS

Mechanism of Action of Renin Inhibitors

- Direct renin inhibitors bind the active site of renin to block conversion of angiotensinogen to angiotensin I, thus decreasing the levels of angiotensin I, angiotensin II, and aldosterone.
- Theoretically, blocking renin should be more effective at inhibiting the RAAS than the use of ACEIs or ARBs. This is the reason a direct renin inhibitor has the potential to be an effective antihypertensive.
- The only renin inhibitor available currently is aliskiren.

Indications for Renin Inhibitors

Aliskiren is approved for the treatment of HTN.

- Aliskiren has BP lowering effects like diuretics, ACEIs, and ARBs, and further lowers BP when used in combination with other agents.
- However, there are restrictions for using a renin inhibitor in combination with an ACEI or an ARB. See section below on important medication interactions.

Special Dosing Information for Renin Inhibitors

- No dose adjustment is needed when CrCl $\geq$ 30 mL/min. No dose adjustments are given by the manufacturer for a CrCl $\leq$ 30 mL/min, yet there is a risk for hyperkalemia and worsening renal function.
- No dose adjustment required for patients on dialysis, however, the risk for hyperkalemia is high.
- No initial dose adjustment required for hepatic impairment.

(Up to Date®, Lexidrug™, 2026)

Select Adverse Effects of Renin Inhibitors

- Adverse effects may include those seen with the use of ACEIs or ARBs and include hypotension, hyperkalemia, angioedema, and renal impairment.
- The most common adverse effect according to product labeling is increased BUN and creatinine ($\leq$ 7%).

(Up to Date®, Lexidrug™, 2026)

Contraindication Highlights for Renin Inhibitors

- Consult manufacturer recommendations for use in children, pregnant women, and nursing women.
- Although aliskiren is approved for treatment of HTN, it is not recommended as initial therapy.
- See section below on important medication interactions and restrictions when using a renin inhibitor with an ACEI or an ARB.

(Jones et al., 2025)

Special Considerations & Monitoring with Renin Inhibitors

BP, renal function, and potassium need to be monitored prior to initiation and periodically throughout therapy with the frequency determined by the patient's clinical status and concomitant medications.

Key Pharmacokinetic & Pharmacodynamic Information for Renin Inhibitors

- Grapefruit juice may decrease the serum concentration of aliskiren. Separation of several hours between the medication and grapefruit juice may decrease the interaction.
- High fat meals decrease the absorption of aliskiren.
- Maximum antihypertensive effect is seen within 2 weeks.

(Lexicomp, 2023; Up to Date®, Lexidrug™, 2026)

Important Medication Interactions with Renin Inhibitors

Aliskiren in combination with an ACEI or an ARB is contraindicated in patients with diabetes or renal impairment (eGFR < 60 mL/min/1.73 m^2) due to increased risk of adverse effects (FDA, 2012, April 20).

Appendix 4 provides additional details regarding renin inhibitors.

MINERALOCORTICOID RECEPTOR ANTAGONISTS

MRAs are also referred to as aldosterone antagonists or aldosterone blockers. Mineralocorticoid receptors are found primarily in the heart, kidneys, vasculature, and brain. Aldosterone is a mineralocorticoid hormone produced in the adrenal cortex. The overactivation of aldosterone, often caused by renovascular HTN results in increased inflammation and fibrosis causing CV and kidney damage secondary to progressive fibrosis.

Activation of the RAAS system, stimulated most often by low BP, low renal perfusion or low sodium levels, results in the formation of angiotensin II. One of the effects of angiotensin II is the release of aldosterone. Aldosterone has several negative effects in HF, HTN and CKD including:

- Retention of sodium and water.
- Loss of magnesium and potassium.
- Activation of the SNS and potentiation of catecholamines (causing vasoconstriction).
- Inhibition of the parasympathetic nervous system.
- Myocardial and vascular fibrosis.
- Endothelial dysfunction and vascular inflammation.
- Promotion of direct remodeling.
- Prothrombotic properties.

(Agarwal et al., 2022; Scott, Menouar, & Dunn, 2023)

Mechanism of Action & Types of MRAs

There are three types of MRAs:

- Nonselective steroidal MRA: Spironolactone.
- Selective steroidal MRA: Eplerenone.
- Selective nonsteroidal MRA: Finerenone.

The mechanism of action of MRAs varies based on whether the agent is selective or nonselective and whether the agent is steroidal or nonsteroidal.

- Spironolactone and eplerenone compete with aldosterone for the receptor site in the distal renal tubules. This results in maintaining potassium and hydrogen ions and increasing the excretion of sodium and water.
- Eplerenone more selectively blocks mineralocorticoid receptors than spironolactone.
- Finerenone, a new MRA, selectively blocks mineralocorticoid receptor mediated sodium reabsorption and overactivation in the kidneys, heart, and blood vessels.
- Blocking the effects of aldosterone is beneficial in treating HF, HTN, and CKD via the following mechanisms:
    - Diuresis is promoted by blocking sodium and water retention caused by aldosterone. This can decrease preload and lower BP.
    - Hypokalemia that can occur with non-potassium sparing diuretics, commonly used in treatment of both HF and HTN, can be prevented by blocking aldosterone.
        - Hypokalemia is a risk factor for cardiac arrhythmias.
        - The use of potassium sparing diuretics with aldosterone blocking effects reduces the risk of arrhythmic death when compared to non-potassium sparing diuretics.
    - Blocking the effects of aldosterone is beneficial to the heart and kidneys.
        - Aldosterone contributes to cardiac and kidney fibrosis.
        - Fibrosis results in end organ damage which leads to the progression of HF and CKD.
    - Blocking the effects of aldosterone is beneficial for blood vessels.
        - Aldosterone contributes to fibrosis in blood vessels, which impairs vasodilation and results in increased afterload.
        - Activation of SNS induced by aldosterone also causes peripheral vasoconstriction, increasing LV afterload.

- Blocking aldosterone can prevent endothelial dysfunction by preventing the effects of aldosterone. Aldosterone decreases production of nitric oxide (a vasodilator) and increases formation of endothelin (a potent vasoconstrictor) in blood vessels, contributing to an increase in afterload.

♦ Even though aldosterone levels fall initially with treatment with an ACEI or an ARB, levels rise again with prolonged treatment. This is called "aldosterone escape". Adding an aldosterone antagonist blocks the effects of aldosterone levels that may rise after prolonged therapy with other drugs.

(Ahmad et al., 2017; Colucci & Pfeffer, 2022; Hilal-Dandan, 2018; Opie & Pfeffer, 2013)

Table 3
Indications for MRAs

Medication	Indications
Spironolactone	▪ Ascites due to cirrhosis: Generally used in combination with furosemide. ▪ HFrEF as part of evidenced based therapy for mortality benefit. ▪ HFpEF with a HF hospitalization or an elevated natriuretic peptide level within the last year [off label]. ▪ Post-MI complicated with reduced EF [off label]. ▪ Chronic HTN (alternative agent): Used for resistant HTN when BP is not at goal on combination therapy of preferred agents. A preferred agent in the treatment of resistant HTN. ▪ Primary aldosteronism. ▪ Acne vulgaris moderate to severe in females [off label]. ▪ Hair loss female pattern [off label]. ▪ Hirsutism in females [off label]: Typically given in combination with oral contraceptives. ▪ Hormone therapy for transgender females (assigned male at birth) [off label]: Used in combination with other agents.
Eplerenone	▪ HFrEF as part of evidenced based therapy for mortality benefit [off label]. ▪ HFpEF with a HF hospitalization or an elevated natriuretic peptide level within the last year [peripheral label]. ▪ Post-MI complicated with reduced EF. ▪ Chronic HTN (alternative agent): Used for resistant HTN when BP is not at goal on combination therapy of preferred agents. Preferred agent in the treatment of resistant HTN. ▪ Primary aldosteronism.
Finerenone	▪ CKD associated with DMT2 to reduce the risk of sustained GFR decline, end stage kidney disease, CV death, nonfatal MI, and hospitalization for HF in adult patients with CKD associated with type 2 diabetes. ▪ HFpEF to reduce HF events and CV death.
(Jones et al., 2025; Rossing et al., 2022a; Solomon et al., 2024; Up to Date®, Lexidrug™, 2026)	

Indications for MRAs

Table 3 summarizes indications for MRAs.

♦ Aldosterone antagonists are also referred to as potassium sparing diuretics.

♦ However, MRAs have indications for reasons beyond any potential diuretic effect, with indications for improved outcomes, including the reduction of mortality in certain clinical circumstances.

♦ Spironolactone and eplerenone have been shown to reduce morbidity, mortality, and hospitalizations for HF. They are recommended in patients with HFrEF and NYHA class II to IV symptoms who have adequate renal function (eGFR is >30 mL/min/1.73 m^2) and no hyperkalemia (Heidenreich et al., 2022).

- ♦ Spironolactone and eplerenone may be considered to decrease hospitalizations in patients with preserved EF, particularly among patients with LVEF on the lower end of this spectrum (Heidenreich et al., 2022).
- ♦ Eplerenone has been shown to reduce the incidence of all-cause mortality, CV mortality, CV hospitalizations, and sudden cardiac death in patients who are post-acute MI complicated with S&S of HF and an LVEF of $\leq$ 40% (Adamopoulos et al., 2009).
- ♦ Kidney Disease: Improving Global Outcomes (KDIGO) 2022 Clinical Practice Guideline on Diabetes Management in CKD suggests the use of a nonsteroidal MRA (finerenone) with proven kidney or CV benefit in patients with T2D, an eGFR $\geq$25 mL/min/1.73 m^2, normal serum potassium concentration, and albuminuria ($\geq$30 mg/g [$\geq$ 3mg/mmol]) despite maximum tolerated dose of RAAS inhibitor (Cheung et al., 2021).
- ♦ As of this writing, finerenone is not yet indicated in the treatment of HFrEF.
  - Clinical trial data demonstrate that there is a significant decrease in time to CV death, nonfatal MI or stroke, and hospitalization for HF in patients with CKD and type II diabetes. However, there is not yet statistical evidence that mortality is impacted in patients with HFrEF.
  - The FINEARTS-HF trial evaluated finerenone in patients with HFmrEF and HFpEF for impact on the composite outcome of worsening HF events and CV death.
    - In this study finerenone reduced the composite endpoint compared to placebo.
    - The driving factor in the reduction of the composite endpoint was the reduction in first or recurrent HF events.
    - As a result of this trial, finerenone was approved for use in the treatment of HFpEF.
  - Finerenone provides a better safety profile as far as hyperkalemia over steroidal MRAs and can be administered at lower levels of GFR while improving renal function. The current steroidal MRAs, while improving mortality in HFrEF, worsen renal function and are often discontinued due to hyperkalemia or worsening renal function

(Chimura et al., 2024; Filippatos et al., 2022; Kintscher & Edelmann, 2023; Solomon et al., 2024)

Special Dosing Information for MRAs

Spironolactone

- ♦ The dose of spironolactone used in HF for mortality reduction is much lower than the dose that is used as a diuretic in treating hepatic ascites.
- ♦ Dose adjustments for spironolactone are recommended when the eGFR is $\leq$ 50 mL/min/1.73 m^2.
- ♦ Below are the recommendations when using the tablet form of the medication in HF treatment.
  - If the eGFR is between 30 and 50 mL/min/1.73 m^2 the starting dose is 12.5 mg every other day.
  - If after 4 weeks renal function is stable, and the K^+ is < 5.0 mEq/L the dose can be doubled every 4 weeks to a maximum recommended dose of 25 mg/day.
  - If the eGFR is < 30 mL/min/1.73 m^2 the medication should not be used because HF clinical trials excluded patients with a creatinine of $\geq$ 2.5 mg/dL.
  - Spironolactone is unlikely to be significantly dialyzed and is not routinely recommended in patients receiving hemodialysis or peritoneal dialysis. However, there is evidence from two small clinical trials that the use is safe.
    - In one trial hyperkalemia occurred more frequently when the dose was 50 mg a day and in the other trial there was an increased frequency of moderate hyperkalemia, but not an increase in severe hyperkalemia.
    - In these 2 small clinical trials the use of spironolactone did not demonstrate CV benefit in patients with end stage renal disease.

(Charytan et al., 2019; Hammer et al., 2019)

Eplerenone

- Renal dosing recommendations when used in the treatment of HF include:
  - No dose adjustments if the eGFR is ≥ 50 mL/min/1.73 m^2.
  - If the eGFR is between 31 and 49 mL/min/1.73 m^2 eplerenone should be started at 25 mg every other day. If after 4 weeks renal function and potassium level are stable, the dose can be doubled at 4 weeks to a maximum recommended dose of 25 mg/day.
  - If the eGFR is < 30 mL/min/1.73 m^2 the medication is not recommended.
- Dose adjustments are not required in chronic HTN when the CrCl is > 50 mL/min. Eplerenone should not be used to treat chronic HTN if the CrCl is < 50 mL/min or if the creatinine is > 2 mg/dL in men or > 1.8 mg/dL in women (manufacturer recommendation). Alternate recommendation when CrCl is < 50 mL/min and the benefit outweighs the risk, is to start at lower dose and carefully monitor.
- Beer's criteria states to use with caution in patients > 65 years of age due to the potential to cause or exacerbate syndrome of inappropriate antidiuretic hormone (SIADH) or hyponatremia.
- Eplerenone is poorly dialyzable.
- There are no dosing adjustments recommended based on hepatic function per the manufacturer's recommendation. There is an increase in systemic exposure when there is moderate hepatic dysfunction.

(Accord Healthcare Inc., 2025; Lexicomp, 2023; Up to Date®, Lexidrug™, 2026)

Finerenone

- The dose of finerenone should be reduced by 50% when the eGFR is between 25 and 59 mL/min/1.73 m^2.
- Finerenone is not recommended for use when the eGFR is < 25 mL/min/1.73 m^2.

(Up to Date®, Lexidrug™, 2026)

Select Adverse Effects of MRAs

- The nonselective steroidal MRA, spironolactone, also blocks androgen receptors and stimulates progesterone receptors, which causes undesirable side effects such as gynecomastia, vaginal bleeding, and sexual dysfunction, thus decreasing patient adherence with therapy.
  - Spironolactone can cause gynecomastia in patients of all ages. This most often affects both breasts. This adverse effect is both time and dose related. The onset is delayed and ranges from 1 to 2 months after the start of therapy to over a year from the start of therapy.
  - Transitioning to eplerenone, which is a selective MRA, may eliminate gynecomastia and other adverse effects related to blocking androgen and stimulating progesterone. The selective aldosterone receptor antagonist, eplerenone, blocks aldosterone but does not cause the undesirable effects of spironolactone, a nonselective steroid MRA.
- The most dangerous adverse effect of aldosterone antagonists is hyperkalemia with the potential to be life threatening, especially when used with an ACEI or an ARB.
  - The highest risk of hyperkalemia occurs when the aldosterone antagonist is initiated at serum K^+ ≥5.0 mEq/L and continued with a serum K^+ ≥5.5 mEq/L.
  - Spironolactone is associated with a greater increase in serum potassium than eplerenone.
  - Finerenone, because it is a selective nonsteroidal MRA, seems to be less likely to cause hyperkalemia. In clinical trial data finerenone led to significantly smaller increases in serum potassium and smaller decreases in GFR than spironolactone with comparable efficacy (Pitt et al., 2015).
- In addition to hyperkalemia, MRAs have the potential adverse effect of hyponatremia. The highest risk is with spironolactone and finerenone.

(Lexicomp, 2023; Up to Date®, Lexidrug™, 2026)

Contraindication Highlights for MRAs

- Consult manufacturer recommendations for use in children, pregnant women, and nursing women.
- A MRA may be contraindicated based on the GFR. Suggested hold criteria include eGFR is $\leq$ 30 mL/min/1.73 m^2 for spironolactone and eplerenone and an eGFR <25 mL/min/1.73 m^2 for finerenone.
- Hyperkalemia at the time of initiation, or a potassium that cannot be maintained at $\leq$ 5.5 mEq/L after initiation are considered contraindications to an MRA.
- MRAs are contraindicated in primary adrenal insufficiency.

(Bayer HealthCare Pharmaceuticals; 2021; Lexicomp, 2023; Pfizer, 2008; Pfizer, 2022b; Up to Date®, Lexidrug™, 2026)

Linking Knowledge to Practice

- ✓ *Diarrhea causing dehydration or other reasons for holding loop diuretic therapy should result in an evaluation of the need to temporarily hold an aldosterone antagonist.*
- ✓ *When a patient with HF develops worsening renal function and/or hyperkalemia it may be more than an adverse medication effect. Worsening renal function and hyperkalemia may be a sign of an acute change in clinical condition or a progression of the patient's heart failure. In addition to holding the patient's aldosterone antagonist, a more complete clinical evaluation is warranted. (Heidenreich et al., 2022)*
- ✓ *In the setting of HF, spironolactone should be temporarily held or the dose adjusted in the setting of worsening renal function or if the serum K^+ is $\geq$ 5.5 mEq/L (Meyer, 2025). While spironolactone is beneficial in HF, hyperkalemia is dangerous and potentially life threatening. The management of a patient on spironolactone requires meticulous follow up to assure both benefit and safety.*

Special Considerations & Monitoring with MRAs

- Spironolactone:
  - Check potassium within a week of starting the medication or within a week of any dose titration.
  - Sodium, renal function, glucose, uric acid, BP, and volume status should be monitored.
  - Spironolactone should be stopped if the potassium level cannot be maintained at < 5.5 mEq/L.
  - In the setting of HF potassium and renal function should be checked 3 days after starting the medication and at the 1-week mark. Potassium and renal function should then be checked monthly for the first 3 months and every 3 months on an ongoing basis.
  - In the setting of HF, the monitoring cycle should be restarted when an ACEI, ARB, or ARNI is added or up titrated.

  (Heidenreich et al., 2022; Maddox, et al., 2021; Pfizer, 2022b; Up to Date®, Lexidrug™, 2026)
- Eplerenone:
  - BP and potassium should be checked before starting or increasing the medication and within 1 week and 1 month after initiating or titrating therapy. Periodic monitoring is then indicated.
  - Potassium and creatinine should be evaluated within 3 to 7 days of starting concurrent therapy with an ACEI, ARB, ARNI, NSAID, or moderate CYP3A inhibitor.
  - Monitoring recommendations in the setting of HF are the same as those for spironolactone.
  - Monitor sodium level closely when initiating or increasing the dose in older adults due to the risk of hyponatremia.

  (Pfizer, 2008; Up to Date®, Lexidrug™, 2026)
- Finerenone:
  - Monitoring should be done more frequently in patients at higher risk for hyperkalemia.
  - Potassium should be checked at baseline, 4 weeks after starting the medication or making any dose adjustments, and periodically during maintenance therapy.

- The GFR should be assessed at baseline and periodically during therapy.

(Bayer HealthCare Pharmaceuticals, 2021; Rossing et al., 2022a; Up to Date®, Lexidrug™, 2026)

> ***Linking Knowledge to Practice***
>
> ✓ *Patients who drink alcohol beyond moderation are at high risk for the development of hyponatremia. These patients will require more frequent evaluations of serum sodium levels when prescribed an aldosterone antagonist.*

Key Pharmacokinetic & Pharmacodynamic Information for MRAs

- ♦ A high calorie or high fat meal increases the bioavailability of spironolactone to approximately 90%.
- ♦ The metabolism of eplerenone is primarily hepatic via CYP3A4.
- ♦ The metabolism of finerenone is primarily hepatic via CYP3A4 (90%).
- ♦ Grapefruit juice may increase the serum concentration of eplerenone and finerenone.

(Bayer HealthCare Pharmaceuticals, 2021; Pfizer, 2008; Pfizer, 2022b; Up to Date®, Lexidrug™, 2026)

Important Medication Interactions with MRAs

- ♦ Potassium sparing diuretics should not be used in combination with other potassium sparing diuretics or MRAs.
- ♦ Potassium sparing diuretics including MRAs enhance the hyperkalemic effect of ACEIs, ARBs, and ARNIs.
- ♦ Spironolactone and eplerenone increase the hyperkalemic effect of cyclosporine and should be avoided in patients taking cyclosporine.
- ♦ CYP3A4 inhibitors may increase the serum concentration of eplerenone and finerenone. CYP3A4 inducers may decrease the serum concentration of eplerenone and finerenone.
- ♦ NSAIDs may decrease the antihypertensive effects of spironolactone and eplerenone and increase the hyperkalemic effect.

(Bayer HealthCare Pharmaceuticals, 2021; Pfizer, 2008; Pfizer, 2022b; Up to Date®, Lexidrug™, 2026)

Appendix 5 provides additional details regarding MRAs.

BETA BLOCKERS

The SNS exerts its CV effects by stimulating α and ß receptors in the heart and/or blood vessels. Refer to the discussion under SNS above for a summary of the effects of α and ß stimulation.

Mechanism of Action & Types of Beta Blockers

Beta blockade results in the following effects:

- ♦ Heart: ↓ HR (sinus bradycardia), ↓ contractility (↓ LV function), ↓ AV conduction, and AV block.
- ♦ Blood vessels:
    - Non-cardioselective agents block the vasodilating ß2 receptors, thus preventing vasodilation in arterioles and veins.
    - This allows α1 receptors to work unopposed, resulting in vasoconstriction.
    - This can worsen angina that occurs secondary to coronary vasospasm. It can also cause claudication in peripheral vascular disease.

- Lungs: Prevents bronchodilation and can cause bronchospasm. Non-cardioselective beta blockers are contraindicated in patients with reactive airway disease.
- Kidney: Decreases renin secretion, thus inhibiting the RAAS.

Types of beta blockers include:

- Nonselective beta blockers: These medications block both β1 and β2 receptors, so the effects include undesired bronchoconstriction and peripheral vascular constriction (because blockade of β2 receptors in peripheral vessels leaves the α vasoconstrictor receptors unopposed).
- Cardioselective beta blockers: These medications primarily block the β1 receptors to avoid the undesired pulmonary and peripheral vascular effects. Cardioselectivity occurs with lower doses of these drugs; at high doses, the β2 receptors are also blocked.
- Vasodilating beta blockers:
  - Some of these medications combine α and β blockade resulting in peripheral vasodilation by blockade of α1 receptors (labetalol, carvedilol).
  - Other vasodilatory mechanisms include stimulation of nitric oxide (nebivolol, carvedilol).
  - Some beta blockers have intrinsic sympathomimetic activity (ISA) in which β2 receptors are mildly stimulated to result in vasodilation (pindolol, acebutolol). Drugs with ISA do not decrease HR or contractility as much as other beta blockers.

Linking Knowledge to Practice

✓ *It is important to remember cardioselective beta blockers are cardioselective at lower doses. However, at higher doses they block β2 and can prevent bronchial and peripheral arterial vasodilation and aggravate bronchospastic disease and peripheral arterial disease.*

✓ *This is the reason why some providers may not prescribe even cardioselective beta blockers to patients with severe reactive airway disease or severe peripheral arterial disease.*

Table 4 lists examples for each classification of beta blocker.

Table 4

Classifications of Beta Blockers

Nonselective Beta Blocker	Cardioselective Beta Blockers	Vasodilating Beta Blockers
▪ Carvedilol: (also vasodilating) ▪ Labetalol: (also vasodilating) ▪ Nadolol ▪ Pindolol: (also ISA) ▪ Propranolol ▪ Sotalol: (also Class III antiarrhythmic) ▪ Timolol	▪ Acebutolol: (also ISA) ▪ Atenolol ▪ Betaxolol ▪ Bisoprolol ▪ Esmolol ▪ Metoprolol succinate ▪ Metoprolol tartrate ▪ Nebivolol: (also vasodilating)	▪ Carvedilol (dilates via α1blockade) ▪ Labetalol (dilates via α1blockade) ▪ Nebivolol (dilates via nitric oxide production)

Indications for Beta Blockers

Arrhythmias

- Beta blockers slow the HR, slow conduction through the AV node, and decrease ventricular irritability in the ischemic myocardium.
- Both supraventricular and ventricular arrhythmias can be treated with beta blockers.

- They are effective in arrhythmias caused by excessive adrenergic stimulation or increased sensitivity to catecholamines, such as acute MI, HF, exercise induced arrhythmias, and postoperative arrhythmias.
- Guidelines for management of supraventricular arrhythmias and atrial fibrillation recommend beta blockers for rate control in atrial fibrillation/flutter, and for treatment of SVT, including SVTs caused by an accessory pathway (Joglar et al.; Page et al., 2016).
- Guidelines for managing ventricular arrhythmias and preventing sudden cardiac death recommend beta blockers as one of the options for treating several ventricular arrhythmias.
    - They are recommended as first-line agents for long QT syndrome and catecholaminergic polymorphic VT.
    - Beta blockers are also recommended for the treatment of polymorphic VT due to myocardial ischemia.
    - They are also used in the management of symptomatic premature ventricular contractions (PVCs) in structurally normal hearts.

  (Al-Khatib et al., 2018)

Linking Knowledge to Practice

✓ *When a HR is elevated, it is very important to understand the reason for the elevated HR.*

✓ *When the HR is elevated due to a tachyarrhythmia, the rhythm will need to be treated either with pharmacological rate control or cardioversion.*

✓ *If the HR is elevated as compensation for low SV, it is important to identify the reason for the low SV.*

✓ *If the patient has compensatory tachycardia from low stoke volume due to volume depletion, the patient needs volume replacement to correct the underlying problem. It would be harmful to a patient with volume depletion to be given a HR lowering medication such as a beta blocker.*

✓ *If the patient has compensatory tachycardia from low stoke volume due to reduced contractility it is important to know if the patient's low contractility is acute or chronic.*

- *If the patient is in acute shock from a STEMI, HR lowering medications such as beta blockers are contraindicated.*
- *However, if the patient has reduced contractility and stable HF or reduced contractility from a MI and is hemodynamically stable, then evidence-based beta blockers can be used as a treatment strategy to favorably impact ventricular function.*

Acute Coronary Syndrome

- Beta blockers are effective in treating unstable angina as well as MI.
- Beta blockers reduce ischemia by reestablishing the balance between myocardial O_2 supply and demand.
    - Myocardial O_2 demand is decreased by the slower HR, decreased contractility, and decreased BP caused by beta blockade.
    - O_2 supply may be increased when a slower HR prolongs diastolic filling time and coronary perfusion time.
- Beta blocker therapy reduces infarct size and decreases complications including reinfarction and life-threatening ventricular arrhythmias. Clinical trials have shown that beta blocker therapy results in a relative risk reduction for sudden cardiac death.
- It is reasonable to use intravenous (IV) beta blockers in patients with STEMI who are hypertensive or have ongoing ischemia in the absence of contraindications.

- ♦ Beta blockers reduce early and late mortality in acute MI regardless of reperfusion status.
- ♦ Guidelines for management of STEMI and for management of NSTE-ACS recommend that oral beta blockers should be initiated in the first 24 hours in patients with STEMI who do not have signs of HF, evidence of low CO state, increased risk for cardiogenic shock, or other contraindications.
- ♦ There is evidence for the continued use of beta blocker therapy for up to 3 years after MI.
- ♦ Beta blockers are often continued indefinitely in patients who are considered high risk.

(Amsterdam et al., 2014; Bohula & Morrow, 2019; Giugliano & Braunwald, 2019; Moliterno & Januzzi, 2017; O'Gara et al., 2013; Opie, 2013a; Patel et al., 2017; Rosenson et al., 2024)

Specific Hold Criteria for Beta Blockers in the Acute Presentation of MI

- STEMI precipitated by cocaine:
  - Concern for exacerbation of coronary artery vasoconstriction or vasospasm by leaving alpha adrenergic stimulation unopposed by blocking β2 receptors.
  - Note: Some studies show beta blockers in the setting of cocaine induced chest pain do not increase the risk of MI or death (Pham et al., 2018).
- Heart blocks (unless pacemaker is in place):
  - 1st degree AV block with PR > 0.24 sec.
  - 2nd or 3rd degree AV block.
- HR < 60 beats per minute (BPM). This is a high-risk feature for cardiogenic shock.
- Systolic BP < 100 mmHg. This is a high-risk feature for cardiogenic shock.
- Moderate LV failure in patient naïve to beta blocker therapy (signs of acute decompensated HF or shock).
- Active asthma or reactive airway disease.

(O'Gara et al., 2013)

Heart Failure

- ♦ Beta blockers decrease the neurohumoral effects of chronic sympathetic stimulation and activation of the RAAS that occurs in HF.
  - Chronic SNS stimulation causes tachycardia, increases myocardial O_2 demands, contributes to cardiac myocyte hypertrophy and ventricular remodeling, promotes arrhythmias, and stimulates the RAAS.
  - In addition, chronic stimulation of beta receptors causes beta receptor downregulation, which decreases the number of beta receptors on the cell membrane and reduces responsiveness to beta stimulation.
- ♦ The benefits of beta blocker therapy in HF include:
  - Lowering of HR.
  - Reduction of circulating vasoconstrictor substances including norepinephrine, renin, and endothelin.
  - Upregulation of beta receptors resulting in an increased number of beta receptors on the cell membrane to restore inotropic and chronotropic myocardial responsiveness.
  - Reduction of MVO_2.
  - Anti-ischemic effects.
  - Improvement of coronary blood flow through lengthening of diastole.
  - Antiarrhythmic effects.
  - Decreased LV volume.

- Improved LVEF.

(Masarone et al., 2021)

◆ Long-term treatment with beta blockers improves symptoms of HF, slows progression of HF, increases LV function, decreases hospitalizations for HF, and improves survival in all NYHA classes of HF (Heidenreich et al., 2022).

◆ Guidelines for the management of HF recommend that oral beta blocker therapy be initiated in all patients with an LVEF of ≤ 40%. This includes those who have never demonstrated signs of HF (Stage B) and those with current or prior symptoms of HFrEF (Stage C and D) to reduce morbidity and mortality unless there are contraindications (Heidenreich et al., 2022).

Linking Knowledge to Practice

✓ *HF guidelines specify that only 3 beta blockers are recommended in patients with an LVEF ≤ 40% to achieve the benefit of decreased mortality and morbidity. The 3 recommended beta blockers are bisoprolol, carvedilol, and sustained-release metoprolol succinate.*

✓ *The above 3 beta blockers are indicated in the treatment of HFrEF because they interrupt the toxic effects of chronic SNS stimulation and reduce mortality even though they have a negative inotropic effect.*

- *However, in the setting of acute decompensated HF in a patient who has not been on a beta blocker, the beta blocker should be held until the patient is euvolemic.*
- *In this setting of acute decompensation, it is not desirable to add a negative inotropic agent.*

✓ *If a patient who is already being treated with a beta blocker is admitted with an acute decompensation, the beta blocker is typically not stopped. However, the dose may need to be reduced.*

✓ *If an inotropic medication is needed, the beta blocker is generally discontinued until the patient stabilizes. If the inotrope is dobutamine (a beta agonist), the concurrent administration of a beta blocker will counteract the $\beta 1$ stimulation of dobutamine.*

Hypertension

◆ BP is determined by CO and SVR. Beta blockers decrease CO by decreasing HR and contractility, and they decrease renin release in the kidney, which results in a decrease in SVR.

◆ Current guidelines for the management of HTN list beta blockers among several classes of drugs that can be used for HTN treatment. However, beta blockers are not recommended as first-line agents unless the patient has ischemic heart disease or HF when beta blockers are used as part of guideline directed medical therapy.

◆ Beta blockers are beneficial in combination with primary drugs (thiazide and thiazide-like diuretics, ACEIs, ARBs, CCBs) in treating HTN but are less effective than other drugs at preventing CV events, especially stroke.

(Opie, et al., 2013; Jones et al., 2025)

Hypertrophic Cardiomyopathy (HCM)

◆ Beta blockers are first-line agents for treatment of symptoms (exertional angina or dyspnea) in patients with nonobstructive HCM (Members et al., 2024).

◆ Beta blockers decrease contractility and prevent tachycardia, both of which help to decrease outflow tract obstruction in HOCM.

◆ Non vasodilating beta blockers should be used in patients with HOCM and symptoms (dyspnea, chest pain, syncope, or near syncope) attributable to LV outflow tract obstruction (Members et al., 2024).

Acute Dissecting Aortic Aneurysm

- ♦ Beta blockers (esmolol and labetalol) are first-line agents used in the initial management of an acute aortic dissection because they decrease HR and the force of myocardial contraction, thus decreasing stress on the aneurysm.
- ♦ Beta blockers are also beneficial when vasodilators such as nitroprusside are used to decrease BP, because they blunt the reflex tachycardia caused by vasodilation.

(Black & Burke, 2022)

> ***Linking Knowledge to Practice***
>
> ✓ *In the treatment of an acute dissecting thoracic aortic aneurysm, HR reduction to a HR of < 60 BPM with IV esmolol or labetalol is recommended PRIOR to the initiation of vasodilators. Once the HR is < 60 BPM if the systolic BP remains > 120 mmHg then vasodilator therapy can be initiated.*
>
> *(Black & Burke, 2022)*

Table 5 lists the CV indications for beta blocker therapy and the mechanism of action for each indication.

Special Dosing Information for Beta Blockers

The following information is based on carvedilol and metoprolol. Consult Appendix 6, manufacturer recommendations or other drug reference for recommendations for each individual beta blocker.

- ♦ No dose adjustments are needed based on renal function.
- ♦ Carvedilol is poorly dialyzed. Metoprolol metabolites are dialyzable, but no dose adjustment is needed.
- ♦ Metoprolol tartrate rather than succinate should be used for initial dosing in the setting of liver cirrhosis. In the setting of any moderate to severe liver dysfunction, lower dosing is recommended. Metoprolol elimination is highly dependent on liver blood flow so liver dysfunction can result in higher bioavailability and prolonged half-life.
- ♦ Special considerations are required when carvedilol is used in patients with mild to moderate hepatic impairment.
  - Initial lower doses should be used.
  - Carvedilol should be stopped when there is MAP < 65 mmHg, AKI, or hyponatremia.
  - Carvedilol is contraindicated in severe hepatic impairment although you may see it used by some experts in select circumstances. If used in the setting of more severe hepatic impairment the same stop criteria for mild to moderate hepatic impairment apply.

(UptoDate®, Lexidrug™, 2026)

Select Adverse Effects of Beta Blockers

Cardiac

- ♦ Bradycardia can occur due to depressed sinus node automaticity leading to exercise intolerance.
- ♦ AV block can develop due to slowing of the conduction though the AV node.
- ♦ Worsening HF can occur due to decreased contractility with higher doses.
  - When initiating a beta blocker, patients may feel some adverse effects for the first few months until beta receptors upregulate.
  - Beta blockers are initiated at low doses and titrated upwards slowly to help patients adjust to any initial adverse effects.
  - Symptoms of HF will ultimately improve as beta blockers achieve their therapeutic effect.

- Despite the potential downside from decreased contractility beta blockers are recommended as guideline directed medical therapy in chronic HFrEF to improve mortality.
- However, in acute decompensated HF a beta blocker should be initiated until the patient has achieved adequate diuresis and is stable.

♦ Hypotension may occur.
- Some beta blockers have additional vasodilating properties and thus lower BP more than beta blockers without vasodilating properties.
- However, even a beta blocker without vasodilating properties has the potential to lower BP through the mechanism of decreasing contractility which can decrease CO.

♦ Abrupt discontinuation of long-term beta blocker therapy can exacerbate angina and increase the risk of sudden death. Beta blockers should be weaned off when discontinued (Podrid, 2026).

Pulmonary

♦ Bronchoconstriction (with nonselective agents or high doses of cardioselective agents) can occur due to β2 blockade which prevents bronchodilation.

♦ Pulmonary edema can occur due to decreased contractility in the setting of depressed LV function.

Linking Knowledge to Practice

✓ *Consider using a cardioselective beta blocker in patients with chronic lung disease who require beta blocker therapy. This will avoid β2 blockade that will prevent bronchodilation.*
✓ *The addition of a cardioselective beta blocker in a patient using an inhaled beta agonist for treatment of lung disease may lead to an increase in inhaler use.*
✓ *Remember high doses of cardioselective beta blockers can still result in bronchoconstriction.*

Peripheral Vascular

♦ SVR increases with the nonselective beta blockers because β2 receptors are blocked.

♦ Cold extremities can develop due to peripheral vasoconstriction.

♦ Worsening claudication occurs due to β2 blockade leaving α1 receptors unopposed. When α1 receptors are unopposed vasoconstriction occurs.

Metabolic

♦ Beta blockers can mask signs of hypoglycemia (tachycardia, sweating, etc.) in patients with diabetes.

♦ Decreased insulin sensitivity occurs with most beta blockers resulting in hypoglycemia.

♦ Carvedilol, however, increases insulin sensitivity in patients with insulin resistance resulting in hyperglycemia.

♦ Nonselective agents decrease the formation of glucose in liver and can delay recovery from insulin-induced hypoglycemia, especially in patients with DMT1.

♦ Nonselective beta blockers increase LDL cholesterol and serum triglycerides.

(Ko et al., 2002; Opie, 2013a; Westfall et al., 2018)

Central Nervous System

♦ The incidence of significant CNS impact is very low and is a true finding in clinical trials much less often than suggested.

- Fatigue is a potential adverse effect occurring in approximately 18 of every 1000 patients.
- Depression has been reported in approximately 6 of every 1000 patients.
- Erectile dysfunction, although not common, has been reported in approximately 5 of every 1000 patients.

(Ko et al., 2002; Opie, 2013a; Westfall et al., 2018)

Table 5

Indications for Beta Blocker Therapy

Use	Mechanism of Action
ACS (Unstable angina, STEMI, NSTE-ACS)	▪ ↓ automaticity in ventricle so ↓ risk of VF early in MI. ▪ Rebalance O_2 supply and demand by ↓ O_2 demands (↓ HR, ↓ contractility↓ BP) and ↑ O_2 supply (↓ HR increases diastolic filling time and coronary perfusion time). ▪ ↓ infarct size, rate of reinfarction, and mortality.
Arrhythmias (A Fib, A flutter, SVT, some VT, congenital long QT syndromes)	▪ ↓ automaticity so ↓ VT, VF. ▪ ↓ AV conduction so can slow ventricular response to atrial fibrillation/flutter and may terminate paroxysmal SVT. ▪ Blunt adrenergic surge that causes Torsade de Pointes in long QT syndrome and catecholaminergic polymorphic VT.
Classic Angina (due to atherosclerotic obstruction of coronary arteries)	▪ ↓ O_2 demand by ↓ HR, ↓ contractility, ↓ BP. ▪ ↑ O_2 supply by ↓ HR which increases diastolic filling and coronary perfusion time.
HF (low dose beta blockade to block neurohormonal SNS response)	▪ ↓ HR = longer diastolic filling time, ↑ coronary perfusion time, ↓ myocardial O_2 demands. ▪ Protect the heart from cardiotoxic effects of high norepinephrine levels that occur in HF causing upregulation of beta receptors. ▪ ↓ renin release so ↓ angiotensin II levels and ↓ SVR.
HTN	▪ ↓ HR = ↓ CO = ↓ BP (BP = CO × SVR). ▪ ↓ contractility = ↓ CO = ↓ BP. ▪ ↓ renin release in kidney causes less angiotensin II and ↓ SVR.
Acute Aortic Dissection	▪ ↓ contractility to reduce stress on the aneurysm. ▪ ↓ HR to blunt reflex tachycardia caused by vasodilators.
Migraine Headaches (H/As)	▪ Inhibits β mediated vasodilatation in cerebral vessels (use is prophylactic, not for treatment of migraines).
Obstructive Cardiomyopathy	▪ ↓ contractility so reduces outflow tract obstruction. ▪ ↓ HR allows longer diastolic filling time so more blood in ventricle to keep outflow tract open.

Linking Knowledge to Practice

✓ *When introducing a beta blocker to the treatment regimen of a patient with DMT2, it is important to educate the patient regarding the potential for the beta blocker to potentiate hypoglycemia. A beta blocker can also mask S&S of hypoglycemia, especially tachycardia.*

✓ *However, carvedilol in patients with HF may worsen hyperglycemia to the point of requiring an adjustment in their antidiabetic medication (UptoDate®, Lexidrug™, 2024).*

✓ *Blood glucose levels should be carefully monitored in patients taking beta blockers.*

Prescribing Pearls for Beta Blockers

- Both beta blockers and ACEIs are used after an ACS to reduce complications immediately post-MI.
  - The first dose of these medications should not be given at the same time. There is a high risk for hypotension early during a MI because the extent and impact of myocardial dysfunction may not be known.
  - Beta blockers have priority over ACEIs early after presentation. An ACEI can be added after a beta blocker once stability is maintained on a beta blocker.
- The BP and HR hold criteria for beta blockers in the setting of MI are different than hold criteria in other clinical conditions. For example:
  - 1) When beta blockers are used for stable angina, the HR goal is often < 60 BPM to optimally decrease MVO2.
  - 2) When beta blockers are used in the treatment of chronic stable HFrEF they are often given when the systolic BP is < 90 mmHg in a patient who is asymptomatic since asymptomatic hypotension is common in HFrEF (Ko et al., 2004; Masarone et al., 2021).
- An advantage of beta blockers in the setting of an MI is the suppression of ventricular arrhythmias. Bigeminal PVCs may result in a HR of < 60 BPM. However, in this situation beta blockers may still be given to suppress the ventricular ectopy.
- Be aware of hospital based preset hold criteria for medications.
  - The hospital may have a standard hold of < 60 BMP for all beta blockers. However, in cardiology a hold of < 50 BMP is often preferred to assure the patient is receiving the medication for mortality benefit.
  - Providers should specify hold criteria with each order based on the clinical goals and patient condition.
- If a patient presents in acute decompensated HF currently on a beta blocker, the beta blocker does not always need to be discontinued on presentation.
  - If the patient is volume overloaded but adequately perfusing the beta blocker should be continued (Masarone et al., 2021).
  - If the patient is hemodynamically compromised and an inotrope is required, then the beta blocker will most likely need to be discontinued until there is no further need for the inotrope.

Contraindication Highlights for Beta Blockers

- Consult manufacturer recommendations for use in children, pregnant women, and nursing women.
- The following are clinical conditions in which beta blockers are contraindicated:
  - Hypotension (symptomatic or systolic BP less than 90 mmHg).
  - Symptomatic or severe bradycardia, sick sinus syndrome.
  - Heart block – 2nd or 3rd degree block unless a pacemaker is present.
  - Pre-excitation tachycardias.
  - Cardiogenic shock.
  - Acute decompensated HF in a patient who is not already on a beta blocker.
  - Angina due to coronary vasospasm.
  - Severe asthma or severe or decompensated bronchospastic disease.
  - Peripheral arterial disease (PAD) with worsening claudication or ischemic pain at rest.

- Severe depression.

(UptoDate®, Lexidrug™, 2026)

Special Considerations & Monitoring with Beta Blockers

- ♦ Beta blockers can mask the presentation of hyperthyroidism by blunting tachycardia.
- ♦ In untreated pheochromocytoma, alpha blockers (either a selective $alpha_1$ blocker or a non-selective alpha blocker) should be given prior to beta blockers.
- ♦ Beta blockers need to be slowly tapered to avoid acute tachycardia, HTN, or ischemia in patients with underlying CAD.
- ♦ It is important to remember that patients taking beta blockers for another indication may have underlying CAD that has not been diagnosed. Anginal symptoms have been reported to begin 12 to 24 hours after abrupt withdrawal.
- ♦ Chronic beta blocker therapy should not be withdrawn prior to major surgery unless there is a compelling reason.
- ♦ HR is an important monitoring consideration.
  - In previous versions of guidelines for the management of NSTE-ACS and chronic angina the target resting HR goal has been between 50 or 55 and 60 BMP) (Braunwald et al., 2002; Gibbons et al., 1999).
  - The most recent guidelines for NSTE-ACS and chronic angina do not specify a target HR when treating a patient with a beta blocker.
- ♦ The ECG should be evaluated for the presence of any AV block exacerbated by beta blockers.
- ♦ Glucose should be carefully monitored in patients with diabetes.
- ♦ Patients should be monitored for adverse nervous system effects including fatigue, dizziness, and depressed mental alertness.
- ♦ Patients with bronchospastic disease or significant PAD typically are not treated with beta blockers due to the concern of blocking β2 receptors resulting in bronchial and peripheral arterial vasoconstriction depending on the dose of beta blocker.
  - However, in some patients, the benefit of a beta blocker may outweigh the risk.
  - These patients need to be monitored for exacerbation of bronchospastic disease or peripheral arterial insufficiency.

(UptoDate®, Lexidrug™, 2026)

Key Pharmacokinetic & Pharmacodynamic Information for Beta Blockers

The following information is based on carvedilol and metoprolol. Consult Appendix 6, manufacturer recommendations or other drug reference for recommendations for each individual beta blocker.

Key considerations for carvedilol include:

- ♦ Hepatic metabolism involves CYP2D6, CYP2CP, CYP3A4, CYP2C19, CYP1A2, and CYP2E1. CYP2D6 poor metabolizers will have higher plasma concentrations.
- ♦ Bioavailability is increased in patients with congestive HF.
- ♦ In HF, plasma concentrations can be increased by up to 100%.
- ♦ Patients with hepatic cirrhosis have a 4-to-7-fold increase in drug concentration.
- ♦ Plasma concentrations may be 40 to 50% higher in the setting of moderate to severe kidney impairment.

◆ In older adults, plasma levels are approximately 50% higher.
(UptoDate®, Lexidrug™, 2026)

Key considerations for metoprolol include:

◆ Metabolism is primarily hepatic via CYP2D6. Poor CYP2D6 metabolizers will have much higher plasma concentrations.

◆ Elimination half-life is prolonged in the setting of hepatic impairment.
(UptoDate®, Lexidrug™, 2026)

Linking Knowledge to Practice

✓ *The physiological rationale for not using beta blockers in the setting of a cocaine-induced MI is the same as for the need to withdraw beta blockers before weaning a patient off clonidine.*
  - *Vasoconstriction and HTN can occur with both cocaine use and clonidine withdrawal secondary to alpha adrenergic stimulation.*
  - *If β2 adrenergic receptors (responsible for peripheral vasodilation) are blocked, the alpha-adrenergic stimulation will be unopposed.*

✓ *The acute withdrawal of beta blockers can lead to ischemic symptoms that can result in acute MI in patients with known coronary disease.*
  - *This is thought to be due to the upregulation of the adrenergic receptors during the blockade of the SNS system with beta blockers (Elliott, 2025).*
  - *With the sudden withdrawal of a beta blocker, beta receptor responsiveness to the adrenergic upregulation can be increased (and is unopposed) which can result in a hyperadrenergic state.*
  - *This is more prominent with short-acting beta blockers than long-acting beta blockers, most notably propranolol.*
  - *Titration of beta blockers is preferred prior to discontinuation. The rate of titration depends on the half-life of the drug and can be accomplished over a relatively short period of time.*

Important Medication Interactions with Beta Blockers

The select medication interactions below are based on information for carvedilol and metoprolol. Please refer to drug specific references for medication interactions specific to other beta blockers.

◆ Beta blockers are frequently used with multiple other classes of CV drugs.

◆ Additive effects can occur between beta blockers and other drugs that slow HR, decrease AV conduction, and depress contractility, especially the non-dihydropyridine CCBs.

◆ Beta blockers are generally not used when a patient is receiving inotropic therapy since beta blockers are negative inotropes. Beta blockers will directly compete with the impact of dobutamine, a beta agonist.

◆ Beta blockers must be withdrawn several days before discontinuing clonidine.
  - The rationale is to have β2 vasodilating receptors available to counteract the increased α1 vasoconstriction that occurs due to increased catecholamine levels when clonidine is discontinued.
  - This reduces the risk of rebound HTN with clonidine withdrawal.

◆ Amiodarone and dronedarone can substantially enhance the bradycardic effect of beta blockers.

◆ Midodrine can enhance the bradycardic effect of beta blockers.

◆ Beta blockers can enhance the HR lowering effect of ivabradine.

◆ Cardioselective beta blockers may enhance the hypoglycemic effect of antidiabetic medications. Non-selective beta blockers may enhance the hypoglycemic effects of insulin.

- Carvedilol may increase the serum concentration of digoxin.
- Beta blockers can enhance the neuromuscular blocking effect of succinylcholine.
- Nonselective beta blockers can diminish the bronchodilation effects of β 2 agonists.
- CYP2D6 inhibitors can increase the serum concentration of metoprolol and carvedilol.

(UptoDate®, Lexidrug™, 2026)

Appendix 6 provides additional details regarding individual beta blockers.

CALCIUM CHANNEL BLOCKERS

Mechanism of Action & Types of CCBs

Mechanism of Action of CCBs

Calcium plays a major role in depolarization of the sinus node and the AV node. Calcium also binds to actin and myosin proteins in cardiac and smooth muscle fibers to facilitate contraction of the heart and of the smooth muscle layer in peripheral blood vessels. CCBs inhibit inward flow of calcium ions in cardiac myocytes, in the SA and AV nodal cells, and through the L-type calcium channel in smooth muscle.
(Elliott & Ram, 2011)

Types of CCBs

Dihydropyridines

- Dihydropyridine type CCBs end in "pine" and have more effect on peripheral blood vessels than on the heart, although there is still the potential for cardiac depression with these drugs.
- Because of their relative vascular selectivity, dihydropyridines are used to treat effort angina and HTN. Nifedipine is the prototype of this group of CCBs.
- Dihydropyridines have more effect on arteries than veins and therefore are better afterload reducers than preload reducers.
- The vascular selectivity of dihydropyridines causes peripheral vasodilation and decreased BP which elicits a reflex increase in HR and contractility; therefore, these agents do not cause bradycardia or have the same negative inotropic effect that non-dihydropyridines do.
- Newer generation non-dihydropyridines, like felodipine and amlodipine, have very little cardiac depressant activity and are better tolerated in patients with HF.

Non-Dihydropyridines

- These drugs have more cardiac effects than peripheral effects.
- Non-dihydropyridines decrease contractility and lower HR.
- Verapamil, and diltiazem are the 2 agents in this class of CCBs; they both decrease HR and AV conduction and are used primarily to treat supraventricular arrhythmias.
- Both drugs also have some peripheral vasodilating effects; diltiazem is often used to prevent spasm in radial artery grafts used in cardiac bypass surgery.

Table 6 outlines the physiological impact of each of the types of CCBs.

Note the similarities in action between verapamil and diltiazem which are the only 2 CCBs used to decrease HR and or slow conduction through the AV node.

Table 6 Physiological Impact of CCBs			
Effect of Medication	**Non-dihydropyridines**		**Dihydropyridines**
	Verapamil	Diltiazem	
Heart Rate	▼▼	▼	▲
Direct AV Nodal Effects	▼▼	▼	none
Contractility	▼▼	▼	▼
Arterial Vasodilatation	▲▲	▲	▲▲▲

The clinical effects of CCBs include:

- Cardiac:
  - Decreased HR (verapamil and diltiazem).
  - Decreased conduction velocity through AV node (verapamil and diltiazem).
  - Decreased contractility (especially verapamil, to a lesser extent diltiazem).
- Vascular:
  - Prevention of contraction of muscular layer in arterial blood vessels (less effect on venous vessels).
  - Coronary vasodilation (prevents coronary vasospasm).
  - Peripheral vasodilation (afterload reduction).

Indications for CCBs

Table 7 summarizes the clinical uses and mechanisms of action for CCBs.

Angina

- CCBs are effective in exertional angina. CCBs help reestablish the balance between myocardial O_2 supply and demand by decreasing HR, decreasing contractility, and by peripheral vasodilation and afterload reduction.
- In vasospastic angina (also called variant angina) the angina is due to coronary artery vasospasm. CCBs increase O_2 supply by causing coronary artery vasodilation and preventing spasm (Eschenhagen, 2018; Opie, 2013b).
- Guidelines for management of stable ischemic heart disease recommend a CCB for relief of angina if beta blockers are contraindicated or not tolerated (Fihn et al., 2012).
- Guidelines for management of unstable angina and non-ST elevation ACS recommend a non-dihydropyridine CCB (verapamil or diltiazem) for continuing or frequently recurring ischemia in patients with contraindications to beta blockers or who do not respond to beta blockers and who have no LV dysfunction or other contraindication to CCB therapy. These guidelines also recommend CCBs for treatment of vasospastic angina (Amsterdam et al., 2014).

Hypertension

See Table 8 for medication specifics for the CCBs used in hypertensive emergencies.

- ♦ The primary mechanism of the CCB antihypertensive effect is a decrease in SVR due to peripheral vasodilation. Some CCBs also decrease HR and contractility, which can contribute to their antihypertensive effect.
- ♦ CCBs can be effective alone or in combination with other antihypertensive agents and are among the first-line drugs recommended for BP control in 2025 HTN Guidelines (Jones et al., 2025).
- ♦ CCBs are particularly effective agents for prevention of stroke and in African Americans and older patients (Opie et al., 2013). Stroke prevention guidelines list CCBs among primary antihypertensive agents in reducing stroke risk (Meschia et al., 2014).
- ♦ Two CCBs, clevidipine and nicardipine, are specifically recommended for potential use in a hypertensive emergency.

Arrhythmias

- ♦ The non-dihydropyridine CCBs, verapamil and diltiazem, are effective in slowing conduction through the AV node and therefore are useful as ventricular rate control drugs in atrial fibrillation/flutter.
- ♦ However, non-dihydropyridine CCBs should not be used in atrial fibrillation with rapid ventricular response when there is evidence of pre-excitation. The reason is due to the potential to shorten the refractory period of the accessory pathway and increase the ventricular rate (Joglar et al., 2024).
- ♦ Atrial tachycardia, multifocal atrial tachycardia, and junctional tachycardia can also be treated with non-dihydropyridine CCBs (Page et al., 2016).
- ♦ CCBs can terminate or possibly prevent AV nodal reentry tachycardia (AVNRT) and the reentry tachycardias due to the presence of an accessory pathway (AVRT) in Wolff-Parkinson-White syndrome (UptoDate®, Lexidrug™, 2026).
- ♦ CCBs are generally contraindicated in acute treatment of VT.
  - IV verapamil can cause hemodynamic collapse if given for VT in patients with previous MI.
  - However, VT originating from the RV outflow tract can sometimes be managed chronically with non-dihydropyridine CCB in patients with structurally normal hearts.
  - Oral and IV verapamil can also be used for idiopathic interfascicular reentrant left VT.

  (Al-Khatib et al., 2018)

> ***Linking Knowledge to Practice***
>
> ✓ *It is important to remember that only 2 CCBs, diltiazem and verapamil, slow HR. The dihydropyridine CCBs may instead cause some increase in HR due to a reflex response to peripheral vasodilation and drop in BP.*
>
> ✓ *The non-dihydropyridine CCBs may be used in the treatment of reentry tachycardias due to the presence of an accessory pathway in WPW which can produce an AVRT (Joglar et al., 2024).*
>
> - *However, they should not be used in patients with WPW who are in atrial fibrillation with evidence of pre-excitation (Joglar et al., 2024).*
> - *In this setting the slowing of conduction through the AV node can result in increased conduction over the accessory pathway, thus increasing the ventricular rate.*

Hypertrophic Cardiomyopathy

- ♦ Verapamil is recommended for the treatment of symptoms in patients with HCM (obstructive or non-obstructive) who do not respond to beta blockers or who have side effects or contraindications to beta blocker (Elliott et al., 2014; Members et al., 2024). Verapamil decreases contractility and prevents tachycardia, both of which help to decrease outflow tract obstruction in HOCM.

- ♦ Dihydropyridine CCBs are contraindicated in HOCM because of their peripheral vasodilating effects. Peripheral vasodilation increases the pressure gradient between the LV and the aorta, which can facilitate collapse of the LV outflow tract.

Special Dosing Information for CCBs

The information below contains some dosing highlights for diltiazem, verapamil (oral), and the dihydropyridines amlodipine and felodipine. Consult Appendix 7, manufacturer recommendations or other drug reference for recommendations for each individual dihydropyridine CCB.

- ♦ No dose adjustments are needed for diltiazem or verapamil based on renal function. However, manufacturer labeling for verapamil recommends close monitoring in patients with severe renal impairment because approximately 70% of the drug is excreted as metabolites in the urine.
- ♦ Diltiazem and verapamil are not significantly dialyzed.
- ♦ Use diltiazem with caution in hepatic disease because it is metabolized by the liver. The half-life of the medication is increased in patients with cirrhosis.
- ♦ Verapamil is given at only 20 to 30% of the normal dose depending on formulation in the setting or cirrhosis or severe hepatic impairment.
- ♦ There is a difference between verapamil regular extended release (ER) formulation and the ER formulation with a delayed onset of action.
  - The regular ER tablets can be used once daily or twice daily when higher doses are needed.
  - The ER formulation with a delayed onset of action is only used once a day (at bedtime) regardless of dose.
- ♦ Amlodipine and felodipine do not require dosing adjustments based on renal function.
- ♦ Amlodipine is poorly dialyzable.
- ♦ In patients with hepatic impairment, amlodipine and felodipine should be started at low doses and titrated slowly. BP should be monitored closely during titration.

((UptoDate®, Lexidrug™, 2026; Schwarz Pharma, 2009; Valeant Pharmaceuticals North America, 2014)

Select Adverse Effects of CCBs

- ♦ Bradycardia can occur due to ↓ sinus rate (verapamil, diltiazem), especially in combination with beta
- ♦ AV block can occur due to ↓ AV node conduction (verapamil, diltiazem), especially in combination with beta blockers.
- ♦ Hypotension can occur due to vasodilation, especially with short acting dihydropyridines.
- ♦ Decompensation of HF can occur due to ↓ contractility, especially with verapamil.
- ♦ Short acting nifedipine causes a precipitous drop in BP and it should not be used to treat acute coronary ischemia. Long acting nifedipine can be used safely to treat effort angina, vasospastic angina, and HTN.
- ♦ Dihydropyridines can cause reflex tachycardia if they cause BP to drop significantly. This is less likely to happen if they are used with beta blockers.
- ♦ Additional side effects include flushing, H/As, peripheral edema, constipation, and aggravation of gastroesophageal reflux.

(UptoDate®, Lexidrug™, 2026)

Contraindication Highlights for CCBs

- ♦ Consult manufacturer recommendations for use in children, pregnant women, and nursing women.

- Dihydropyridines are not recommended in severe aortic stenosis, obstructive cardiomyopathy, unstable angina (impending infarction) and preexisting hypotension (Lexicomp, 2023).
- Dihydropyridines are also generally contraindicated in HFrEF but if needed for angina or BP control, amlodipine is the preferred agent.
- Non-dihydropyridines (verapamil and diltiazem) are contraindicated in bradycardia, 2nd or 3rd degree heart block and sick sinus syndrome (unless a pacemaker is present), HFrEF, hypotension, VT, and in atrial fibrillation with evidence of pre-excitation.

(UptoDate®, Lexidrug™, 2026)

Linking Knowledge to Practice

- ✓ *Although beta blockers decrease contractility they have been shown to reduce mortality in patients with HFrEF by blocking the adverse effects of SNS stimulation.*
- ✓ *CCBs blockers also decrease contractility; however, they have not been shown to reduce mortality in HFrEF and thus they are contraindicated in patients with HFrEF except for amlodipine which has not been shown to worsen mortality in HFrEF.*

(Heidenreich et al., 2022)

Special Considerations & Monitoring with CCBs

- Liver function should be monitored with diltiazem.
- Liver function and renal function should be monitored with verapamil.
- The non-dihydropyridines should not be used in combination with a beta blocker in high-risk patients (history of 2nd or 3rd degree AV block, sinus node dysfunction, or HFrEF) unless the patient has a pacemaker in place.
- Patients taking CCBs should be monitored for peripheral edema. This adverse effect is dose dependent and usually occurs within 2 to 3 weeks of starting therapy.
- BP should be monitored with all CCB. HR and AV conduction should be monitored in patients taking verapamil and diltiazem.

(UptoDate®, Lexidrug™, 2026)

Table 7

Indications and Mechanisms of Action of CCBs

Use	Mechanism of Action
Angina: Coronary Spasm Classic Angina (All agents)	▪ Prevent vasoconstriction by ↓ amount of calcium available for contraction; this results in coronary vasodilation. ▪ Coronary vasodilation = ↑ collateral blood flow to ischemic areas. ▪ ↓ MVO_2 by ↓ HR, ↓ contractility, and ↓ afterload.
HTN (All agents)	▪ **BP = CO × SVR.** ▪ ↓ CO by ↓ contractility, ↓ SVR by vasodilation.
Arrhythmias: SVT (Verapamil/Diltiazem)	▪ Slow AV conduction so ↓ ventricular response to atrial fibrillation/flutter. ▪ Can terminate AV nodal active arrhythmias AVNRT and AVRT.
HCM (Verapamil)	▪ ↓ contractility decreases outflow tract obstruction. ▪ ↓ HR allows longer diastolic filling time so more blood in ventricle ↓ outflow tract obstruction. ▪ Dihydropyridines are contraindicated because of their peripheral vasodilating effects.

Table 8 CCBs Used in Hypertensive Emergency	
Nicardipine	**Clevidipine**
▪ Initial dose 5 mg/hour (hr). ▪ Titrate every 5 to 15 minutes by 2.5 mg/hr. ▪ Max dose 15 mg/hr. ▪ Contraindicated in advanced aortic stenosis. ▪ Lower end of dose range in elderly. ▪ Use central line or large peripheral line. Change peripheral site every 12 hours to minimize venous irritation.	▪ Initial 1 to 2 mg/hr. ▪ Double every 90 seconds till BP approaches target; then increase by smaller increments every 5 to 10 minutes. ▪ Each 1 to 2 mg/hr increase results in an additional 2 to 4 mg reduction in systolic BP. ▪ Max infusion volume approximately 21 mg/hr x 24 hours due to lipid load restriction. ▪ Invert vial gently several times to achieve uniformity of emulsion. ▪ Cannot use in soy/egg allergies. ▪ Contraindicated: defective lipid metabolism; acute pancreatitis (formulated 20% fat emulsion). ▪ Lower end of dosing in elderly.
(Jones et al., 2025; UptoDate®, Lexidrug™, 2024)	

Key Pharmacokinetic & Pharmacodynamic Information for CCBs

- Diltiazem, verapamil, and felodipine undergo hepatic metabolism with an extensive first-pass effect.
- For diltiazem, verapamil, and felodipine clearance is decreased in the setting of hepatic impairment. The half-life will prolong and the area under the curve may increase.
- The area under the curve also increases in amlodipine in patients with moderate to severe HF.
- In older adults:
  - The bioavailability of verapamil may be higher, and the half-life may be prolonged.
  - Clearance decreases and plasma concentrations increase with felodipine.
  - The area under the curve may increase 40 to 60% with amlodipine.
- Grapefruit juice may increase the serum concentration of diltiazem and verapamil. Grapefruit is known to increase the concentration of felodipine.

(UptoDate®, Lexidrug™, 2026)

Important Medication Interactions with CCBs

- Verapamil and diltiazem have an additive effect on ↓ HR and ↓ AV conduction when used with beta blockers, amiodarone, dronedarone, and digoxin.
- All CCBs will have an additive effect on BP when used with other vasodilators/antihypertensives.
- Verapamil and diltiazem are moderate inhibitors of CYP3A4. As a result, they may increase the concentration of medications metabolized by enzyme CYP3A4 producing multiple medication interactions.
- Verapamil and diltiazem can increase statin levels, and some statins (e.g. simvastatin) can increase the level of diltiazem.
- Verapamil and diltiazem can increase the concentration of dofetilide, finerenone, ivabradine, and ranolazine.
- CYP3A4 inducers can decrease the concentration of CCBs.
- CYP3A4 inhibitors can increase the concentration of CCBs.

- ♦ There are multiple medications that are CYP3A4 inhibitors and thus there are multiple potential drug interactions especially with diltiazem and verapamil.

(Sadovsky, 2002; Sunwoo et al., 2019; UptoDate®, Lexidrug™, 2026)

> ***Linking Knowledge to Practice***
>
> ✓ *Beta blockers and the non-dihydropyridine CCBs (verapamil and diltiazem) have the same effects on the heart: they both decrease HR and contractility.*
> - *Both types of drugs are used to treat angina and HTN; therefore, many patients are on both a beta blocker and a CCB and may experience additive effects of these drugs.*
> - *Watch for bradycardia, AV block, and hypotension in patients taking both a beta blocker and a non-dihydropyridine CCB.*
> - *If combination therapy is not tolerated, the CCB is usually discontinued, and the beta blocker is continued due to the positive mortality benefits of beta blockers.*
>
> ✓ *Drug induced bradycardia can be an indication for pacing.*

Appendix 7 provides additional details regarding individual CCBs.

SODIUM-GLUCOSE COTRANSPORTER 2 INHIBITORS

- ♦ Sodium-glucose cotransporter 2 inhibitors (SGLT2Is), the "gliflozins", were introduced in 2013 as a new classification of medications used in the treatment of DMT2. These agents are designed to treat DMT2 by increasing blood glucose excretion from the body.
- ♦ SGLT2Is do not work through traditional treatment methods aimed at increasing insulin availability, improving sensitivity to insulin, or delaying the delivery and absorption of carbohydrates from the gastrointestinal track.
- ♦ Data obtained from CV outcomes trials demonstrated SGLT2Is improved outcomes in patients with CV disease and HF. As a result, SGLT2Is are now indicated not only for the treatment of DMT2 but also for the treatment of CV disease, HF, and CKD in patients both with and without DMT2.

Historical Overview: Diabetes Medications and CV, HF, and Renal Outcomes

- ♦ In December 2008, the FDA established a practice of requiring pharmaceutical companies to complete CV outcome trials on all oral agents released for the treatment for DMT2 (Cefalu et al., 2018).
  - This mandate was the result of the post-marketing concerns that the thiazolidinedione rosiglitazone was associated with worsening CV outcomes (Nissen & Wolski, 2007).
  - CV outcome trials have since demonstrated that SGLT2Is are not only safe but that they also improve CV outcomes.
- ♦ In 2013, canagliflozin was the first SGLT2I approved for the treatment of DMT2 (Johnson & Johnson, 2013). Since that time five additional SGLT2Is have been approved for the treatment of adults with DMT2. These agents are dapagliflozin, empagliflozin, ertugliflozin, bexagliflozin, and sotagliflozin.
- ♦ In 2016, the FDA expanded the indications for empagliflozin beyond the treatment of DMT2 to include the use of this medication for the reduction of the risk of CV death in adults with DMT2 and established CV disease (FDA, 2016, December 2).
- ♦ In 2018, the FDA also expanded canagliflozin's indication. The expanded indication included the use of this medication for the reduction of major adverse CV events including heart attack, stroke, and death in adults with DMT2 who have established CV disease (Johnson & Johnson, 2018).
- ♦ SGLT2Is are also indicated in the treatment of HFrEF.

- Clinical trial data have demonstrated a reduction in the composite outcome of CV death or hospitalization for worsening HF with dapagliflozin and empagliflozin (McMurray et al., 2019; Packer et al., 2020).
- In 2020, dapagliflozin was the first SGLT2I approved by the FDA to reduce the risk of CV death and HF hospitalization in adults with HFrEF with and without DMT2 (FDA, 2020a, May 5). This was the first use of an SGLT2I as a treatment strategy for HF and the first indication for an SGLT2I in patients without DMT2.
- In 2021, the FDA expanded the indications for empagliflozin to include treatment of adults (with and without DMT2) living with HFrEF (Boehringer Ingelheim, 2021).

♦ SGLT2Is are also associated with an improvement in renal function, especially in those with CKD secondary to DMT2 who have albuminuria.
- As a result, there are new clinical indications for SGLT2Is in the treatment of patients with CKD who have persistent albuminuria despite being on maximally tolerated ACEI or ARB.
- Benefit has been shown in patients with or without DMT2.

(EMPA-Kidney Collaborative Group, 2023; Heerspink et al., 2020)

♦ More recently, the EMPEROR-Preserved clinical trial demonstrated that patients with HFpEF taking empagliflozin had superior outcomes over those taking placebo.
- This clinical trial demonstrated statistically significant improvement in outcomes in the empagliflozin group including a lower risk of CV death, hospitalization for HF, or emergent/urgent HF visits requiring IV therapy.
- Additionally, the total number of hospitalizations requiring ICU care and the need for vasopressors or inotropes were fewer in the empagliflozin group.
- These outcomes were similar in patients with and without DMT2.

(Anker et al., 2021; Packer, Butler et al., 2021)
- As a result, the FDA granted the manufacturer's request for empagliflozin to have "Breakthrough Therapy" designation for HFpEF and in February of 2022 empagliflozin became the first SGLT2I approved to improve outcomes in patients with HFpEF with and without DMT2 (Boehringer Ingelheim, 2021; FDA, 2022, February 24).

♦ Subsequently, in 2023 dapagliflozin and the newest SGLT2I, sotagliflozin, received FDA approval to improve CV outcomes (CV mortality, hospitalizations for HF, urgent HF visits) in patients with HFpEF in addition to HFrEF with and without DMT2 (Brooks, 2023; FDA, 2023, May 26).

Mechanism of Action of SGLT2Is

♦ SGLT2 is a protein that is a member of a group of sodium dependent glucose transporters.

♦ Glucose is normally filtered from the blood at the level of the glomerulus in the Bowman's Capsule.
- The filtrate leaves the Bowman's Capsule and enters the proximal tubule of the nephron.
- In the proximal tubule SGLT2 is expressed causing approximately 90% of the filtered glucose to be reabsorbed and returned to the circulation for use by the body.
- SGLT1 is responsible for reabsorption of the additional 10% of the filtered glucose further along in the proximal tubule.
- As a result of the work of SGLT1 and SGLT2 in the proximal tubule the urine will be free of glucose in healthy persons.
- In a patient with DMT2 the SGLT2 transporter reabsorbs higher than normal amounts of blood glucose which contributes to the persistent elevation in serum blood glucose.

(Moses et al., 2014; Desouza et al., 2015)

♦ SGLT2Is are unique in the treatment of DMT2 since the mechanism of action is not impacted by the availability or action of insulin. The mechanism of action is impacted by blood glucose levels.

♦ Patients with DMT2 have a higher-than-normal filtered glucose load.

- The administration of an SGLT2Is reduces the reabsorption of the filtered glucose by approximately 55%, resulting in an increased renal excretion of glucose that produces glucosuria.
- The increased renal excretion of glucose lowers blood glucose level in the body.

♦ The high glucose load in the urine causes an increase in urine osmolality.
- As a result of increased urine osmolality, osmotic diuresis occurs as water is pulled into the filtrate to compensate for the increase in the large glucose molecules.
- The pulling of water into the filtrate helps maintain normal urine osmolality.

> ***Linking Knowledge to Practice***
>
> ✓ *Patients taking SGLT2Is should not experience hypoglycemia in the absence of other agents known to cause hypoglycemia. These agents include insulin, sulfonylureas, and meglitinides.*
>
> ✓ *SGLT2Is eliminate filtered glucose. As blood glucose levels decrease so does the amount of filtered glucose thus preventing an over reduction in blood glucose.*
>
> *(Samuel & Lee, 2017)*

Indications for SGLT2Is

The indications for SGLT2Is are expanding as clinical trials continue to produce new evidence. It is important to know that not all SGLT2Is have the same indications.

See Table 9 for the history of approved indications for SGLT2Is.

DMT2 Treatment

♦ Canagliflozin, dapagliflozin, empagliflozin, ertugliflozin, and bexagliflozin are indicated as an adjunct to diet and exercise to improve glycemic control in adults with DMT2. At the time of this writing sotagliflozin prescriber information does not list DMT2 as an indication (AstraZeneca Pharmaceuticals, 2024; Boehringer Ingelheim International, 2023; Janssen Pharmaceutical Companies, 2023; Lexicon Pharmaceuticals, 2023; Merck & Co., 2021; Theracos Bio, 2023).

♦ The following are expected effects of SGLT2Is in patients with DMT2:
- Reduction of fasting plasma glucose concentrations.
- Hemoglobin A1c (A1c) reduction of 0.6 to 1.0%.
- Greater reduction in A1c when used in combination with metformin, a GLP1 receptor agonist, sulfonylureas, pioglitazone, or insulin.

(Samuel & Lee, 2017)

DMT2 with Established CV Disease or CV Risk Factors for Purpose of Risk Reduction

♦ Empagliflozin is approved to reduce the risk of CV death in adults with DMT2 and established CV disease (Boehringer Ingelheim International, 2023).
- The EMPA-REG OUTCOME trial studied patients with DMT2 who had established CV disease.
- The results demonstrated a 38% relative risk reduction in death from CV causes in patients taking empagliflozin compared to placebo. There was also a 32% reduction in death from any cause in patients taking empagliflozin compared to placebo.

(Zinman et al., 2015)

♦ Canagliflozin is approved to reduce the risk of major adverse CV events in adults with DMT2 and established CV disease (Janssen Pharmaceutical Companies, 2023).
- The CANVAS trial studied adults with DMT2 and a history of CV disease.
- The trial demonstrated a 14% relative risk reduction in CV events in those taking canagliflozin over the placebo group.

(Neal et al., 2017)

- ♦ Dapagliflozin is approved to reduce the risk of hospitalization for HF in patients with DMT2 and established CV disease or multiple CV risk factors (AstraZeneca Pharmaceuticals).
  - In the DECLARE-TIMI 58 trial dapagliflozin demonstrated a 27% relative risk reduction for HF hospitalization in patients with DMT2 who had or were at risk for having CV disease.
  - The only improved CV outcome in the study was the reduction of hospitalizations for HF.

  (Wiviott et al., 2019)
- ♦ Sotagliflozin is approved to reduce the risk of CV mortality, hospitalization for HF, and urgent HF visits in adults with DMT2, CKD, and other CV risk factors (Lexicon Pharmaceuticals, Inc., 2023).
  - The SCORED clinical trial evaluated the use of sotagliflozin versus placebo in patients with DMT2, CKD (with and without albuminuria), and risk for CV disease.
  - Study data demonstrated a 25% relative risk reduction favoring sotagliflozin over placebo in the composite endpoint evaluating CV death, hospitalization for HF, and urgent HF visits.

  (Bhatt et al., 2021a)

HFrEF for Outcome Improvement

- ♦ Dapagliflozin and empagliflozin have been approved to reduce the risk of CV death and HF hospitalization in adults with HFrEF.
- ♦ This indication for HFrEF includes patients with and without DMT2.

(AstraZeneca Pharmaceuticals, 2024; Boehringer Ingelheim International, 2023)

- The DAPA-HF Trial randomized symptomatic HFrEF patients, both with and without DMT2, to dapagliflozin or placebo. All patients were on standard HF medications.
  - The primary outcome was a composite of worsening HF (hospitalization or an urgent visit resulting in IV therapy for HF) or CV death.
  - Patients randomized to dapagliflozin experienced a 26% reduction in the primary outcome compared to the placebo group. Additionally, the patients who received dapagliflozin experienced a 30% relative risk reduction for the occurrence of a first worsening HF event.
  - The results were similar in those with DMT2 and those without.

  (McMurray et al., 2019)
- In the EMPEROR-Reduced Trial, symptomatic HFrEF patients, both with and without DMT2, were randomized to treatment with placebo or empagliflozin. All patients were on standard therapy for HF.
  - The primary outcome was a composite of CV death or hospitalization for worsening HF. Participants receiving empagliflozin experienced a 25% reduction in the primary outcome compared to those taking placebo.
    - This benefit was consistent in those with and without DMT2.
    - The benefit was realized within 12 to 18 days of beginning treatment and was sustained throughout the clinical trial.
  - Additionally, the empagliflozin group experienced a lower rate of HF hospitalizations requiring ICU care, vasopressor therapy, inotropic therapy, or mechanical or surgical intervention.
  - The risk of inpatient or outpatient worsening of HF was reduced in the group receiving empagliflozin.
  - The patients randomized to empagliflozin also experienced an improvement in NYHA functional class.

  (Packer et al., 2020; Packer et al., et al., 2021)

HFpEF for Outcome Improvement

- ♦ Empagliflozin, Dapagliflozin and Sotagliflozin have all been approved to reduce CV mortality, hospitalization for HF, and urgent HF visits in patients with HFpEF.

This indication is in those with and without DMT2.
(AstraZeneca Pharmaceuticals, 2024; Boehringer Ingelheim International, 2023; Lexicon Pharmaceuticals, Inc., 2023)

- ♦ Empagliflozin was the first SGLT2I approved to reduce the risk of CV death and HF hospitalization in patients with HF regardless of LVEF or the presence or absence of diabetes (FDA, 2022, February 24). This approval for use in HFpEF is important because historically there have been limited treatment options for HFpEF.
  - The EMPEROR-Preserved clinical trial demonstrated the superiority of empagliflozin over placebo in patients with HFpEF.
  - Empagliflozin demonstrated a 23% reduction in the combined risk of CV death, hospitalization for HF, or emergent/urgent HF visits requiring IV therapy compared to placebo.
  - The empagliflozin group experienced a 29% reduction in the total number of hospitalizations requiring ICU care, and the need for vasopressors or inotropes was reduced by 27%.
  - Additionally, the treatment group was more likely to have a better NYHA functional class. This impact was seen after just 12 weeks of treatment and maintained for at least 2 years.
  - The outcomes were consistent regardless of diabetes status.

  (Anker et al., 2021; Packer et al., 2021)
- ♦ Dapagliflozin demonstrated statistically significant lower rates of worsening HF or CV death than placebo in the DELIVER clinical trial which evaluated patients with HFmrEF and HFpEF with and without diabetes (Solomon et al., 2022). The 18% relative risk reduction resulted in additional FDA approval of dapagliflozin to improve outcomes in patients with HF and an LVEF > 40%.
- ♦ Sotagliflozin also received FDA approval in 2023 for use in patients with HF regardless of LVEF to improve HF outcomes.
  - In the SOLOIST-WHF trial the primary end point of total number of deaths from CV causes, HF hospitalization, and urgent visits for HF were lower in the sotagliflozin group compared to the placebo group.
  - The sotagliflozin group experienced a 33% relative risk reduction in the primary outcome compared to the placebo group.
  - Interestingly all patients in the SOLOIST-WHF had DMT2, yet the indication is for HF patients regardless of diabetes status.
  - Sotagliflozin, an inhibitor of SGLT1 and SGLT2, does not have approval for the treatment of diabetes mellitus in the United States.

  (Bhatt et al., 2021)

Guideline Recommendations for SGLT2Is in Heart Failure

- In 2022 the AHA, ACC, and HFSA published updated guidelines for the treatment of HF and in 2024 the ACC published an Expert Consensus Decision Pathway for the Treatment of HFrEF.
- Key recommendations from these publications are:
  - In patients with symptomatic chronic HFrEF, SGLT2Is are recommended to reduce hospitalization for HF and CV mortality, irrespective of the presence of DMT2 (Class 1A recommendation).
  - In patients with HFmrEF SGLT2Is can be beneficial in decreasing HF hospitalizations and CV mortality (Class 2A recommendation).
  - In patients with HFpEF, SGLT2Is can be beneficial in decreasing HF hospitalizations and CV mortality (Class 2A recommendation).
  - The SGLT2Is that have been approved to meet these indications, as of this writing include empagliflozin, dapagliflozin and sotagliflozin.

(Heidenreich et al., 2022; Maddox et al., 2024)

CKD (with or without Diabetes Mellitus) for Outcome Improvement

- Dapagliflozin has been approved to reduce the risk of sustained GFR decline, end stage kidney disease, CV death, and hospitalization for HF in adults with CKD at risk of progression (AstraZeneca Pharmaceuticals, 2024).
  - The DAPA-CKD trial evaluated the effect of dapagliflozin in patients with and without diabetes and with CKD (eGFR 25 to 75 mL/min/1.73 m^2) who also met specified albuminuria criteria.
  - The primary outcome was a composite of a sustained decline in the eGFR of at least 50%, end stage kidney disease (ESKD) (transplant, dialysis, or a sustained eGFR of < 15 mL/ min/1.73 m^2), or death from renal or CV causes.
  - The patients in the trial randomized to dapagliflozin experienced a 39% reduction in the primary outcome over those in the placebo group.
  - The results were similar in patients with and without DMT2.

  (Heerspink et al., 2020)
- Empagliflozin was approved in 2023 by the FDA based on the results of the EMPA-Kidney trial to reduce the risk of sustained decline in GFR, ESKD, CV death and hospitalization in adults with CKD at risk of progression (Boehringer Ingelheim International, 2023; Up to Date®, Lexidrug™, 2024).
  - The EMPA-Kidney clinical trial evaluated the effect of empagliflozin in patients with CKD and an eGFR of > 20 but < 45 mL/min/1.73 m^2 or who had an eGFR of ≥ 45 but < 90 mL/min/1.73 m^2 with a urinary albumin-to-creatinine ratio of at least 200.
  - The trial included patients with and without DMT2. The primary outcome was the progression of kidney disease or death from CV causes. The primary outcome occurred more frequently in the placebo group (16.9%) versus the empagliflozin group (13.1%) (P<0.001).

  (EMPA-Kidney Collaborative Group, 2023)
- SGLT2Is are not currently indicated for use in the treatment of patients with CKD secondary to polycystic kidney disease.
  - Patients with polycystic kidney disease were excluded from clinical trials that evaluated the renal benefits of SGLT2Is in patients with CKD.
  - However, patients with polycystic kidney were not excluded from CV safety trials involving SGLT2Is nor from SGLT2I trials evaluating CV benefit. Additional data is needed to determine the benefit of SGLT2Is in slowing the progression of CKD in patients with polycystic kidney disease (Afsar et al., 2022).

DMT2 with Diabetic Nephropathy (DKD) for Outcome Improvement

- Canagliflozin is approved to reduce the risk of ESKD, doubling of serum creatinine, CV death, and hospitalization for HF in adults with DMT2 and diabetic nephropathy with urinary albumin excretion >300 mg/day (Janssen Pharmaceutical Companies, 2023).
- The CREDENCE Trial evaluated the impact of canagliflozin on patients with DMT2 and albuminuric CKD. Albuminuric CKD was defined as an eGFR of 30 to < 90 mL/min/1.73 m^2 and albuminuria (albumin-to-creatinine ratio > 300 to 5000).
  - The primary outcome was a composite of ESKD, doubling of serum creatinine, or death from a renal or CV cause.
  - All patients were treated with a RAAS inhibitor.
  - The primary outcome occurred 30% less often in the patients receiving canagliflozin.
  - Additionally, the canagliflozin group had a lower rate of CV death, MI, and stroke (20% reduction), and a lower rate of hospitalization for HF (39% reduction).
  - The renal specific outcomes (composite of ESKD, a doubling of the creatinine level, or death from renal cause) were 34% lower in the canagliflozin group.

  (Perkovic et al., 2019)

Table 9 FDA Approval History of SGLT2 Inhibitors						
FDA Approval	**Cana-gliflozin**	**Dapa-gliflozin**	**Empa-gliflozin**	**Ertu-gliflozin**	**Bexa-gliflozin**	**Sota-gliflozin**
DMT2: To improve glycemic control as an adjunct to diet and exercise.	2013 ✓	2014 ✓	2014 ✓	2017 ✓	2023 ✓	
DMT2: To reduce risk of CV death, MI, and stroke.	2018 ✓	2019 ✓	2016 ✓			
DMT2 with HFrEF and CV Disease: To reduce risk of HF hospitalization.		2019 ✓				
HFrEF with or without DMT2: For the treatment of HFrEF.		2020 ✓	2021 ✓			
ANY HF with or without DMT2: To reduce CV mortality, HF hospitalization and urgent HF visits.		2023 ✓	2022 ✓			2023 ✓
CKD at risk for progression of CKD with or without DMT2: To reduce risk of kidney function decline, kidney failure, CV death, and HF hospitalization.		2021 ✓	2023 ✓			
DMT2 with CKD or other CV risk factors: To reduce the risk of CV death, HF hospitalization, and urgent HF visits.						2023 ✓
DMT2 with DKD and established CV disease: To reduce the risk of heart attack, stroke, or CV death.	2019 ✓					
(FDA releases for SGLT2Is, Manufacturers prescribing information for SGLT2Is, and Up to Date®, Lexidrug™, 2024)						

Special Dosing Information for SGLT2Is

Dosing Adjustments Based on Hepatic Function

- Bexagliflozin, canagliflozin, dapagliflozin, ertugliflozin, and sotagliflozin are not recommended in patients with severe hepatic dysfunction because they were not studied in these patients.
- The manufacturer of empagliflozin states no dose adjustment is required for hepatic dysfunction. There is increased systemic exposure of the medication in the setting of hepatic dysfunction, but the changes are not considered clinically significant.

(UptoDate®, Lexidrug™, 2024)

Dosing Adjustments Based on Renal Function

- ♦ Canagliflozin, dapagliflozin, and empagliflozin are highly protein bound and are unlikely to be dialyzable. They should be avoided in patients requiring any type of RRT.
- ♦ Bexagliflozin, sotagliflozin, and ertugliflozin are not recommended in patients needing dialysis because they have not been studied in patients requiring dialysis.

(UptoDate®, Lexidrug™, 2024)

Table 10 outlines dosing adjustments based on renal function for each medication and based on indication.

Table 10

Renal Dose Adjustments for SGLT2Is

SGLT2I	For DMT2	For CKD / DKD	For HF
Canagliflozin	▪ eGFR 30 to < 60: 100 mg/day. ▪ Hold eGFR < 30 due to lack of efficacy.	▪ DKD: If eGFR < 25 to 30 do not initiate, if already taking may continue at 100 mg/day.	N/A
Bexagliflozin	▪ No adjustment needed for eGFR ≥ 30. ▪ Hold eGFR < 30 due to lack of efficacy.	N/A	N/A
Dapagliflozin	▪ Hold eGFR < 45 due to lack of efficacy.	▪ CKD & DKD: No dose adjustment if eGFR ≥ 25. ▪ CKD & DKD: If eGFR < 25 do not initiate, but if already taking may continue at 10 mg/day.	▪ No dose adjustment if eGFR 25 or greater. ▪ If eGFR < 25 do not initiate, but if already taking may continue at 10 mg/day.
Empagliflozin	▪ No adjustment needed for eGFR > 30. ▪ Hold eGFR < 30 due to lack of efficacy.	▪ CKD: No adjustment needed for eGFR ≥ 20; do not initiate therapy if eGFR < 20. ▪ DKD: Some experts continue off label use at 10 mg/day if eGFR < 30.	▪ Benefits of 10 mg/day have been shown in patients with eGFR ≥ 20.
Ertugliflozin	▪ No adjustment needed for eGFR ≥ 45. ▪ Hold eGFR < 45 due to lack of efficacy.	N/A	N/A
Sotagliflozin	N/A	▪ Indicated in patients with DMT2 and CKD for CV risk reduction. ▪ No dosing adjustment provided by manufacturer for eGFR < 25; in clinical trials medication was stopped for eGFR ≤ 15.	▪ No dosing adjustment provided by manufacturer for eGFR < 25; in clinical trials medication was stopped for eGFR < 15.

Table specific abbreviation: eGFR = eGFR mL/min/1.73 m^2
(AstraZeneca Pharmaceuticals, 2024; Boehringer Ingelheim International, 2023; Janssen Pharmaceutical Companies, 2023; Lexicon Pharmaceuticals, Inc., 2023; Merck & Co., Inc., 2021; Theracos Bio, 2023; Up to Date®, Lexidrug™, 2024)

Advanced Concept Focus:
Renal Function and SGLT2Is

- ♦ There is an anticipated reversible decline in the GFR (up to 30% reduction) with the initiation of an SGLT2I. The GFR is expected to return to baseline with the continuation of therapy (de Boer et al., 2022; Lam & Shaikh, 2021; Sridhar et al., 2020).
- ♦ Although there is a reversible decline in the GFR with the start of an SGLT2I, clinical trial data demonstrated lower rates of AKI in the patients taking SGLT2Is compared to the control groups (Bailey et al., 2022; de Boer et al., 2022; Lam & Shaikh, 2021; Sridhar et al., 2020).
- ♦ It remains important, however, that SGLT2Is are not initiated in the setting of hypovolemia or hypotension; and that hypovolemia and hypotension are avoided while the patient is on therapy. Hypovolemia and hypotension are both risk factors for the development of prerenal AKI, especially in the setting of SGLT2I therapy.
- ♦ SGLT2Is are not as effective in lowering the A1c at a lower GFR. However, even at a lower GFR they still play a very important role in improving clinical outcomes in those with DMT2, especially in those with DMT2 and CKD.
- ♦ The ADA in collaboration with KDIGO agree that in patients with DMT2 and CKD the addition of an SGLT2I (even if the A1c is already at goal) is important to reduce the progression of CKD and to improve HF and CV outcomes.
  - SGLT2Is should be started in patients with diabetes and CKD if the eGFR is $\geq$ 20 mL/min/1.73 m^2 and there are no other contraindications (de Boer et al., 2022).
  - The guideline recommendation for starting an SGLT2I in patients with DMT2 and CKD if the eGFR is $\geq$ 20 mL/min/1.73 m^2 is consistent with the manufacturer recommendations for empagliflozin.
  - However, manufacturer recommendations for dapagliflozin list an eGFR of 25 mL/min/1.73 m2 for initiation of therapy.
  - Manufacturer recommendations for sotagliflozin recommend no dose adjustments for an eGFR $\geq$ 25 mL/min/1.73 m^2 and do not provide recommendations for eGFR of < 25 mL/min/1.73 m^2. In clinical trials involving sotagliflozin the medication was stopped when eGFR was < 15 mL/min/1.73 m^2.

  (Up to Date®, Lexidrug™, 2024)
  - The ADA and KDIGO consensus document states that once an SGLT2I has been initiated at an eGFR of $\geq$ 20 mL/min/1.73 m^2 the drug can be continued if the eGFR trends below 20 mL/min/1.73 m^2 (de Boer et el., 2022).

Linking Knowledge to Practice

✓ *The GFR criteria for holding an SGLT2I will be different based on the specific SGLT2I that is prescribed and the indication for which the SGLT2I is being used.*

✓ *It is important to understand that an SGLT2I will lose its effectiveness in lowering the A1c as renal function declines. However, continuing the medication in a patient with DMT2 and declining renal function for other clinical benefits will not cause harm.*

Select Adverse Effects of SGLT2Is

Hypotension

- ♦ A systolic BP reduction is expected in patients taking an SGLT2I secondary to osmotic diuresis.
- ♦ This BP reduction is considered an additional beneficial effect of the medication unless the patient has high risk features (volume depletion or diuretic use) for the development of hypotension.

- ♦ SGLT2Is should not be initiated in patients at risk for developing hypotension. This includes patients with acute medical illness or those who require aggressive diuretic therapy.

> ***Linking Knowledge to Practice***
>
> ✓ *In addition to reducing serum blood glucose levels and A1c, SGLT2Is have secondary effects, many that have proven to be beneficial.*
>
> ✓ *Systolic BP is reduced secondary to osmotic diuresis and natriuresis.*
> - *There is a systolic BP decrease of 5 to 6 mmHg and diastolic BP decrease of 1 to 2 mmHg.*
> - *The higher the BP at initiation the greater the expected reduction in BP.*
>
> ✓ *Body weight is reduced secondary to osmotic diuresis and increased glucosuria.*
> - *Increased glycosuria results in a loss of approximately 240 to 320 consumed calories.*
> - *There is also a reduction of adipose tissue.*
>
> ✓ *Hematocrit increase secondary to reduction in plasma volume.*
>
> ✓ *Uric acid levels are reduced secondary to reduced urate reabsorption.*
> - *Patients with DMT2 often have elevated uric acid levels related to insulin resistance.*
> - *This increases risk for HTN, CV disease, and CKD.*
>
> ✓ *Triglycerides are reduced secondary to increased lipoprotein lipase activity and there is a mild increase in LDL cholesterol. However, most patients taking an SGLT2I are already taking a statin which can be used to manage this mild increase in LDL cholesterol.*
>
> *(Bonora et al., 2020; Garber et al., 2020; Samuel & Lee, 2017; Up to Date®, Lexidrug™, 2024)*

Risk for Bone Fractures

- ♦ There are reports of increased rates of fracture in patients with DMT2 taking canagliflozin.
- ♦ The CANVAS trial reported an increased fracture risk in those taking canagliflozin compared to those taking placebo, although the incidence of those with bone fractures was small (Neal et al., 2017). However, the same findings have not been replicated in additional trials studying canagliflozin (CANVAS-R and the CREDENCE trials) (Neal et al., 2017, Perkovic et al., 2019).
- ♦ When prescribing an SGLT2I, especially canagliflozin, the patient risk factors for fracture should be evaluated including chronic inflammatory disease, steroid use, malabsorption disorders, fall risk, and bone loss (Jackson & Moseley, 2020).
  - The increased fractures in the CANVAS trial occurred in those who were older, had a prior history risk of CV disease, a lower GFR, and higher diuretic use (Watts et al., 2016).
  - The increased risk of fracture in the CANVAS trial may have been associated with an increased fall incidence in the canagliflozin group. The increased falls risk, especially in the elderly, may be secondary to volume depletion that results in orthostatic hypotension (Jackson & Moseley, 2020).
- ♦ In a meta-analysis evaluating thirty-eight randomized control trials studying canagliflozin, dapagliflozin and empagliflozin, the fracture event rates were similar between the study groups and the control groups. The authors also found no significant difference in fracture rates among the 3 agents (Tang et al., 2016).
- ♦ It is appropriate to evaluate bone health in patients prior to initiation of SGLT2Is, including risk for falls, and risk for fractures (Jackson & Moseley, 2020).

Risk for Genitourinary Tract Infections

There has been a reported increased incidence of urinary tract infections (UTIs), and genital mycotic (fungal) infections associated with the use of SGLT2 inhibitors (Bundhun & Huang, 2018; Devi et al., 2017; Feng et al., 2019; Zhang et al., 2021).

Urinary Tract Infection

- People with DMT2 are at increased risk for UTI due to increased glucosuria, increased adherence of bacteria to uroepithelial cells, and compromise of the immune system.
- There have been reports of pyelonephritis and other severe UTIs with the use of SGLT2Is (Pishdad, Auwaerter, and Kalyani; 2024). SGLT2Is increase the amount of glucose expelled through the urinary tract starting with the first dose.
- The increased incidence of UTI associated with the use of SGLT2Is in early clinical trials was higher in women and in those with a history of recurrent UTIs (Geerlings et al., 2014).
- While this increased incidence of UTIs was seen across most of the early clinical trials, 2 separate meta-analyses involving ertugliflozin showed there was no increased risk of UTI (Patel et al., 2020; Zhang et al., 2021).
- An additional meta-analysis of 86 randomized clinical trials involving 50,880 patients demonstrated the risk of UTI was not increased in patients taking dapagliflozin, empagliflozin, or canagliflozin in comparison with those taking placebo or an alternative antidiabetic agent, except for with dapagliflozin at the higher 10 mg dose (Puckrin et al., 2018).
- Prescribers should evaluate the risk for UTI prior to the initiation of an SGLT2I and should monitor for UTIs occurring during therapy. Patients should receive education about S&S of UTIs and should be instructed to seek prompt treatment if S&S occur.

Genital Mycotic Infections

- Female sex and a previous history of recurrent genital mycotic infections (≥ 3 per year) are risk factors for the development of these infections (Puckrin et al., 2018; Engelhardt et al., 2021).
- Genital mycotic infections, including vulvovaginal candidiasis have been reported in 10 to 15% of women taking SGLT2Is (DeSantis, 2021).
- A meta-analysis of 86 randomized clinical trials involving 50,880 patients taking dapagliflozin, empagliflozin, or canagliflozin in comparison with those taking placebo or an alternative antidiabetic agent reported a 3-fold increase in genital infections in those taking SGLT2Is compared to those taking another oral diabetic agent, and a 4-fold increase in genital mycotic infections in those taking SGLT2Is compared to placebo (Puckrin et al., 2018).
- In both a meta-analysis and a pooled analysis there was an increased risk of genital mycotic infections in patients taking ertugliflozin compared to patients receiving placebo. There was a higher rate reported in women compared to men. And there was a higher rate in uncircumcised males over circumcised males.

(Patel et al., 2020; Zhang et al., 2021).

- A systematic evaluation of population based observational studies also confirmed an increased risk of genital mycotic infections with the use of SGLT2Is (Caparrotta et al., 2021).
- Prescribers should consider avoiding the use of SGLT2Is in women with a history of severe or recurrent genital mycotic infections (Engelhardt et al., 2021).

Fournier Gangrene

- Fournier gangrene is an extremely rare life-threatening necrotizing fasciitis of the perineum caused by a bacterial infection.
- The infection usually begins with a break in the skin in the perineal area, allowing bacteria to move into the surrounding tissues and invade the fascia under the skin surrounding the muscles, nerves, fat, and blood vessels of the perineum.

- Patients with diabetes are already at higher risk for the development of this serious disorder due to increased glucosuria. Additional risk factors include obesity, peripheral vascular disease, alcoholism, and immunosuppression.
- The FDA issued a Medication Guide stating that cases of rare but serious infection of the genitals and around the genitals (Fournier gangrene) were reported in patients taking SGLT2Is (FDA, 2018, August 28).
  - In a review of 15 years of data from the FDA's Adverse Events Reporting System (FEARS), a voluntary reporting system, the incidence of Fournier gangrene associated with the use of SGLT2Is rose. The reporting of Fournier gangrene increased after the above FDA warning was released which likely contributed to the increased incidence in the 15-year review.
  - Also, the number of patients taking SGLT2Is has increased exponentially since first approved in 2013 with reports of 1.7 million new patients on SGLT2Is in 2017 alone.

  (Bloomgarden et al., 2019)
- However, it is unclear if SGLT2Is further increases the risk of Fournier gangrene in patients already at risk. No association was observed between SGLT2Is and Fournier gangrene in any of the large SGLT2I clinical trials (Lam & Shaikh, 2021).
  - The Declare TIMI-58 trial reported only one case of Fournier gangrene in the group receiving dapagliflozin and five reported cases of Fournier gangrene in the placebo group (Wiviott et al., 2018).
  - In a review of the IBM Marketscan claims data base of a large population the researchers found no evidence that there is an increased risk of Fournier gangrene with SGLT2Is compared to dipeptidyl peptidase-4 (DPP-4) inhibitors (Yang et al., 2019).

Linking Knowledge to Practice

✓ *Patients with DMT2 who have hyperglycemia and obesity are at an increased risk for infection prior to starting treatment with an SGLT2I. Optimization of diabetes care including glycemic control and weight loss can help reduce with risk of infection for all patients with DMT2.*

✓ *Educating patients taking SGLT2Is on useful personal hygiene practices may help reduce the incidence of genital mycotic infections and UTIs.*

✓ *Instructions such as rinsing the genital area with water after each void and at bedtime can be helpful. The use of prepackage flushable hygiene wipes is encouraged. Cotton underwear in females may also help mitigate the risk of vaginal candidiasis.*

(Engelhardt et al., 2021)

Linking Knowledge to Practice

✓ *Fournier gangrene occurs more often in men than women and scrotal pain is the predominant symptom.*

(Huayllani et al., 2022)

Risk for Amputation

- Lower extremity amputations are a rare adverse event associated with the use of SGLT2Is.
- Combined data from the CANVAS and CANVAS-R studies showed an increased incidence of amputation in those randomized to canagliflozin over the placebo group. Amputation was primarily at the level of the toe or metatarsal (Neal et al., 2017). Risk factors for amputation included age ≥ 65 years, prior amputation, PAD, CAD, neuropathy, diabetic foot ulcers, and no engagement in preventative foot care (Rossing et al., 2022b).

- ♦ In five previous clinical trials evaluating the efficacy and safety of canagliflozin in the treatment of DMT2, amputation was not identified as an adverse event (Rosiak et al., 2014).
- ♦ The CREDENCE trial evaluating renal outcomes in patients taking canagliflozin did not show any difference in the rate of amputation between patients randomized to canagliflozin or placebo (Perkovic et al., 2019).
- ♦ Miyashita and colleagues completed a meta-analysis of five clinical trials evaluating SGLT2Is and the incidence of amputation. The authors concluded that the incidence of amputation did not increase with the use of an SGLT2Is and that there was no difference in the rate of amputation noted between dapagliflozin, canagliflozin and empagliflozin (Miyashita et al., 2020).
- ♦ Yuan and colleagues evaluated the real-world use of SGLT2Is in comparison to patients on other antidiabetic agents. In this evaluation of over 118,000 patients there was no evidence of an increased risk of below the knee amputation in those taking an SGLT2I. When evaluating the risk in those taking canagliflozin, again there was no increase in rate of amputation in the canagliflozin group (Yuan et al., 2018).
- ♦ In 2020 the FDA, after reviewing additional trials, removed the United States (US) Boxed Warning regarding the amputation risk associated with the use of canagliflozin (FDA, 2020b, August 6).
- ♦ Data from seven Phase 3 clinical trials evaluating ertugliflozin demonstrated more amputations in the ertugliflozin groups compared to the placebo group, however the difference was not statistically significant.
- ♦ The prescribing information for canagliflozin and ertugliflozin cautions that prior to initiation of these agents, patients should be evaluated for risk factors for lower extremity amputation including prior amputation, peripheral vascular disease, neuropathy, and diabetic foot ulcers.
- ♦ The ACC has stated that SGLT2Is can be used safely in patients with peripheral vascular disease (Maddox et al., 2024).

Risk for Diabetic Ketoacidosis (DKA)

- ♦ In May of 2015 and again December of 2015 the FDA published warnings regarding the risk of ketoacidosis in patients taking SGLT2Is.
- ♦ Ketoacidosis was identified in patients with only mild elevations of blood glucose and even in patients with normal glucose levels.

(FDA, 2015, December 5; FDA, 2015, May 15)

- ♦ Ketoacidosis in the setting of a normal blood glucose level is called euglycemic diabetic ketoacidosis (eDKA).
  - The risk for the development of eDKA (DKA with blood glucose < 250 mg/dL), while rare, has been seen in patients with DMT2 who are in starvation states.
  - Risk factors for a state of starvation are decreased carbohydrate intake, fasting, severe acute illness, and excessive alcohol intake.
  - Since SGLT2Is have been introduced eDKA has become more prevalent (Bamgboye et al., 2021).
  - Clark and colleagues evaluated 647 admissions for DKA over a 4-year period. They noted that 6.6% of the cases occurred in patients taking SGLT2Is. Of those patients with DKA who were taking an SGLT2I, 69.8% had eDKA, and of those with eDKA nearly 62% had started the SGLT2I within the previous 6 months (Clark et al., 2021).
- ♦ Patients taking SGLT2Is who develop DKA present with lower blood glucose levels secondary to the persistent glucosuria produced by the medication.
  - Patients may present in DKA with a blood glucose level < 250 mg/dl.
  - When blood glucose is < 250 mg/dl DKA is often not suspected, resulting in delayed treatment.

- The risk of eDKA has been reported as high as 9% in patients with DMT1 (Plewa et al., 2020), and as a result SGLT2Is are do not have an approved indication for treating DMT1 in the United States at the time of this writing.

Advanced Concept Focus:
Euglycemic DKA (eDKA)

- When an SGLT2I removes glucose from the body via the urinary tract and serum glucose levels are reduced, the pancreatic beta cells decrease insulin production.
- The relative loss of blood glucose stimulates glucagon secretion from the alpha cells, increasing blood glucose levels.
- With depressed insulin production and an increase in glucagon production there is a lower ratio of insulin to glucagon in the body.
- If circumstances exist where there is inadequate insulin to carry blood glucose into the cells for use by the body, the process of lipolysis begins, and free fatty acids are increased.
- The body will shift to fat metabolism for fuel which results in fatty acids being broken down into ketone bodies and as a result ketoacidosis develops.
- When the cells of the body experience starvation (lack of glucose in the cells) the compensatory process is to move to fat metabolism for fuel.
  - In a patient taking an SGLT2I there are situations which can place the patient at risk for their cells to go into a starvation state and thus develop eDKA.
  - These situations include those where there is increased catecholamine production and situations where there is decreased food or carbohydrate intake.
  - Increased catecholamine production results in increased blood glucose levels which further alter the insulin to glucagon ratio.
  - Situations that increase catecholamine production and subsequent blood glucose release include high stress situations, and severe illness such as sepsis.
    - In these situations, the SGLT2I continues to remove blood glucose from the body and thus insulin release gets suppressed and, as a result the body does not have an adequate amount of insulin to carry the catecholamine induced excess blood glucose into the cells.
    - Since excess glucose is not moved into the cells for fuel, the process of lipolysis begins, and free fatty acids are broken down into ketone bodies.
  - Decreased food / carbohydrate intake occurs in situations such as being NPO (nothing by mouth), or a change in dietary pattern to a low carbohydrate diet.
    - With decreased food intake and lower blood glucose levels, insulin production is inhibited.
    - In these situations, there is not enough blood glucose available for cell metabolism and cell starvation begins again moving to fat metabolism through the process of lipolysis.
- The following situations place the patient at high risk for eDKA either because of decreased carbohydrate intake or increased catecholamine production: periods of fasting, low carbohydrate diets, dehydration, acute illness, excessive alcohol intake, bariatric surgery, and other major surgical procedures.
- The risk of developing eDKA is highest in those taking SGLT2Is and insulin.
- eDKA may be more prevalent in those with lower body mass index and decreased glycogen stores.
- Patient counseling for those prescribed SGLT2Is should include the following instructions:
  - SGLT2Is should not be taken on sick days or on days when the patient is not eating or drinking normally.
  - The following should be avoided: heavy alcohol use, very low carbohydrate diets, and ketogenic diets.

- ♦ SGLT2Is should be held for 3 days (4 days with ertugliflozin) prior to any surgery that requires an NPO status (FDA, 2022, March 15).
- ♦ SGLT2Is can be restarted postoperatively when the patient is feeling well and able to consume a normal diet (FDA, 2022, March 15).
- ♦ Patients taking both insulin and an SGLT2I should be counseled against reducing or omitting insulin at their own discretion because this practice can increase the risk for the development of eDKA.
- ♦ eDKA is suspected when the blood glucose is < 250 mg/dL, pH < 7.3, and serum bicarbonate < 18 mEq/L. Serum and urine ketones will be present. An abnormal anion gap is also expected.
- ♦ Kussmaul respirations occur to blow off carbon dioxide (CO_2) as a compensatory response to metabolic acidosis.
- ♦ If Kussmaul respirations or a fruity odor of breath is present this indicates a more severe level of metabolic acidosis.
- ♦ The onset of eDKA is often insidious, delaying recognition.
  - It is important to recognize potential S&S including malaise, dyspnea, loss of appetite, nausea and vomiting (N&V).
  - If these S&S are present the following should be evaluated: blood pH, serum ketones (beta-hydroxybutyric acid) and urine ketones.
  - Patients should be counseled to recognize these S&S of eDKA and self-test at home for ketones by urine dipstick.
  - If the urine is positive for ketone production, the patient should implement the STICH protocol (outlined in the box below).
    - ▪ The STICH Protocol was developed for patients with DMT1 taking SGLT2Is (which is off label in the United States).
    - ▪ It has also been found to be useful in patients with insulin dependent DMT2 taking SGLT2Is when eDKA is suspected.
- ♦ SGLT2Is should be stopped when eDKA is suspected and should continue to be held until eDKA is fully resolved.
- ♦ SGLT2Is may potentially be reintroduced once risk factors for eDKA have been resolved.

(Goldenberg et al., 2016; Kalra & Gupta, 2016; Plewa et al., 2020)

STICH Protocol for eDKA

- o **ST**: Stop the SGLT2I.
- o **I**nsulin: Bolus utilizing short acting insulin while also consuming the carbohydrates listed in the next step below.
- o **C**onsume 30 to 60 grams (g) of carbohydrates.
- o **H**ydrate with 200 to 500 mL (8 to 16 ounces) of fluids (water). This should be repeated every 1 to 2 hours.
- o Notify provider of eDKA.
- o Repeat above steps every 1 to 2 hours.
- o Repeat ketone assessment every 3 to 4 hours.
- o Seek medical assistance if ketosis does not resolve or symptoms of worsening eDKA develop.
- o Symptoms of worsening eDKA include abdominal pain, nausea, vomiting, fatigue and/or dyspnea.
- o When providing instructions to the patient on the STICH protocol, the diabetes provider should recommend a specific insulin dose and amount of carbohydrate.

(Garg et al., 2018)

Linking Knowledge to Practice

- ✓ *A starvation state can lead to ketoacidosis. Patients can trigger a starvation state by fasting or substantially lowering their carbohydrate intake. Also, during periods of severe acute illness patients may not be able to maintain an adequate oral intake or they may experience vomiting.*
- ✓ *Excessive alcohol intake can also lead to ketosis. Acetic acid is produced when alcohol is metabolized, and acetic acid has the potential to be further converted to acetyl-CoA and used in the metabolic pathway that leads to the formation of ketone bodies.*
  - *Severe ketosis related to alcohol use usually occurs once drinking has stopped due to the development of N&V.*
  - *During active alcohol consumption the metabolism of alcohol produces substances that inhibit peripheral lipolysis and as a result there is a limit to the fatty acid that can be delivered to the liver.*
  - *However, once alcohol levels begin to fall there are increased levels of norepinephrine and cortisol in response to withdrawal. Norepinephrine and cortisol act synergistically with the hormonal response to a fasting state and this substantially increases lipolysis.*

(Mehta & Emmet, 2023)

Risk for Hypoglycemia

- ♦ Hypoglycemia can occur if an SGLT2I is used in conjunction with other antidiabetic agents that can cause hypoglycemia. The most common agents associated with hypoglycemia in the treatment of DMT2 are insulin, sulfonylureas and meglitinides.
- ♦ Hypoglycemia is not an expected adverse reaction in patients taking SGLT2Is who do not have DMT2.
  - SGLT2Is decrease the renal threshold for glucose excretion, and this results in glucosuria. However, glucose excretion does not occur to the point of causing hypoglycemia.
  - The normal renal threshold for glucose excretion is approximately 180 mg/dL in patients without diabetes. When this threshold is reached there is renal excretion of glucose. This results in glucosuria and lower serum blood glucose.
  - The renal threshold for glucose excretion in patients with DMT2 is higher at approximately 240-250 mg/dL.
  - When a patient is on an SGLT2I the renal threshold for glucose excretion is lowered. This means glucosuria will occur at a lower blood glucose level than normal for patients with and without diabetes.
  - SGLT2Is reduce serum glucose levels and in response to lower serum glucose levels the production of glucosuria slows. Blood glucose levels in the normal range will inhibit further glucose excretion via the urinary tract.

(Palmer & Clegg, 2023)

Contraindication Highlights for SGLT2Is

- ♦ Consult manufacturer recommendations for use in children, pregnant women, and nursing women.
- ♦ A history of serious hypersensitivity to the drug or any component of the drug formulation is a contraindication for each SGLT2I. Cases of angioedema and anaphylaxis have been reported in patients taking an SGLT2I (UptoDate®, Lexidrug™, 2025).
- ♦ In the United States the FDA has not approved any SGLT2Is for use in the treatment of DMT1. There are some small trial and anecdotal reports of off label use in patients with DMT1 (El Hage, Kashyap, and Rao, 2019).
- ♦ SGLT2Is should be avoided in patients requiring any type of RRT (UptoDate®, Lexidrug™, 2025).

Special Considerations & Monitoring with SGLT2Is

- Monitor renal function at baseline and periodically during treatment.
  - There is an expected reversible decline in GFR with the initiation of an SGLT2I.
  - Don't initiate in the setting of AKI until acute injury is resolved. Don't initiate in patients at high risk for AKI. This includes patients with hypotension or volume depletion.
  - If AKI develops while a patient is taking an SGLT2I the medication should be temporarily stopped until the AKI and risk factors for AKI are resolved. Volume loss associated with glucosuria and natriuresis can contribute to worsening prerenal AKI (Lu et al., 2021).
  - The dose may need to be lowered or stopped with a decline in renal function depending on the SGLT2I that is being used and the indication for which the SGLT2 is being given.
- Monitor for the development of UTIs or genitourinary infections while on therapy.
- Monitor for S&S of possible Fournier gangrene.
  - S&S include tenderness or swelling of the genitals or the area from the genitals to the rectum that is associated with a fever (temperature > 100.4 Fahrenheit).
  - Remind patients each visit that these S&S require immediate reporting and emergency treatment.
- Monitor for adequate peripheral perfusion at each visit. There is no longer a US Boxed Warning for increased risk of lower extremity amputations, however, it is recommended to evaluate for worsening PAD and to stop the SGLT2 inhibitor in patients who have S&S of worsening PAD.
  - Teach patients the importance and the components of routine preventative foot care.
  - Instruct patients to monitor for and report S&S of infection, including osteomyelitis.
  - Reportable S&S include new pain or tenderness, or sores or ulcers involving the lower limbs.
- Educate patients on the risk of DKA and eDKA as discussed above.
- There are special considerations in patients undergoing bariatric surgery:
  - SGLT2Is should be held 3 to 5 days prior to bariatric surgery to avoid the risk of eDKA.
  - Absorption of the medication may be altered after gastric bypass or sleeve gastrectomy surgery.
  - SGLT2Is should not be reinitiated after surgery until all postoperative fluid requirements and volume status goals have been achieved.
  - DMT2 may be in remission post-bariatric surgery and the SGLT2I may not be resumed if its purpose was for the treatment of DMT2.

(UptoDate®, Lexidrug™, 2024)

Key Pharmacokinetic & Pharmacodynamic Information for SGLT2Is

- Peek action with most SGLT2Is is 1 to 2 hours with the longest being 2.5 to 4 hours with Sotagliflozin.
- SGLT2Is can be taken with or without food. When taken with food there is a minor delay in the peek action, but this has not been found to impact the pharmacodynamics of these medications.
- Once an SGLT2I is stopped the effect of decreasing the renal threshold for glucose excretion through the urinary tract will decrease over time.
  - Much of the medication impact will be minimized in 3 days.
  - However, there are reports of continued glucosuria up to 10 days after discontinuation of the SGLT2Is with late reports of eDKA (Wang & Isom, 2020).

(UptoDate®, Lexidrug™, 2024)

Important Medication Interactions with SGLT2Is

- For all SGLT2Is there is a recommendation to consider modifying insulin and sulfonylureas before starting the SGLT2I.

- ♦ Sotagliflozin is a P-glycoprotein / ABCB1 inhibitor and as a result may increase the concentration of other medications. Review medication interactions before prescribing.
- ♦ Fosphenytoin, phenytoin, phenobarbital, primidone, rifampin, and ritonavir can decrease the concentration of canagliflozin requiring a higher dose of canagliflozin.

(UptoDate®, Lexidrug™, 2024)

Diabetes Foot Care Essentials

- Patients should be instructed to wear footwear that fits properly to prevent both injury and skin breakdown.
- Patients should routinely see a podiatrist for comprehensive foot care.
- Patients should be instructed to inspect their feet daily for injury or skin breakdown because neuropathy can mask the pain associated with injury and skin breakdown.
- Patients should perform daily skin cleansing and should apply topical moisturizer daily to prevent dryness and fissures. Autonomic neuropathy diminishes sweat secretion placing patients at risk for cracking of the skin.
- Patients should stop smoking because up to 40% of diabetic ulcers involve ischemia (Edmonds et al., 2021).
- Patients should be instructed to report skin lesions immediately so treatment if needed can begin immediately.

Prescribing Pearls for SGLT2 Inhibitors

Part 1 Adjustments in Diabetic Regimen in Patients with DMT2 Prior to Initiation

- A sulfonylurea or meglitinide dose should be reduced by 50% or discontinued completely prior to initiating an SGLT2I to avoid the risk of hypoglycemia (Lam & Shaikh, 2021).
- The insulin dose should be stable prior to initiation of an SGLT2I and in some situations the dose may need to be decreased.
  - Patients with an elevated A1c, obesity, or large insulin needs may not need any insulin adjustments.
  - In patients with A1c of ≤ 7-8.5% insulin reduction may be needed to prevent hypoglycemia.
    - An initial reduction of 10 to 20% of the total insulin dose is recommended.
    - Prandial insulin should be adjusted first if the patient is on both prandial insulin and a long-acting agent.
    - The initial reduction in prandial insulin should not be more than 20% the baseline dose. Dose reductions of greater than 20% from the patient's baseline prandial dose can increase the risk of DKA.
    - If the patient is only on a long-acting agent, the initial insulin reduction should be no greater than 10%.

  (Gomez-Peralta et al., Gomez-Peralta et al., 2017; Lam & Shaikh, 2021; Ma et al., 2023)
- If you are a provider and are initiating an SGLT2I for a CV, HF, or renal benefit in a patient with DMT2, you must collaborate with the provider who is managing the patient's DMT2.
  - You need to determine what, if any, adjustments will be needed in the patient's other medications being used to treat DMT2.
  - This is especially important if the patient is being treated with insulin, a sulfonylurea, or a meglitinide because these medications will need to be adjusted to avoid hypoglycemia.

Prescribing Pearls for SGLT2 Inhibitors

Part 2 Assessment of BP and Volume Status Prior to Initiation

- Assess volume status and BP.
- Consider adjusting the dose of antihypertensive agents or diuretics prior to initiation of SGLT2Is to avoid hypotension and hypovolemia.
- Patients at high risk for hypotension and hypovolemia include the elderly and those taking diuretics, ACEIs, and ARBs.
- Consider a reduction in dose of diuretic by 50% with the initiation of an SGLT2I.
  - Subsequent adjustments can be made based on urine output response to the SGLT2I (Gomez-Peralta et al., 2017; Lam & Shaikh, 2021).
  - In patients taking diuretics for HF, daily weight monitoring and reporting of weight gain should be stressed during this adjustment period.
- Consider reducing the dose of antihypertensive medications if the patient is at high risk for hypotension or on the lower end of a normal BP.
  - Some authors recommend adjusting the antihypertensive agents with initiation of the SGLT2I if the BP is < 140/80 mmHg.
  - Most patients should be on a maximally tolerated dose of a RAAS blocker consistent with how patients were treated in the clinical trials that evaluated the use of SGLT2Is for improvement in renal and CV outcomes (Lam & Shaikh, 2021).
  - Additionally, RAAS inhibition is a treatment standard in patients with HTN, DMT2 and HTN, and in patients with albuminuria. An ACEI or an ARB is recommended to be continued when an SGLT2I is added to therapy for the treatment of DMT2 and CKD (Rossing et al., 2022b).
  - Patients should be encouraged to participate in home BP monitoring and documentation.
- Carefully assess fall risk prior to initiation.
  - Assess for orthostatic hypotension.
  - This is especially important for patients who are frail to help mitigate the risk of falls and subsequent fractures.

Appendix 8 provides additional details regarding individual SGLT2Is.

DIURETICS

Diuretics work within the tubular structure of the nephron to alter sodium reabsorption and excretion with a net result of increased loss of water and electrolytes, thus reducing intravascular volume, decreasing preload, and lowering BP. For these reasons diuretics are used to treat HF and HTN.

Three types of diuretics that are commonly used in clinical practice are loop diuretics, thiazide and thiazide-like diuretics, and potassium sparing diuretics. These three types of diuretics are called natriuretic diuretics. They work by decreasing sodium reabsorption at different places within the tubular structure of the nephron. As a result, there is an increase in urinary sodium and water.

Another type of diuretic is an aquaretic diuretic that targets and inhibits water reabsorption rather than sodium reabsorption. Aquaretic medications block vasopressin receptors in the connecting tubule and collecting duct (Brater & Ellison, 2023).

Loop Diuretics

Commonly used loop diuretics include furosemide, torsemide and bumetanide. In a meta-analysis, torsemide improved functional class and reduced intermediate term readmissions in patients with HF compared to furosemide. However, torsemide did not reduce mortality risk compared to furosemide (Miles et al., 2019). In a combined systematic review and meta-analysis comparing loop diuretics, torsemide significantly reduced BNP levels and edema compared to other agents, however there was no difference in terms of hospital readmissions and mortality (Eid et al., 2021).

Figure 8 shows the location of action of various diuretics.

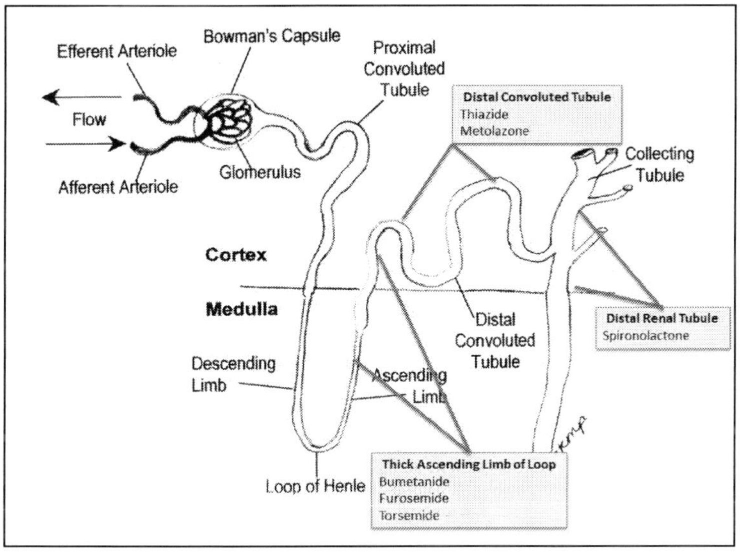

Figure 8: Site of Action for Diuretics

Mechanism of Action & Types of Loop Diuretics

- Loop diuretics work in the ascending limb of the Loop of Henle to inhibit reabsorption of sodium, chloride, and potassium back into the blood, and cause excretion of sodium, chloride, potassium, calcium, magnesium, phosphate, and water in urine.
- Loop diuretics cause natriuresis but are less likely to cause hyponatremia because they impair urine concentrating ability and water is excreted more than sodium. This is referred to as hypotonic renal loss. See the Advanced Concept Focus section below on diuretic induced hyponatremia.
- There is some evidence that furosemide causes peripheral venous vasodilation and thus symptom relief before the diuretic effect occurs. Most experts believe the venous vasodilation is because of the release of prostaglandins by the veins. However, furosemide may also cause peripheral arterial vasoconstriction which is an unwelcome hemodynamic effect (Jhund, McMurray, & Davie, 2000).

Linking Knowledge to Practice

✓ *The following loop diuretic doses are equivalent:*
- *Furosemide 40 mg.*
- *Torsemide 20 mg or (10 to 20 mg).*
- *Bumetanide 1 mg.*
- *Ethacrynic acid 50 mg.*

Table 11 summarizes and compares the different loop diuretics.

Advanced Concept Focus:

Diuretic Mechanisms of Action

- Cells that transport sodium contain pumps (Na-K-ATPase pumps). These pumps return reabsorbed sodium back into circulation.
- These pumps maintain a low concentration of sodium and a high concentration of potassium inside the cell. The low concentration of sodium inside the cell facilitates the process of sodium that has been filtered out of the blood entering the cells.
- Sodium cannot freely cross the lipid layer of the cell membrane. A carrier or sodium channel is required for sodium to enter the cell. Each major nephron segment has one or more sodium entry mechanisms, and it is on these mechanisms that diuretics work.
- Most filtered sodium (60 to 65%) is reabsorbed back into circulation in the proximal tubule. Water is also reabsorbed along with sodium.
  - This is the site where acetazolamide, a carbonic anhydrase inhibitor, works.
  - While this is the site of much sodium reabsorption, acetazolamide does not have high diuretic efficacy because the excess fluid removed from the proximal convoluted tubule can be reabsorbed later, primarily in the loop of Henle and to a much lesser degree in the distal convoluted tubule.
- Loop diuretics work in the ascending loop of Henle to reduce sodium and chloride reabsorption. However, some of the extra sodium and chloride intended for excretion can be reabsorbed in the distal convoluted tubule.
  - This is one of the factors that contributes to diuretic resistance that is sometimes seen with the use of loop diuretics.
  - However, the capacity to reabsorb in the distal tubule and collecting duct are limited and therefore effective natriuresis usually occurs with loop diuretics even though there is the potential for sodium and water reabsorption in the distal tubule.
- Thiazide and thiazide-like diuretics inhibit sodium reabsorption primarily in the distal convoluted tubule and can be used to combat diuretic resistance when it occurs in people on chronic loop diuretic therapy.
  - However, when used alone, thiazides have a weaker diuretic response because the distal convoluted tubule reabsorbs a smaller proportion of the sodium and chloride that have been filtered out of the blood.
  - Some thiazides such as chlorothiazide also inhibit sodium reabsorption to some degree in the proximal convoluted tubule because they partially inhibit carbonic anhydrase.
  - Also, as with other diuretics, the effectiveness of thiazides can be impacted by what happens downstream where there is the potential for sodium and chloride reabsorption to occur in the collecting tubule and the collecting duct.
- When administered at maximum doses loop diuretics bind sodium reentry into the cells that contain pumps and return sodium back into circulation. As a result, 20 to 25% of the sodium that is filtered out during glomerular filtration gets excreted in the urine.
- Even when thiazide and thiazide-like diuretics are given at their maximum dose, they can only inhibit the reabsorption of about 3 to 5% of the sodium and chloride that have been filtered.
- The process of inhibiting the reabsorption of sodium and chloride in the ascending loop of Henle by loop diuretics also inhibits the reabsorption of calcium and leads to increased calcium excretion. Calcium handling in the ascending loop of Henle is tied to the handling of sodium and chloride so that when there is a decrease in the reabsorption of sodium and chloride, there is a parallel decrease in the reabsorption of calcium.

- ♦ Thiazides also impact calcium because the distal convoluted tubule is an important site for active calcium reabsorption and in this area of the tubular system the calcium reabsorption is independent of sodium reabsorption. Thiazide and thiazide-like diuretics increase the reabsorption of calcium in both the distal tubule and in the proximal tubule.
- ♦ Thiazide and thiazide-like diuretics also impact the handling of water, and this contributes to the risk for the development of hyponatremia. The distal convoluted tubule is part of the diluting segment of the tubular system and when sodium and chloride are blocked at this location it impairs the ability to dilute urine. More information about thiazides and how they increase the risk for hyponatremia is discussed in the Advanced Concept Focus section below on diuretic induced hyponatremia.

(Brater & Ellison, 2023)

Indications for Loop Diuretics

- ♦ Loop diuretics are the first-line agents used for the immediate relief of symptoms in acute pulmonary edema and for volume overload in chronic HF.
  - Diuretics reduce fluid volume and ventricular preload, therefore relieving symptoms of pulmonary and systemic congestion in HF. Loop diuretics are preferred for the management of HF due to their rapid onset of action and more potent diuretic effect.
  - Guidelines for management of HF recommend the use of diuretics in patients with symptoms of fluid retention in combination with other evidence-based medications shown to reduce mortality.
  - The use of diuretics alone is not associated with a reduction in mortality, however, controlled trials with diuretics showed their effects to include improved symptoms, quality of life, and exercise tolerance

(Colucci & Sterns, 2022; Heidenreich et al., 2022)

- ♦ Per the guideline for the prevention, detection, evaluation, and management of high BP in adults, loop diuretics are also preferred over thiazides for treatment of HTN in the setting of CKD disease when the eGFR is below 30 mL/min/1.73 m^2 (Jones et al., 2025). There is emerging evidence that thiazides may also be used in the setting of advanced CKD. This evidence is discussed below with thiazide and thiazide-like diuretics.
- ♦ Ascites secondary to cirrhosis is an additional indication for loop diuretics (UptoDate, Lexidrug™, 2025).

Special Dosing Information for Loop Diuretics

Outpatient

- ♦ If the patient is diuretic naïve start furosemide 20 to 40 mg once or twice daily. The effective dose of diuretic must be determined. If there is no response to a dose of 20 mg of furosemide the dose needs to be increased to 40 mg.
- ♦ When GFR is normal the maximum single dose is a furosemide equivalent of 40 to 80 mg. In the setting of renal insufficiency, the maximum single dose is much higher and may be up to 200 mg.
- ♦ In outpatients with HF, the patient is usually started on low dose diuretic therapy until urine output increases and weight decreases. In the outpatient setting the weight loss goal is 0.5 to 1.0 kilograms (kg)/day. Since daily labs are not being monitored the amount of diuresis needs to be controlled.
- ♦ With appropriate counseling and coaching, patients can be safely educated to adjust their loop diuretic dose in the outpatient setting.
- ♦ Once euvolemia is achieved the dose of diuretic should be adjusted to the minimum dose needed to sustain euvolemia.
- ♦ The subcutaneous (SQ) form of furosemide can be used in outpatient environments.

One use includes home SQ furosemide as a strategy to help manage HF.

- SQ furosemide is delivered with a preprogrammed infuser that gives 30 mg over the first hour followed by 12.5 mg/hr over the next 4 hours for a total of 80 mg over a 5-hour period.
- This method of administration is not recommended for long-term use. Patients should be transitioned back to oral therapy as soon as possible.

(Colucci & Sterns, 2025, Heidenreich et al., 2022, UptoDate, Lexidrug™, 2026)

Inpatient

- ♦ The initial dose of loop diuretic should be given IV early upon arrival to the hospital (in the ED or immediately after admission).
- ♦ Furosemide IV is usually the first-line agent and initial dose is between 1 and 2.5 times the patient's home total daily dose in the furosemide equivalent. The maximum effective single dose ranges from 80 mg to 200 mg depending on renal function.
- ♦ If the initial dose does not result in effective diuresis the dose should be doubled. It is not effective to increase the frequency of a dose that does not achieve diuresis.
- ♦ IV furosemide is given every 8 to 12 hours. An alternative to every 8 to12 hour dosing is a continuous infusion.
  - A continuous infusion should only be started after a patient has responded to a bolus dose.
  - The bolus dose at which a patient had a diuretic effect will determine the infusion rate.
  - A continuous drip should be started immediately after an effective bolus dose.
- ♦ In a systematic review and meta-analysis there were no clear differences in outcomes between furosemide given in bolus doses versus continuous infusion (Shastri et al., 2022).
- ♦ The dose of loop diuretics should be increased until urine output increases, weight decreases, and there is an improvement in symptoms.
- ♦ Monitoring the response is important when making decisions about increasing or decreasing the dose.
  - Indications of adequate / effective diuresis:
    - ▪ BNP or NT-pro BNP reduction.
    - ▪ Improvement in orthopnea.
    - ▪ Reduction in level of jugular venous pulsation elevation.
  - Indications of over diuresis (volume contraction):
    - ▪ Hypotension.
    - ▪ Dizziness.
    - ▪ Orthostatic hypotension.
    - ▪ Renal insufficiency.

  (Colucci & Sterns, 2022; Heidenreich et al., 2022; Hollenberg et al., 2019; UptoDate, Lexidrug™, 2026)
- ♦ When transitioning IV furosemide back to oral furosemide therapy, use 1 to 2 times the 24-hour IV or SQ dose and give the oral medication in 1 to 2 doses per day (UptoDate, Lexidrug™, 2026).
  - However, when transitioning from IV back to oral bumetanide or torsemide the oral dose should be the same as the IV dose, as opposed to 1 to 2 times higher, because these agents have greater oral bioavailability.
  - Patients with renal dysfunction benefit from dividing their 24-hour dose into 2 or 3 doses.
- ♦ Diuretic therapy should be prescribed at hospital discharge either to continue diuresis to target weight or to maintain euvolemia. Evidence from the OPTIMIZE-HF registry showed a reduced 30-day all-cause mortality and hospitalization for HF in older patients when diuretic therapy was prescribed at discharge compared to no diuretic therapy after a hospitalization for HF (Faselis et al., 2020).

Table 11

Comparison of Sulfonamide Loop Diuretics

Bumetanide	Furosemide	Torsemide
▪ Oral bioavailability 80 to 100%. ▪ Max recommended 24-hour dose: 10 mg/day. ▪ Max effective single dose: 3 to 10 mg. ▪ Onset 30 to 60 minutes oral; 2 to 3 minutes IV. ▪ Peak 1 to 2 hours oral; 15 to 30 minutes IV. ▪ Duration 4 to 6 hours oral; 2 to 3 hours IV.	▪ Oral bioavailability 47 to 64%. ▪ Max recommended 24-hour dose: 600 mg/day oral; 960 mg/day IV drip. ▪ Max effective single dose: 80 to 200 mg. ▪ Onset 30 to 60 minutes oral; IV 5 minutes. ▪ Peak 1to 2 hours oral; 30 minutes IV. ▪ Duration 6 to 8 hours oral; 2 hours IV. ▪ Can be given SQ in the form of Furoscix (see below).	▪ Oral bioavailability ≈ 80%. ▪ Max recommended 24-hour dose: 200 mg/day. ▪ Max effective single dose: 50 to 100 mg. ▪ Onset within 1 hour oral. ▪ Peak 1 to 2 hours oral. ▪ Duration 6 to 8 hours oral. ▪ IV form discontinued 2008.

(Sidhu & Puckett, 2023; UptoDate, Lexidrug™, 2026). Additional table specific abbreviations: max = maximum
Higher doses may be needed in patients with more advanced CKD (eGFR < 30 mL/min/1.73 m^2).
Ethacrynic acid: For volume overload it is reserved for patients who develop a hypersensitivity reaction to one of the sulfonamide loop diuretics. There is a higher incidence of ototoxicity compared to the other loop diuretics.

Transitioning from Oral to IV Diuretics & From IV to Oral Diuretics

- If a patient is taking bumetanide 1 mg 2 times daily at home and presents to the hospital with a HF exacerbation and evidence of volume overload on physical exam, the initial bolus of IV furosemide should be between 80 and 200 mg. The furosemide equivalent of bumetanide is 80 mg for 24 hours since 1 mg of bumetanide is the equivalent of 40 mg of furosemide; and the recommendation is for the initial bolus to be 1 to 2.5 times the daily home oral maintenance dose.
- If a patient has been receiving IV furosemide 40 mg every 8 hours and is now ready to transition to oral therapy the 24-hour total oral dose would be a furosemide equivalent ranging between 120 and 240 mg daily, which is 1 to 2 times the IV dose. If the patient has any renal dysfunction the total dose should be given in 2 to 3 divided doses/day. In this example options for oral therapy might include furosemide 60 mg 2 times daily or 80 mg 3 times daily based on volume status and renal function. If transitioning to oral torsemide the patient should receive the equivalent the 24-hour IV furosemide dose which would be 60 mg of torsemide per 24 hours which would most often be given in a divided dose such as 30 mg 2 times daily.

(Colucci & Sterns, 2022; Hollenberg et al., 2019; UptoDate, Lexidrug™, 2026)

Select Adverse Effects of Loop Diuretics

Significant

- ♦ Loop diuretics can potentially lead to the development of AKI due to volume depletion and the development of hypovolemia.
  - The risk is higher in those who are older, critically ill, or who have underlying comorbid conditions which result in decreased renal blood flow.
  - The risk is also higher when loop diuretics are used at higher doses or in combination with nephrotoxic medications.
- ♦ Loop diuretics cause electrolyte loss that can lead to hypokalemia, hypocalcemia, and hypomagnesemia.

These electrolyte imbalances can predispose patients to cardiac arrhythmias. The risk increases with higher doses and when the patient has concurrent fluid loss from vomiting or diarrhea.

- ♦ Loop diuretics have been associated with hearing loss and tinnitus.
  - This is most often reversible within 24 hours of administration, although permanent loss has been reported.
  - This adverse effect is dose related. The medication induced impact on the Na-K-2CL co-transporter in the inner ear impacts the ionic composition of cochlear fluids.
  - There is less risk of ototoxicity with bumetanide compared to furosemide.
- ♦ Furosemide and bumetanide have been associated with immediate or delayed hypersensitivity reactions.
  - Immediate reactions may include urticaria, angioedema, and anaphylaxis.
  - Delayed reactions most often involve a skin rash but there have been rare more severe reactions including Stevens-Johnson syndrome, acute generalized exanthematous pustulosis, and toxic epidermal necrolysis.

(UptoDate, Lexidrug™, 2026)

Focused Electrolyte / Metabolic / Endocrine Adverse Effects of Loop Diuretics

- ♦ Hypovolemia (over diuresis).
- ♦ Hypochloremic alkalosis (contraction alkalosis).
- ♦ Hypokalemia, hypomagnesemia, hypocalcemia.
- ♦ Hyponatremia in the setting of HF when used with an MRA.
- ♦ Hyperuricemia (gout).
- ♦ Increased serum cholesterol and triglycerides (furosemide and torsemide).

(UptoDate, Lexidrug™, 2026)

Contraindication Highlights for Loop Diuretics

- ♦ Consult manufacturer recommendations for use in children, pregnant women, and nursing women.
- ♦ FDA approved product labeling states that a hypersensitivity to sulfonamide containing drugs is a contraindication. However, the scientific basis of this cross sensitivity has been challenged.
- ♦ SQ furosemide is contraindicated in anuria, ascites, or hepatic cirrhosis.
- ♦ Anuria is generally considered a contraindication to the continued use of furosemide.

(UptoDate, Lexidrug™, 2026)

Special Considerations & Monitoring with Loop Diuretics

- ♦ Electrolytes and renal function are monitored daily while in the hospital.
- ♦ Electrolytes and renal function are monitored regularly in the outpatient setting.
  - Monitoring should include after initiation and with any dose increase.
  - A disproportionate rise in BUN to creatinine with a stable GFR suggests a prerenal etiology, therefore, no further diuresis is indicated.
  - An increase in CVP (intravascular volume overload) can also worsen GFR.
    - Diuresis should <u>not</u> be stopped prematurely because of small changes in creatinine.
    - The decision to continue diuresis should be made based on S&S of congestion.
    - Diuresis should continue when there is clinical evidence of intravascular volume overload.
- ♦ The serum CO_2 should be evaluated for the presence of contraction alkalosis.

- Volume status should be carefully evaluated including the level of jugular venous pulsation at 30 to 45° (evaluation of the RV) and the presence of orthopnea or bendopnea (evaluation of the LV).

(Colucci & Sterns, 2022; Heidenreich et al., 2022)

Key Pharmacokinetic & Pharmacodynamic Information for Loop Diuretics

- Loop diuretics have a relatively rapid onset and relatively short duration of action.
- They are often referred to as "high ceiling" diuretics because the dose is up titrated to achieve an effective result.
- Loop diuretics are considered potent diuretics compared to thiazide and thiazide-like diuretics because they work in the ascending loop of Henle and can excrete 20 to 25% of the sodium that is filtered out during glomerular filtration (Lexicomp, 2023).

> ***Linking Knowledge to Practice***
>
> ✓ *Outpatients can be educated to increase their loop diuretic dose based on weight gain and other parameters associated with fluid retention. However, it is also important to educate patients about when to hold diuretics such as with a decrease in oral intake or when experiencing vomiting or diarrhea.*
>
> ✓ *While there is the potential for renal insufficiency, particularly with excess use of diuretics, there is also evidence that unresolved elevated venous pressure leads to worsening renal function. An accurate assessment of the patient's volume status is very important when making diuretic decisions to protect the kidneys.*
>
> ✓ *Persistent congestion at the time of discharge has been associated with higher rates of rehospitalizations and mortality (Heidenreich et al., 2022). RNs and APRNs need to assure that results of daily weights, I&Os, physical exam, BNP levels, and results of diagnostic tests show evidence of adequate decongestion prior to discharge.*
>
> ✓ *Decongestion in a HF patient requires more than the use of diuretics. All guideline directed therapies need to be optimized to achieve optimal volume status.*
>
> ✓ *Orthostatic BP assessment on the day of discharge is a tool to prevent readmissions by identifying patients who may be volume depleted and at high risk for falls at home.*

Important Medication Interactions with Loop Diuretics

- Furosemide cannot be given in combination with ethacrynic acid due to increased risk of ototoxicity.
- NSAIDs can decrease the effectiveness of loop diuretics and loop diuretics may enhance the nephrotoxic effects of NSAIDs.
- Loop diuretics may diminish the therapeutic effects of antidiabetic medications.

(UptoDate, Lexidrug™, 2026)

Advanced Concept Focus:

Diuretic Resistance

Diuretic resistance is defined as the lessening of the maximal diuretic effect limiting sodium and chloride excretion. Diuretic resistance is associated with renal impairment, increased risk of re-hospitalization, and mortality. Poor diuretic efficiency = increased risk of death.

Below are the causes and specific strategies that can be used in overcoming diuretic resistance:

- Consumption of excessive amounts of dietary sodium: An exceedingly high sodium intake that exceeds the acute sodium loss induced by diuretic therapy will result in diuretic resistance.

- Oral bioavailability: HF and food intake prolong time to peak concentration.
- Hypoalbuminemia: Loop diuretics are 95% protein bound. Low albumin reduces the availability of loop diuretics for facilitated diffusion.
- NSAIDS and uremic toxins: These competitively inhibit drug transport across proximal tubular epithelial cells.
- Hypochloremia: Decreased serum chloride plays a critical role in neurohormonal activation and renal salt sensing because chloride reduces renin release.
- Braking phenomenon:
  - This is present when there is a diminished diuretic effectiveness with each successive dose. This effect can be observed within hours.
  - The mechanism is unclear, but sodium loss leads to upregulation of proximal and distal tubule transporters.
    - Distal tubule sodium transport has immense potential to weaken the effect of loop diuretics, thus the rationale for the use of thiazide or thiazide-like diuretics with loop diuretics in this situation.
    - The use of a thiazide or thiazide-like diuretic (e.g., metolazone) in combination with a loop diuretic inhibits compensatory distal tubular sodium reabsorption, leading to enhanced natriuresis.
  - However, use caution when considering a thiazide or thiazide-like diuretic. In one study of patients hospitalized with HF, the addition of metolazone to enhance the effectiveness of loop diuretics was found to increase the risk for hypokalemia, hyponatremia, worsening renal function, and mortality (Brisco-Bacik et al., 2018).
- Tubular remodelling: This results in distal tubular hypertrophy that causes enhanced sodium reabsorption.
- CKD: CKD results in reduction of overall diuretic induced sodium excretion because of a reduced and diminished filtered load of sodium. The administration of loop diuretic multiple times a day combats this problem.
- Heart failure: HF decreases the peak effect of the diuretic due to increased proximal tubular reabsorption of sodium. More frequent dosing as opposed to dose escalation can be used to achieve maximal sodium excretion.
- The addition of low dose dopamine to diuretic therapy in the setting of reduced GFR did not improve outcomes in a study that included patients with all EFs, but a subset analysis showed increased urine output and weight loss in patients with low LVEF (Chen et al., 2013). Low dose dopamine may be considered a strategy to enhance diuresis in patients with low EF to avoid the use of inotropes.

(Rangaswami et al., 2019; Heidenreich et al. 2022)

Linking Knowledge to Practice

- ✓ *An elevation in the serum CO_2 may indicate a metabolic alkalosis or contraction alkalosis associated with diuretic therapy.*
- ✓ *The serum CO_2 on a chemistry panel correlates with the HCO_3 (bicarbonate) on the arterial blood gas.*
- ✓ *However, without a blood pH you cannot assume that an elevated CO_2 on the chemistry panel means there is a metabolic alkalosis, even in the setting of aggressive diuresis.*
- ✓ *The serum CO_2 can also be elevated as a compensatory mechanism for respiratory acidosis. Volume overload warranting diuretics can be a cause or contributing factor to ventilatory failure which results in respiratory acidosis.*

Prescribing Pearls for Loop Diuretics

- Loop diuretics cause significant natriuresis during the number of hours the medication is active.
- After the duration of action sodium excretion falls to very low levels. The fluid loss from the initial dose of diuretic leads to activation of both the RAAS and the SNS and as a result angiotensin II, aldosterone, and norepinephrine all promote sodium reabsorption.
- For example: If furosemide is given as a one-time daily dose there will be substantial natriuresis for 6 hours from the time given and then very low levels of sodium excretion for the remaining 18 hours of the day.
- However, there will not be a net sodium loss if the patient is consuming a diet high in sodium.
- There are 3 options for dealing with this sodium chloride retention after diuretic use:
  - Patient adherence to a reduced sodium diet.
  - Giving the diuretic 2 or 3 times a day.
  - Increasing the diuretic dose.
- The preferred option is a reduced sodium diet because it also helps minimize potassium loss associated with loop diuretics. A low sodium diet stimulates renal reabsorption of sodium chloride and because of complex physiological processes in the renal tubules, potassium secretion is limited.
- The least preferred option is to increase the dose of the diuretic because of the risk of hypovolemia.

(Brater & Ellison, 2023)

Thiazide and Thiazide-like Diuretics

Mechanism of Action & Types of Thiazide & Thiazide-like Diuretics

- There are thiazide diuretics (also referred to as thiazide type) and thiazide-like diuretics.
- When the term "thiazides" is used, it is referring to both thiazide and thiazide-like diuretics.
- Thiazide-like diuretics are longer acting. Thiazide-like diuretics are the ones used in most of the clinical trials addressing CV outcomes.
- However, the use of thiazide-like diuretics has been somewhat limited due to lack of convenient formulations.
- Thiazide and thiazide-like diuretics inhibit reabsorption of sodium and chloride in the distal tubule to cause excretion of sodium, chloride, and water in urine.
- They have a delayed onset but longer duration of action than loops.
- Thiazides are called "low ceiling" diuretics because the maximal response is reached at relatively low doses.
- They are less potent in their diuretic effect compared to loops.
- Thiazide and thiazide-like diuretics lose effectiveness in their ability to cause diuresis and lower BP as GFR declines.

(UptoDate, Lexidrug™, 2026)

In Table 12 each diuretic is identified as either a thiazide diuretic or a thiazide-like diuretic.

Indications for Thiazide & Thiazide-like Diuretics

Indication differences exist between loop and thiazide and thiazide-like diuretics. Table 12 outlines the indications for thiazide and thiazide-like diuretics.

Advanced Concept Focus:

Thiazide, Thiazide-Like, and Loop Diuretics in the Treatment of HTN

Role of Thiazide and Thiazide-Like Diuretics in Treatment of HTN

- Thiazide and thiazide-like diuretics are one option for a first-line agent in the treatment of HTN. Other options for first-line agents include ACEIs, ARBs, or CCBs.
- In hypertensive patients with CKD (eGFR < 60 mL/min/1.73 m^2) and albuminuria of > 30 mg/g, RASS inhibition with either (but not both) an ACEI or ARB is recommended as first line therapy. RASS inhibition has demonstrated a reduction in CV disease and delayed progression of CKD. An MRA, thiazide or thiazide-like diuretic is recommended as additional therapy if the target BP is not achieved. Target systolic BP goal in those with CKD and HTN is SBP < 120 mmHg (Cheung et al., 2021).
- However, a thiazide or thiazide-like diuretic is often preferred in patients with edema, osteoporosis, or calcium nephrolithiasis with hypercalciuria.
- Thiazide or thiazide-like diuretics or CCBs, as opposed to ACEIs or ARBs, are recommended as initial antihypertensive agents in black patients without HF or CKD because black patients are less responsive to medications blocking the RAAS.
- Guidelines for management of HTN recommend thiazide or thiazide-like diuretics as an option for most patients with uncomplicated HTN, either alone or combined with other antihypertensive drugs. Thiazide and thiazide-like diuretics can be effective when used alone and they enhance the effectiveness of all other antihypertensive drugs when used in combination.

(Jackson, 2018; Jones et al., 2025; Mann & Flack, 2024)

Preferred Thiazide and Thiazide-Like Diuretics in Treatment of HTN

- Chlorthalidone has often been recommended over hydrochlorothiazide as a preferred thiazide type diuretic in treating HTN because of its prolonged half-life and evidence from previous nonrandomized studies that demonstrated fewer adverse CV events with the use of chlorthalidone compared to hydrochlorothiazide (Cheung et al., 2021; Dorsch et al., 2011; Ernst et al., 2011; Whelton et al., 2018). Results of a meta-analysis also demonstrated slight superiority in BP control with chlorthalidone (Dineva et al., 2019).
- However, in a large observational cohort study chlorthalidone was not associated with significant CV benefits when compared with hydrochlorothiazide and instead was associated with greater risk of renal and electrolyte abnormalities (Hripcsak et al., 2020). It was suggested that the follow up period in this study was too short to account for potential CV benefits with chlorthalidone (Messerli, Roush, & Oparil, 2020).
- In a more recent prospective randomized trial of more than 13,000 patients chlorthalidone was not associated with a lower occurrence of major CV events or non–cancer-related deaths compared to hydrochlorothiazide (Ishani et al., 2022). It is important to note that the dose of chlorthalidone in this study was only 12.5 mg and this lower dose rather than 25 mg may have limited the benefits of chlorthalidone according to some experts (Mann & Flack, 2024).
- Some experts continue to recommend either chlorthalidone or indapamide because of their more potent antihypertensive effect and their longer duration of action resulting in a lower nighttime BP when taken in the morning (Mann & Flack, 2024).

Diuretics in the Treatment of HTN in Patients with Advanced CKD

- Loop diuretics are not routinely used in the treatment of HTN because of their shorter half-life. There are no outcome data for the use of loop diuretics in the treatment of HTN in patients with and without CKD (Cheung et al., 2021).

- ♦ Loop diuretics, however, have historically been preferred over thiazide and thiazide-like diuretics for treatment of HTN in the setting of CKD when the eGFR is below 30 mL/min/1.73 m^2 (Jones et al., 2025). This is because thiazide and thiazide-like diuretics lose efficacy in both BP control and diuresis effectiveness as GFR declines. However, chlorthalidone, metolazone, and indapamide appear to remain more effective than other agents at an eGFR of < 30 mL/min/1.73 m^2 (Cheung et al., 2021).
- ♦ In a study in patients with advanced CKD and poorly controlled HTN, chlorthalidone was more effective than placebo in lowering BP. In this study patients were already taking a mean of 3.4 antihypertensives and 60% of patients were on a loop diuretic at baseline (Agarwal et al., 2021).
- ♦ In most patients with CKD a combination of 3 medications will be needed to achieve a BP at goal. One of the 3 agents will be a diuretic. The choice between a loop and thiazide diuretic will depend on the patient's renal function and volume status.
- ♦ In treating HTN in patients with CKD it is important to know that the KDIGO 2021 Clinical Practice Guideline for the Management of Blood Pressure in CKD recommends a target systolic BP of < 120 mmHg systolic.
  - This target for systolic BP is lower than what is recommended in other guidelines such as those published by the ACC and AHA. The reason for the lower target BP in patients with CKD is because it reduces CV events and all-cause mortality in patients with CKD.
  - This intensive level of BP control is not considered to be renoprotective, yet it is recommended because most patients with CKD are more likely to experience a CV event than to develop ESKD.

(Cheung et al., 2021)

Table 12

Indications for Thiazide and Thiazide-like Diuretics

Chlorothiazide: **Thiazide diuretic**	▪ Edema or general volume overload: Used as an adjunct to loop diuretics. ▪ Chronic HTN: Used alone or in combination with other agents*.
Hydrochlorothiazide (HCTZ): **Thiazide diuretic**	▪ Edema or general volume overload: Used as an adjunct to loop diuretics. ▪ Chronic HTN: Used alone or in conjunction with other agents*. ▪ Nephrogenic diabetes insipidus (DI) caused by lithium [off label]: Used along with amiloride. HCTZ causes a paradoxical antidiuretic effect due to complex physiological processes, some of which are not fully understood. ▪ Calcium nephrolithiasis (kidney stones) [off label]: Thiazide and thiazide-like diuretics raise serum calcium and thus reduce urinary calcium.
Chlorthalidone: **Thiazide-like diuretic**	▪ Edema or general volume overload: Used as an adjunct to loop diuretics. ▪ Chronic HTN: Used in conjunction with other agents*. ▪ Calcium nephrolithiasis (kidney stones) [off label]: Thiazide and thiazide-like diuretics raise serum calcium and thus reduce urinary calcium.
Indapamide: **Thiazide-like diuretic**	▪ Edema or general volume overload: Used as an adjunct to loop diuretics. ▪ Chronic HTN: Used in conjunction with other agents*. ▪ Calcium nephrolithiasis (kidney stones) [off label]: (Thiazide and thiazide diuretics raise serum calcium and thus reduce urinary calcium).
Metolazone: **Thiazide-like diuretic**	▪ Edema or general volume overload: Used as an adjunct to loop diuretics.

* Other agents are usually an ACEI or an ARB or a dihydropyridine CCB.
(UptoDate, Lexidrug™, 2026)

> ***Linking Knowledge to Practice***
>
> ✓ *Thiazides are <u>not</u> the preferred diuretic in the setting of a volume overload because of their limited ability to cause diuresis based on the location in the tubules where they work.*
>
> ✓ *Thiazide and thiazide-like diuretics can be used to enhance the effectiveness of loop diuretics in the setting of volume overload.*
>
> ✓ *Thiazide and thiazide-like diuretics are effective in the treatment of straightforward HTN because in this setting substantial fluid loss is not needed.*
>
> ✓ *Because thiazides increase calcium reabsorption, they can be used to treat nephrolithiasis (renal calculi) secondary to excess calcium in the urine (hypercalciuria) (Zisman, 2024).*

Special Dosing Information for Thiazide & Thiazide-like Diuretics

See Table 13 for special renal dosing considerations for each agent.

- ♦ Several agents have diminished effectiveness in the presence of renal failure. Chlorthalidone, metolazone, and indapamide appear to remain more effective than chlorothiazide at an eGFR of < 30 mL/min/1.73 m^2 (Cheung et al., 2021).
- ♦ There is no dose adjustment recommended for hepatic dysfunction, but thiazide and thiazide-like diuretics should be used cautiously in patients with liver disease. Metolazone is contraindicated in hepatic coma or precoma (Up to Date®, Lexidrug™, 2026).

Select Adverse Effects of Thiazide & Thiazide-like Diuretics

Significant

- ♦ Electrolyte abnormalities:
  - Hypokalemia and hypomagnesemia: These are also adverse effects of loop diuretics.
  - Hyponatremia: Seen more commonly with thiazides compared to loop diuretics. See the Advanced Concept Focus section below on thiazide induced hyponatremia.
  - Hypercalcemia: This adverse effect is not seen with loop diuretics. Loop diuretics can cause hypocalcemia.
- ♦ Hyperuricemia and precipitation of gout.
- ♦ Hypersensitivity reactions (immediate and delayed).
  - Maculopapular skin rashes, to rare severe cutaneous rashes.
  - Interstitial nephritis and interstitial pneumonitis.
- ♦ Photosensitivity with a cumulative effect increases the risk of basal and squamous cell skin cancer.
- ♦ Acute myopia or acute angle-closure glaucoma (generally reversible) related to medications that are sulfa derivatives (hydrochlorothiazide, chlorthalidone, indapamide).

(UptoDate, Lexidrug™, 2026)

Additional Adverse Effects

- ♦ Orthostatic hypotension secondary to volume depletion.
- ♦ Hypochloremic alkalosis (contraction alkalosis).
- ♦ Hyperglycemia and glycosuria.
- ♦ Increased serum cholesterol and triglycerides (hydrochlorothiazide, chlorothiazide).
- ♦ Photosensitivity.

- ♦ Exacerbation of SLE (metolazone, hydrochlorothiazide, chlorothiazide, indapamide, & metolazone).

(UptoDate, Lexidrug™, 2026)

Table 13

Special Renal Dosing Information for Thiazide and Thiazide-like Diuretics

Chlorothiazide: Thiazide diuretic	▪ Medication is considered ineffective with a CrCl of < 30 mL/min unless used in combination with a loop diuretic. ▪ It is not recommended to be used in patients with a CrCl of < 10 mL/min due to lack of efficacy.
Hydrochlorothiazide (HCTZ): Thiazide diuretic	▪ No dose adjustment is needed if CrCl is > 10 mL/min. ▪ There is a diminished diuretic effect when CrCl is < 30 mL/min but there may be some preserved antihypertensive effect. ▪ The patient may need to switch to a loop diuretic if volume overload is present or if BP is not at goal. ▪ It is not recommended to be used in patients with a CrCl of < 10 mL/min due to lack of efficacy.
Chlorthalidone: Thiazide-like diuretic	▪ No dose adjustment is needed if CrCl is > 10 mL/min. ▪ There is a diminished diuretic effect when CrCl is < 30 mL/min but there may be some preserved antihypertensive effect. ▪ The patient may need to switch to a loop diuretic if volume overload is present or if BP is not at goal. ▪ It is not recommended to be used in patients with a CrCl of < 10 mL/min due to lack of efficacy.
Indapamide: Thiazide-like diuretic	▪ This medication does not require dose adjustments based on GFR. ▪ However, the diuretic effect will diminish with an eGFR < 30 mL/min/1.73 m^2, although there may still be antihypertensive effects.
Metolazone: Thiazide-like diuretic	▪ This medication does not require dose adjustments based on GFR. ▪ See ***Linking Knowledge to Practice*** box below for additional dosing information.
(UptoDate, Lexidrug™, 2026)	

Contraindication Highlights for Thiazide & Thiazide-like Diuretics

- ♦ Consult manufacturer recommendations for use in children, pregnant women, and nursing women.
- ♦ Anuria and hepatic coma or precoma are generally considered contraindication to thiazides.
- ♦ Hydrochlorothiazide, chlorthalidone and chlorothiazide are not recommended to be used in patients with a CrCl of < 10 mL/min due to lack of efficacy.
- ♦ Hydrochlorothiazide is not recommended to be used with hemodialysis or peritoneal dialysis due to lack of efficacy.

(UptoDate, Lexidrug™, 2026)

Advanced Concept Focus:

Diuretic Induced Hyponatremia

- ♦ Urinary concentrating ability is impaired with loop diuretics because the inhibition of sodium reabsorption interferes with the creation of a hyperosmotic gradient in the medullary interstitium. The interstitium is normally highly concentrated.

This allows water to be reabsorbed in the medullary collecting tubule in the setting of antidiuretic hormone (ADH), and this results in the normal excretion of concentrated urine.

- Because loop diuretics have impaired concentrating ability, water is excreted more than sodium, and this is referred to hypotonic renal loss.
- As a result of the hypotonic renal loss (the loss of more water than sodium), loop diuretics can be used to treat hyponatremia in patients who are euvolemic or hypervolemic.
- In the setting of a loop diuretic there is a reduced responsiveness to ADH because of the change in the medullary hyperosmotic gradient. Diuretics can also increase ADH levels if they induce hypovolemia. Since ADH does not have its normal effectiveness, there is a limit to water retention, and the development of hyponatremia will be limited under otherwise normal circumstances.
- Loop diuretics have a shorter duration of action, and this also contributes to the reduced risk of hyponatremia.
- Loop diuretics can be associated with hyponatremia in the setting of HF because HF is a risk factor for hyponatremia.
- When hyponatremia develops in the setting of a loop diuretic, the hyponatremia is more likely due to sodium loss than to the retention of free water.
- Thiazide and thiazide-like diuretics act in the distal tubule located in the cortical area of the kidney and do not interfere with the medullary osmotic gradient.
- Thiazides interfere with the maximal dilution of urine by blocking sodium chloride reabsorption in the distal tubule which is the primary diluting site in the kidney.
  - This means more sodium chloride is excreted, and this decreases the amount of free water clearance by the kidneys.
  - This is the number one contributor to thiazide induced hyponatremia.
- With thiazide and thiazide-like diuretics the excretion of sodium is increased while the excretion of water is decreased.
- With thiazides there can be impaired water excretion due to several factors:
  - Volume depletion and other factors such as nausea can stimulate ADH, leading to stimulation of thirst and increased water intake as well as increased water reabsorption resulting in the production of concentrated urine.
  - Thiazide and thiazide-like diuretics do not interfere with the ability of ADH to cause water retention which contributes to the development of hyponatremia.
  - Thiazides may be associated with an inappropriate secretion of ADH in euvolemic patients and if so, this usually happens quickly after starting the diuretic.
  - Thiazides can also exacerbate hyponatremia in patients with SIADH from another cause.
  - Thiazide and thiazide-like diuretics may be associated with water retention independent of ADH. They can result in direct upregulation of the aquaporin–2 receptors in the renal tubules resulting in increased water permeability in the collecting duct leading to increased water reabsorption independent of the presence of ADH.
  - About 50% of patients who develop thiazide induced hyponatremia have a genetic polymorphism that impacts what occurs in the renal collecting duct. As a result, water reabsorption is activated in the collecting duct even though there is suppression of ADH.
- At higher doses thiazides can lead to a decrease in both intravascular volume and GFR, and this stimulates proximal reabsorption of fluid which reduces the amount of fluid delivered to the diluting sites. As a result, there is less free water available for excretion. Higher doses of thiazide and thiazide-like diuretics increase the risk for hyponatremia.

- In the setting of increased water reabsorption due to ADH and increased sodium and potassium excretion from the diuretic, there is excess renal loss of potassium and sodium compared to water.
  - The sodium and potassium concentration in the urine can be higher than in the plasma and this type of sodium and potassium loss is referred to as hypertonic loss. The loss of this type of hypertonic fluid can promote hyponatremia.
  - Patients with thiazide induced hyponatremia often have excess potassium in the urine. This is called kaliuria with a fractional excretion of potassium > 13%.
- Hypokalemia, secondary to a thiazide diuretic, causes sodium to move into the cell and potassium to leave the cell.
  - This intracellular shift of sodium may contribute to thiazide induced hyponatremia.
  - The role of hypokalemia however is not entirely clear because hyponatremia with thiazides can occur in the absence of hypokalemia. It is thought that the relationship between hypokalemia and hyponatremia is more pronounced at higher doses of thiazide and thiazide-like diuretics.
- Hyponatremia appears to be more common with the thiazide-like diuretic chlorthalidone than with hydrochlorothiazide.
- The potassium sparing diuretics spironolactone, eplerenone and amiloride enhance urinary loss of sodium in the cortical distal tubule and when combined with a thiazide they increase the risk of hyponatremia.
- There are additional patient factors that contribute to the development of hyponatremia with the use of thiazide and thiazide-like diuretics:
  - Both a low sodium diet and a low or low normal baseline sodium level are risk factors for the development of thiazide induced hyponatremia.
  - Older age is associated with a smaller amount of muscle mass and with a decreased ability to excrete free water.
    - This is true even in healthy persons and this places patients at risk of hyponatremia caused by an excess water load.
    - Age > 60 is a risk factor for the development of hyponatremia.
  - Patients may have a reduced GFR which is a contributing factor to hyponatremia in older adults. A severely reduced GFR is also a contributing factor to salt wasting nephropathy discussed below.
  - Patients with multiple comorbid conditions are at a higher risk for the development of hyponatremia.
    - Comorbid conditions that place the patient at especially high risk include HF, liver disease, and malignancy.
    - Other comorbid conditions placing the patient at risk include CKD, respiratory disease, depression, and dementia.
  - Persistent N&V are common causes of hyponatremia.
  - Decreased dietary protein can limit the excretion of electrolyte free water. This is also a contributing factor to salt wasting nephropathy discussed below.
  - There is a tendency toward polydipsia in patients taking thiazides. Research has shown that patients with a history of thiazide induced hyponatremia will gain weight rather than lose weight when the patient is rechallenged with a single dose of a thiazide. This finding suggests that there may be an underlying polydipsia in this population.
  - Those who consume an excessive amount of beer are at risk for hyponatremia due to the low solute content of beer and often poor dietary solute intake that results in reduced solute delivery to the kidneys and subsequent impaired ability to remove water.
  - A fluid intake of > 1.5 to 2.0 liters/day predisposes a patient to thiazide induced hyponatremia. This is because the patient will have to excrete more free water to maintain a normal sodium level.

    - However, an increase in water intake does not typically cause hyponatremia unless there is also impaired water excretion such as with older age or reduced renal function.
    - The amount of free water retained in a patient will be the highest in those with both a high-water intake and a low sodium intake.
  - Concurrent use of other medications such as NSAIDs, selective serotonin reuptake inhibitors, serotonin and norepinephrine reuptake inhibitors, tricyclic antidepressants, and even benzodiazepines increase the risk of hyponatremia. These medications can alter water homeostasis.
  - The concurrent use of medications that cause dry mouth and therefore lead to increased water intake can also predispose the patient to hyponatremia.
  - Lower body mass in female patients is also a risk factor for the development of hyponatremia.
  - Older age and NSAIDs result in a reduction in renal prostaglandins. Renal prostaglandins inhibit ADH so a reduction of them can lead to free water retention and hyponatremia.

- Thiazides are the most common reason for drug induced hyponatremia. To avoid thiazide related hyponatremia, thiazide and thiazide-like diuretics should not be used in patients with a history of thiazide induced hyponatremia and only low doses should be used in patients with risk factors for hyponatremia. Hydrochlorothiazide 12.5 mg is an example of a low dose thiazide diuretic.

- Patients presenting with thiazide related hyponatremia can present with a clinical picture of either extracellular volume depletion or of SIADH.
  - When a patient has extracellular volume depletion the following findings are generally present: increased BUN to creatinine ratio, increased uric acid levels, and a urine sodium < 20 mmol/L after stopping the thiazide or thiazide-like diuretic.
  - When a SIADH picture is present the patient will have a low to normal BUN to creatine ratio, decreased uric acid levels, and the urine sodium will be > 20 to 40 mmol/L.
  - A serum uric acid level can differentiate between extracellular volume depletion and SIADH.
    - Uric acid level < 4 mg/dL = SIADH state.
    - Uric acid level > 4 mg/dL = Extracellular volume depletion.
    - Patients can also present with a mixed clinical picture.

- Acute hyponatremia develops within 48 hours and produces the symptoms of N&V, H/As, and even seizures.

- Chronic hyponatremia, even if mild, can result in fatigue, cognitive impairment, gait abnormalities resulting in falls and fractures, and increases mortality risk.

- Strategies to treat thiazide induced hyponatremia include restricting free water, replacing potassium losses, stopping diuretic therapy, and changing to a loop diuretic.

- In patients with chronic severe hyponatremia, there is an increased risk of developing osmotic demyelination syndrome with rapid sodium correction if hypokalemia is also present. It has been suggested that hypokalemia be treated first in this situation.

- Complications of severe hyponatremia include cerebral edema directly caused by hyponatremia and the risk of central pontine myelinolysis (a component of osmotic demyelination syndrome) from the rapid over correction of hyponatremia.

(Sterns, 2023a; Liamis et al., 2016; Mann, 2008; Sica, 2004)

Special Considerations & Monitoring with Thiazide & Thiazide-like Diuretics

Patient monitoring with thiazide and thiazide-like diuretics includes the following components:

- Fluid balance.
- BP, including orthostatic BPs.
- Renal function.

- Electrolytes: high risk for hyponatremia and hypokalemia; also, at risk for hypomagnesemia.
- Uric acid: high risk for hyperuricemia.

Key Pharmacokinetic & Pharmacodynamic Information for Thiazide & Thiazide-like Diuretics

- In patients with altered kidney function some thiazide and thiazide-like diuretics may accumulate, plasma concentrations may be increased, and the half-life may be prolonged.
- Hydrochlorothiazide is not dialyzable. Indapamide is not significantly dialyzable.

(UptoDate, Lexidrug™, 2026)

Important Medication Interactions with Thiazide & Thiazide-like Diuretics

- Thiazide and thiazide-like diuretics can enhance the risk of digoxin toxicity by producing hypokalemia and hypomagnesemia (Wang et al., 2010).
- Thiazide and thiazide-like diuretics can enhance the QT prolonging effect of medications.
- Thiazide and thiazide-like diuretics can enhance the nephrotoxic effect of NSAIDs and NSAIDs can diminish the therapeutic effect of thiazide and thiazide-like diuretics.
- Thiazide and thiazide-like diuretics can enhance the hypercalcemic effects of Vitamin D analogs.
- Corticosteroids and beta-2 agonists can enhance the hypokalemic effect of thiazide and thiazide-like diuretics.
- Bile acid sequestrants may decrease absorption and diuretic response of thiazide and thiazide-like diuretics.
- When used in combination with loop diuretics there can be a greater hypotensive effect.

(UptoDate, Lexidrug™, 2026)

Linking Knowledge to Practice

- ✓ *When used with a loop diuretic to promote diuresis the frequency of dosing depends on the patient's diuretic needs.*
  - *The patient may need metolazone every other day, 2 times a week, 1 time a week or much less frequently.*
  - *It is rare for metolazone to be used daily.*
  - *If ordered daily after discharge or as an outpatient there should be a limit to the consecutive number of days.*
- ✓ *Anytime metolazone is prescribed in the outpatient setting there needs to be close follow up monitoring of the patient's volume status, vital signs, and electrolytes.*
  - *Patients need to be instructed to report a weight loss that is too rapid when taking metolazone.*
  - *The provider should determine how much weight loss is too much and when the metolazone should be held.*
- ✓ *If a patient experiences too rapid of diuresis, the metolazone is typically held for a period of time as opposed the medication being continued at a lower dose.*
- ✓ *It is very important that patients know they <u>cannot</u> independently decide to increase the frequency of metolazone.*
  - *Patients with HF are often taught how to safely adjust their dose of loop diuretic.*
  - *However, metolazone should never be increased without permission from a provider responsible for the patient's fluid status because of the risk of adverse effects including hypovolemia and hyponatremia.*

Linking Knowledge to Practice

✓ *Remember that although loop diuretics and thiazide and thiazide-like diuretics have many similar effects, they also have some important differences regarding expected adverse effects.*
- *Loop diuretics cause a loss of calcium and a risk for hypocalcemia, while thiazides increase calcium levels and can be used in the treatment of hypocalcemia.*
- *Thiazides may be used in clinical conditions where there is a need to reduce the amount of calcium excreted in the urine.*

✓ *Both loop diuretics and thiazides cause a loss of sodium, but thiazide and thiazide-like diuretics have a higher risk of hyponatremia because loop diuretics cause a loss of water to a greater degree than a loss of salt. The loss of water is called aquaresis and the loss of sodium is called natriuresis.*
- *Hyponatremia is a common potential adverse effect of thiazide and thiazide-like diuretics.*
- *However, loop diuretics can be used in the treatment of euvolemic or hypervolemic hyponatremia.*

Advanced Concept Focus:
Salt Wasting Nephropathy

Normal Physiological Processes

- Suppression of thirst and ADH occurs anytime water is ingested or absorbed that causes even a slight hypotonic state.
- This results in the excretion of electrolyte poor water because sodium is reabsorbed without water in the water impermeable ascending loop of Henle and distal convoluted tubule.
- As a result of the above, any water load will be rapidly excreted in dilute urine.
- The maximum urine volume in normal individuals eating a regular diet is > 10 liters per day.
- The normal kidney can dilute urine to an osmolality at least as low as 100 milliosmole (mOsm)/kg and often as low as 50 mOsm/kg.
- A typical diet in the United States generates about 900 mOsm of solute daily ($^1/_2$ urea from dietary protein and $^1/_2$ sodium and potassium salts).
- Excretion of 900 mOsm of solute at a concentration of 50 mOsm/kg will result in 18 liters of electrolyte poor urine. For diets lower in salt, potassium, and protein the ability to excrete large amounts of urine will be less.
- The ability to excrete free water is relatively intact in patients with mild to moderate kidney impairment and this allows normonatremia to be maintained.
- However, there is still a great amount of protection against hyponatremia because the fluid intake in most healthy persons is < 2 to 2.5 liters per day.

(Sterns, 2023b)

Processes in Advanced Kidney Disease

- In advanced renal impairment (eGFR < 15 mL/min/1.73 m^2) the minimum urine osmolality rises to as high as 200 to 250 mOsm/kg despite the appropriate suppression of ADH.
- In advanced renal impairment the functioning nephrons produce osmotic diuresis (by increasing solute excretion), and this results in the inability to dilute the urine.
- Impairment of the free water excretion (described above) can lead to the development of hyponatremia.
- Water retention in advanced kidney disease will lower serum osmolality. However, the lowered osmolality is offset at least partially by an increase in BUN.

- Therefore, the measured serum osmolality will be normal or even increased in the setting of hyponatremia. Under normal circumstances hyponatremia is almost always hypoosmolar.

(Sterns, 2023b)

Potassium Sparing Diuretics

Mechanism of Action & Types of Potassium Sparing Diuretics

There are two groupings of potassium sparing diuretics based on their mechanism of action.

Amiloride and Triamterene

- Amiloride and triamterene block the sodium channels in the late distal convoluted tubule and the collecting duct and this inhibits sodium reabsorption back into the blood. The result is a reduction in intracellular sodium which leads to potassium retention and a decreased excretion of calcium, magnesium, and hydrogen.
- Since the sodium uptake capacity is weak in the late distal convoluted tubule and the collecting duct the effects of amiloride are considered weak in terms of natriuresis, diuresis, and antihypertensive response.

(UptoDate®, Lexidrug™, 2026)

Spironolactone and Eplerenone

- Spironolactone and eplerenone compete with aldosterone for the receptor site in the distal renal tubules. This results in maintaining potassium and hydrogen ions and increasing the excretion of sodium, chloride and water. These medications may also block the effect of aldosterone on smooth muscle.
  - Spironolactone and eplerenone are also called aldosterone antagonists (blockers) or MRAs because they are used for reasons other than their impact for diuresis. These agents have indications for mortality benefit in certain clinical conditions including HFrEF and post-MI complicated by reduced EF.
  - These medications are discussed in more detail in the above section on medications that block the RAAS.
- Another MRA is finerenone, but it does not have a clinical indication for use as a diuretic and is not discussed here. It is discussed in the above section on medications that block the RAAS.

Indications for Potassium Sparing Diuretics

The indications for potassium sparing diuretics are listed in Table 14.

Special Dosing Information for Potassium Sparing Diuretics

Amiloride

- Per the manufacturer labeling the medication should be used with caution in patients with diabetes mellitus or in patients with a serum creatinine > 1.5 mg/dL or a BUN > 30 mg/dL. Also, the medication is contraindicated in patients with anuria, acute or chronic renal insufficiency, or diabetic nephropathy.
- An alternative recommendation is to use 50% of the normal dose when the CrCl is between 10 and 50 mL/min.
- Beers Criteria recommends avoiding use in adults > 65 years of age and with a CrCl < 30 mL/min due to the risk of hyperkalemia and hyponatremia.

- The 2025 guideline for management of HTN in adults published by the ACC and the AHA recommends not using when the patient has CKD with an eGFR of < 45 mL/min/ 1.73 m^2.
- Amiloride should not be used when the CrCl clearance is < 10 mL/min.
- Use with caution with hepatic impairment. No dose adjustments are required.

(American Geriatrics Society Beers, 2023; Jones et al., 2025; UptoDate®, Lexidrug™, 2026)

Triamterene

- Per the manufacturer label there are no dose adjustments for mild to moderate renal impairment. Use is contraindicated in severe renal impairment, progressive kidney disease, or anuria.
- The 2025 guideline for management of HTN in adults published by the ACC and the AHA recommends not using when the patient has CKD with an eGFR of < 45 mL/min/ 1.73 m^2.
- The Beers Criteria recommends avoiding the use of triamterene in adults > 65 years of age with a CrCl < 30 mL/min due to the risk of hyperkalemia and hyponatremia.
- Use is contraindicated with severe hepatic impairment. There is no manufacturer recommendation for mild to moderate impairment due to lack of clinical studies in this patient population.

(American Geriatrics Society Beers, 2023; Jones et al., 2025; Lexicomp, 2023; UptoDate®, Lexidrug™, 2026)

Spironolactone

- When used for HTN, ascites due to cirrhosis, or primary aldosteronism there are no recommendations for dose adjustments based on renal function per the manufacturer label due to lack of clinical trials. The medication should be used with caution. See the above section on MRAs for dose adjustment requirements when spironolactone is being used to treat HF.
- The elimination half-life of spironolactone and its metabolites is prolonged in the setting of abnormal hepatic function. Spironolactone should be started at a low dose and titrated slowly.
- In hepatic ascites, spironolactone is typically used along with furosemide in a ratio of 100 mg of spironolactone to 40 mg of furosemide. The dose of spironolactone can be as high as 400 mg/day.

(UptoDate®, Lexidrug™, 2026)

Select Adverse Effects of Potassium Sparing Diuretics

- The primary adverse effect of potassium sparing diuretics is hyperkalemia.
- There is a US Boxed Warning for hyperkalemia for both amiloride and triamterene. Both agents can cause a potassium level of 5.5 mEq/L and thus potassium levels need to be monitored closely. The risk of hyperkalemia is up to 10% with amiloride.
- The risk for the development of hyperkalemia is greatest in patients with renal impairment, older age, and diabetes mellitus.

(UptoDate®, Lexidrug™, 2026)

Linking Knowledge to Practice

✓ *Potassium supplements should not be used in patients taking potassium sparing diuretics unless there is persistent hypokalemia while taking a potassium sparing diuretic. In this case the patient may warrant a nephrology consult to evaluate the cause of the persistent hypokalemia.*

✓ *In any patient with persistent hypokalemia, it is important to check the patient's magnesium level. Hypomagnesemia is a cause of hypokalemia.*

Table 14 Indications for Potassium Sparing Diuretics	
Medication	**Indications**
Amiloride	▪ Chronic HTN (as an alternative agent): Not recommended for initial management of HTN. Can be used as an option for resistant HTN although spironolactone is generally preferred. ▪ Ascites [off label]. ▪ Hypokalemia due to chronic stable renal potassium wasting such as with a renal tubulopathy, or chronic kaliuretic (substance that enhances potassium excretion) diuretic use [off label]. May be more effective and better tolerated than potassium supplementation.
Triamterene	▪ Edema due to HF, cirrhosis of the liver, nephrotic syndrome, secondary hypoaldosteronism, or idiopathic edema. ▪ Although indicated for HF, other diuretics are preferred in clinical management guidelines. ▪ Chronic HTN (as an alternate agent): Not recommended for initial management of HTN. ▪ There are several significant drug interactions that limit its use.
(Lexicomp, 2023; UptoDate®, Lexidrug™, 2026; Jones et al., 2025)	

Contraindication Highlights for Potassium Sparing Diuretics

- Consult manufacturer recommendations for use in children, pregnant women, and nursing women.
- Hyperkalemia (potassium > 5.5 mEq/L).
- See contraindications based on renal and hepatic function under special dosing information above.

(UptoDate®, Lexidrug™, 2026)

> ***Linking Knowledge to Practice***
>
> ✓ *When used to treat ascites in a patient with liver cirrhosis the dose of spironolactone will be substantially higher than the doses used to treat HF.*
>
> ✓ *When using spironolactone to treat ascites in a patient with liver cirrhosis, even minor alterations in fluid and electrolyte balance can trigger a hepatic coma.*

Special Considerations & Monitoring with Potassium Sparing Diuretics

- Amiloride and triamterene:
  - Potassium monitoring should be the highest after initiation and with any dose adjustment.
  - Additional monitoring should also occur during periods of acute illness.
- Spironolactone:
  - When this medication is mandatory, interventions may be needed to keep potassium at a safe level.
  - Potential interventions include a low potassium diet, concurrent use of loop diuretics, use of a GI cation exchanger such as patiromer or zirconium cyclosilicate, and sodium bicarbonate ($NaHCO_3$) to correct any metabolic acidosis.

(UptoDate®, Lexidrug™, 2026; Weinstein et al., 2021)

Key Pharmacokinetic & Pharmacodynamic Information for Potassium Sparing Diuretics

- The peak beneficial effect of triamterene may not be seen until several days after the start of therapy.
- The half-life elimination of amiloride is greatly increased when the CrCl is < 50 mL/min.
- The terminal half-life of spironolactone is increased in patients with ascites from cirrhosis.

(UptoDate®, Lexidrug™, 2026)

Important Medication Interactions with Potassium Sparing Diuretics

- Potassium sparing diuretics should not be used in combination with other potassium sparing diuretics.
- Potassium sparing diuretics enhance the hyperkalemic effect of ACEIs, ARBs, and ARNIs.
- Potassium sparing diuretics increase the hyperkalemic effect of cyclosporine and isocarboxazid and should be avoided in patients taking cyclosporine.

(UptoDate®, Lexidrug™, 2026)

> ***Linking Knowledge to Practice***
>
> ✓ *The potassium sparing diuretics spironolactone and eplerenone are also used in low doses in patients with HFrEF for the purpose of reducing mortality. In this setting, a diuretic effect is not the primary goal although spironolactone can be used in higher doses to enhance diuresis especially in the setting of right sided volume overload.*
>
> ✓ *To reduce ascites secondary to cirrhosis spironolactone is used in higher doses and it is therefore frequently given in conjunction with a loop diuretic to prevent hyperkalemia.*
>
> ✓ *In HFrEF the initial dose of spironolactone is 12.5 mg to 25 mg/day with a maximum target dose of 50 mg/day (UptoDate®, Lexidrug™, 2026). In ascites due to cirrhosis the initial dose is typically 100 mg/day titrated to the usual maximum dose of 400 mg/day (Shah, 2025; UptoDate®, Lexidrug™, 2026).*

Aquaretic Diuretics

Mechanism of Action & Types of Aquaretic Diuretics

- The vasopressin V2 receptor (also known as the AVPR2 receptor) is primarily involved in the diuretic response. The V2 receptors are in the distal tubule, connecting tubule, and collecting ducts. It's activation results in an antidiuretic effect and the release of coagulation factors. Activation of the V1 receptor (also known as the AVPR1a receptor and previously known as the V1a receptor) induces vasoconstriction. Activation of the V3 receptor (previously known as the V1b receptor) results in increased secretion of adrenocorticotropic hormone (ACTH) and increased insulin secretion.
- Vasopressin receptor antagonists block the V2 receptor and produce water excretion without affecting sodium and potassium excretion. This loss of electrolyte free water will raise the serum sodium. However, thirst increases substantially when these medications are used, and this limits the ability to raise the serum sodium level.
- Tolvaptan is an oral vasopressin receptor antagonist that blocks primarily the V2 receptor.
  - There are two oral forms of tolvaptan under the names of Jynarque and Samsca.
  - Jynarque is the form of tolvaptan used to slow the progression of disease in patients with autosomal dominant polycystic kidney disease.
  - Samsca is the form of tolvaptan used to treat hyponatremia, most commonly in HF patients.
- Conivaptan is an IV vasopressor receptor antagonist that blocks the V2 and V1 receptors.

(García-Álvarez & Arboleda-Salazar, 2023; Robben et al., 2004; UptoDate, Lexidrug™, 2026)

Indications for Aquaretic Diuretics

- Tolvaptan (as trade name Samsa) is indicated for hyponatremia in patients who are either euvolemic or hypervolemic. It is not recommended in acute hyponatremia.
  - Tolvaptan is not approved for the treatment of serious neurological symptoms and in Phase III studies an exclusion criterion was serum sodium < 120 mEq/L.
  - There are limitations to the use of tolvaptan in the setting of SIADH due to both the concern for overly rapid correction of hyponatremia and the concern for hepatotoxicity.

- ♦ Tolvaptan (as trade name Jynarque) is indicated to slow disease progression in patients with autosomal dominant polycystic kidney disease.
- ♦ Conivaptan is indicated for hyponatremia in patients who are either euvolemic or hypervolemic.
- ♦ Conivaptan is not recommended for acute hyponatremia although it can be considered in SIADH in combination with other therapies such as hypertonic saline for severe symptomatic hyponatremia; or it may be considered alone or in combination therapy in mild to moderate hyponatremia.

(Sterns, 2023c; UptoDate, Lexidrug™, 2026)

Special Dosing Information for Aquaretic Diuretics

- ♦ Tolvaptan (Samsa) must be initiated and titrated in the hospital. The medication is given in a once daily oral dose. Serum sodium must be stable prior to discharge. Use is limited to 30 days due to risk of hepatotoxicity.
- ♦ Conivaptan is an IV medication. An initial loading dose is given, followed by a continuous infusion over 24 hours, and is continued for 2 to 4 days. The total duration of therapy cannot exceed 4 days.

(UptoDate, Lexidrug™, 2026)

Select Adverse Effects of Aquaretic Diuretics

- ♦ The most common adverse effects of tolvaptan include increased thirst or polydipsia, polyuria, diarrhea, nausea, dry mouth, dizziness, and fatigue.
- ♦ The most common adverse effects of conivaptan include orthostatic hypotension, hypokalemia, reaction at the injection site, and fever.
- ♦ Tolvaptan (Samsa) and conivaptan have the potential of too rapidly over correcting sodium leading to osmotic demyelination syndrome and permanent neurological damage.
- ♦ There are safety concerns with tolvaptan.
  - In a multicenter clinical trial studying the impact of the medication on the progression of polycystic kidney disease, there was a 2.5-fold increase in liver enzymes with tolvaptan compared to placebo.
  - Liver function studies should be done immediately in any patient on tolvaptan that reports S&S of liver injury including fatigue, anorexia, right upper quadrant tenderness or pain, dark urine, or jaundice.
  - Due to safety concerns tolvaptan use is limited to a maximum of 30 days in any patient. It is not to be used at all in patients with liver disease, including cirrhosis, due to the risk of liver failure or death.

(Sterns, 2023c; UptoDate, Lexidrug™, 2026)

Contraindication Highlights for Aquaretic Diuretics

- ♦ Consult manufacturer recommendations for use in children, pregnant women, and nursing women.
- ♦ Tolvaptan and conivaptan are contraindicated in hypovolemic hyponatremia and in the setting of anuria. Conivaptan are tolvaptan are contraindicated with concurrent use of strong CYP3A4 inhibitors.
- ♦ Tolvaptan (Samsa) should not be used to treat autosomal dominant polycystic kidney disease outside of the FDA approved Risk Evaluation and Mitigation Strategy (REMS) due to the risk of liver toxicity.
- ♦ Conivaptan should be used with caution in moderate to severe hepatic impairment.
  - The dose may need to be reduced in the setting of hepatic impairment.
  - Tolvaptan may increase the risk for hepatotoxicity including toxicity that is fatal.

(Sterns, 2023c; UptoDate, Lexidrug™, 2026)

Special Considerations & Monitoring with Aquaretic Diuretics

- Tolvaptan needs to be initiated and reinitiated in the hospital.
  - The initial goal is to raise sodium by 4 to 6 mEq/L in 24 hours with a maximum rise of 8 mEq/L in 24 hours. Sodium raised by more than 12 mEq/L over 24 hours can result in permanent neurological damage from osmotic demyelination syndrome.
  - Slower rates of sodium correction should be considered in high-risk patients with hyponatremia. High risk patients include those with alcoholism, advanced liver disease, or severe malnutrition.
- The appropriate dose of tolvaptan needs to be determined while the patient is still in the hospital. Strict urine output measurement is important while in the hospital to determine the amount of water loss created by tolvaptan. Patients need to be able to replace their water loss each day to be safely discharged home.
- The following should be monitored when using tolvaptan (Samsa):
  - Serum sodium.
  - Rate of increase in serum sodium.
  - Volume status.
  - Potassium: Monitoring is important if potassium is > 5.0 mEq/L before treatment or if the patient is on medications that raise potassium. Tolvaptan may increase the risk for hyperkalemia in patients taking potassium sparing diuretics.
  - S&S of liver toxicity.
- Tolvaptan availability in the form of Jynarque is restricted under a REMS and prescribers must be registered. Tolvaptan in the form of Samsa is not restricted under REMS unless it is being used to treat autosomal dominant polycystic kidney disease.
- The following should be monitored when giving conivaptan.
  - Serum sodium and neurological status: Discontinue medication if the rate of sodium increase is too fast.
  - Vital signs and volume status: If hypotension or hypovolemia occur, they should be corrected, and the dose needs to be reduced if the indication for therapy remains.
  - Potassium: Hypokalemia is reported in the range of 10 to 22%.

(Sterns, 2023c; UptoDate, Lexidrug™, 2026)

Key Pharmacokinetic & Pharmacodynamic Information for Aquaretic Diuretics

- Tolvaptan metabolism is almost entirely via CYP3A4.
- Conivaptan undergoes hepatic metabolism via CYP3A4.
- Tolvaptan exposure may be doubled when taken with grapefruit juice and thus it should be avoided.

(UptoDate, Lexidrug™, 2026)

Important Medication Interactions with Aquaretic Diuretics

- Conivaptan is a moderate CYP3A4 inhibitor. As a result, it may increase the concentration of medications metabolized by enzyme CYP3A4 producing multiple medication interactions.
- Strong CYP3A4 inducers may decrease the serum concentration of tolvaptan and should be avoided.
- Strong CYP3A4 inhibitors may increase the serum concentration of tolvaptan and conivaptan and should be avoided.
- Tolvaptan and conivaptan may increase the serum concentration of digoxin.
- Tolvaptan can increase the hyperkalemic effects of potassium sparing diuretics.

(UptoDate, Lexidrug™, 2026)

Appendix 9 provides additional details regarding individual diuretics.

> ***Linking Knowledge to Practice***
>
> ✓ *When tolvaptan is started in the hospital it is vital for patient safety to obtain a strict I&O.*
>
> ✓ *Patients will lose electrolyte free water and there must be documentation that the patient is able to replace this free water loss with appropriate fluid intake.*
>
> ✓ *Patients should not be discharged home if there is not documentation of adequate fluid intake that covers free water loss.*
>
> ✓ *The patient cannot be on tolvaptan if there is not an adequate response to thirst.*

INTRAVENOUS FLUIDS

- Fluid in the body is found in 3 compartments: 1) intracellular, 2) interstitial, and 3) intravascular. The interstitial and the intravascular fluids combined are referred to as extracellular fluid. Most of the fluid in our bodies is located inside the cells.
- Healthy adults generally require 30 to 40 mL/kg of water each 24 hours (Ismail & Elbaih, 2020). In a 70 kg adult this translates to 2.1 to 2.8 liters per day. Fluid requirements will vary based on clinical factors such as renal and cardiac function and patient factors such as frailty.
- IV fluids are used frequently in clinical practice to restore circulating volume, treat cellular hydration, correct sodium abnormalities, and repair acid base imbalances.
- IV fluids are considered isotonic, hypotonic, or hypertonic. If a solution is hypertonic or hypotonic there will be a change in cell volume. Hypertonic solutions draw water out of cells and hypotonic solutions result in excess water entering the cells.

Principles of IV Fluid Administration

- IV fluids should be treated like all other medications. There are indications, contraindications, and adverse effects.
- The 3 indications for IV fluids include:
  - Resuscitation.
  - Replacement.
  - Maintenance.
- There are four distinct phases of fluid resuscitation in a critically ill patient:
  - Rescue: The purpose of this phase is to save the life of a patient in shock. It includes rapid boluses which typically occur over a period of minutes.
  - Optimization: This phase occurs while the patient is still unstable and aims to rescue organs and optimize tissue perfusion. This phase typically continues for hours. In this phase the patient's response to IV fluids should be carefully evaluated to minimize excess fluids that don't provide a clinical benefit.
  - Stabilization: This phase occurs in stable patients and usually lasts for days. The goal is to support organ function. IV fluids should be minimized as patients resume oral intake.
  - De-escalation: In this phase, vasoactive medications are weaned. Treatments are aimed at achieving a negative fluid balance. This phase can last for days to weeks.

  (Vincent & De Backer, 2013)
- IV fluids are only one component of resuscitation. Vasoactive medications to help increase venous return or increase cardiac contractility may also be indicated.

- Once IV fluids are ordered it is important to recognize when fluid status has been optimized and when IV fluids can or should be discontinued. It is important to evaluate end organ function in addition to intravascular volume.
- Hypervolemia is a potential complication of IV fluids and patients may require diuretics to correct the hypervolemia after IV fluids have been stopped.
- All resuscitation fluids can lead to interstitial edema. Crystalloids are commonly associated with the development of interstitial edema.
  - This is particularly true when the patient receiving the IV fluid is in an inflammatory state such as what occurs with sepsis.
  - The endothelial layer that determines membrane permeability varies among different vascular organs. Membrane integrity can be disrupted resulting in a leaky state.
  - Fluid that enters the interstitial space is returned to circulation primarily via the lymphatic system.
- It is important to carefully monitor the patient's volume status when IV fluids are being administered, especially in resuscitation because volume overload is associated with adverse effects.
  - In the PICARD study patients with AKI who had fluid overload were less likely to have recovery of their renal function. Fluid overload at the time of AKI diagnosis and at the time of initiation of RRT was associated with increased mortality at 30 and 60 days. Fluid overload in this study was defined as > 10% accumulation (Bouchard et al., 2009).
  - In patients with severe sepsis or septic shock every 1-liter increase in cumulative fluid balance 72 hours after ICU admission was associated with increased hospital mortality in all patients regardless of the presence of AKI or a history of CKD (Neyra et al., 2016).

(Myburgh & Mythen, 2013; Tinawi, 2021)

Linking Knowledge to Practice

✓ *It is important to monitor the patient receiving IV fluids for a positive cumulative fluid balance because excess volume is associated with adverse clinical effects including increased mortality.*

✓ *Always remember that nursing interventions such as accurate I&Os and daily weights are powerful tools for improving patient outcomes.*

Crystalloids

Crystalloids can be isotonic, hypotonic, or hypertonic compared to plasma. The half-life of crystalloids is 20 to 40 minutes in patients who are conscious. In the setting of dehydration or NPO status the half-life becomes longer (Tinawi, 2021).

Isotonic Crystalloids

- An isotonic solution has approximately the same concentration of salt and solute as the blood and cells in the body. As a result, isotonic fluids have a similar osmolality compared to body fluids. Normal plasma osmolality is 280-295 mOsm/L.
- Cell volume will stay constant when isotonic fluids are administered.
- Isotonic solutions are indicated when there is a need to restore intravascular volume. However, not all the volume ends up in the intravascular space.
  - It is important to know how much of each liter of IV fluid stays in the vascular space.
  - When 1 liter of an isotonic fluid such as 0.9% normal saline (NS) or lactated Ringers (LR) is given to an 80 kg lean man, approximately 250 mL will stay in the vascular space if there is no capillary leak. The other 750 mL will enter and reside in the interstitial space.

- If 1 liter 0.45% NS were to be given to the same person only 167 mL would stay in the vascular space, and if 1 liter of D5W were given only 83 mL would stay in the vascular space.

♦ In patients who are volume depleted and have a normal serum sodium, LR or 0.9% NS are usually the first-line agents to restore volume.

♦ In patients who are hypotensive due to volume depletion, an isotonic solution is given regardless of the patient's serum sodium. Once the patient is hemodynamically stable, the IV fluid can be changed to correct the serum sodium.

(Tinawi, 2021)

Linking Knowledge to Practice
✓ *Isotonic crystalloids are given for the purpose of restoring intravascular volume, yet not all the fluid given remains in the intravascular space. For example, for every 1 liter of 0.9% NS given only about 250 mL remains in the intravascular space. The other 750 mL will reside in the interstitial space.*
✓ *Intravascular pressure can increase with isotonic crystalloids and in a patient with cardiac failure this can result in pulmonary edema.*
✓ *Additionally, interstitial edema develops as a complication of crystalloid therapy. If a patient has a condition such as sepsis where the capillaries are leaky there will be an increased amount of interstitial edema.*

Table 15 compares isotonic crystalloids.

0.9% NS

♦ NS contains only water, sodium, and chloride. See Table 15 for the properties of 1 liter 0.9% NS. The pH of 0.9% NS is acidic.

♦ Normal plasma sodium is approximately 140 mEq/L. However, plasma is 93% water with the remainder consisting of lipids and protein. Normal sodium in plasma water is approximately 151 mEq/L. Each liter of 0.9% NS contains 154 mEq of sodium.

♦ There is always the potential for salt and water overload with the administration of large amounts of 0.9% NS.

♦ 0.9% NS does not contain potassium or other electrolytes. When used as a maintenance IV potassium can be added to 0.9% NS if needed. Other electrolytes such as magnesium, phosphorus, and calcium may need to be replenished.

♦ 0.9% NS has the following indications:
  - Expansion of extracellular fluid volume in the setting of hypovolemia.
  - Restoration of normal BP in the setting of hypotension.
  - Treatment of chloride sensitive metabolic alkalosis.
  - Correction of hyponatremia that is associated with hypovolemia.

♦ 0.9% NS is the only IV fluid recommended to be used with the transfusion of red blood cells (Blumberg et al., 2018; Lotterman & Sharma, 2023).

♦ However, the following is written in the manufacturer recommendations for Plasma-Lyte A (discussed below). Plasma-Lyte A is compatible with blood or blood components.
  - It may be administered prior to or following the infusion of blood through the same administration set (i.e., as a priming solution), added to or infused concurrently with blood components, or used as a diluent in the transfusion of packed erythrocytes.

- Plasma-Lyte A Injection and 0.9% Sodium Chloride Injection, USP are equally compatible with blood or blood components (Baxter, 2007).

◆ Observational studies have raised concerns about the adverse effects of large amounts of 0.9% NS during resuscitation.
  - Administration of large amounts of 0.9% NS leads to an elevated serum chloride and the patient can develop hyperchloremic metabolic acidosis. The chloride content in 0.9% NS is higher than the chloride in plasma. Normal plasma chloride is 98 to 106 mEq/L and the amount of chloride in 1 liter of 0.9% NS is 154 mEq.
    - This is a non-ion gap metabolic acidosis.
    - The acidosis is not caused by the acidic pH of normal saline, but rather 0.9% NS dilutes the normal buffer system that is found in plasma. 0.9% NS, unlike LR does not have a buffer base. Additionally, the volume expansion that occurs with 0.9% NS administration leads to a decreased reabsorption of bicarbonate in the proximal tubule.
    - Metabolic acidosis can then result in hyperkalemia because potassium shifts from the intracellular space to the extracellular space.
  - The high chloride content in 0.9% NS has also been associated with inflammation and chloride mediated renal and splanchnic vasoconstriction. A hyperchloremic state may also interfere with coagulation and T cell immune function. Adverse outcomes associated with 0.9% NS include AKI and even death (Ismail & Elbaih, 2020; Semler et al., 2018).

◆ 0.9% NS in small volumes (2 liters or less) does not have the same toxicity associated with large volume saline administration (Blumberg et al., 2018).

◆ When 0.9% NS is used for fluid resuscitation in the setting of shock the patient will often have lactic acidosis. By successfully restoring circulating volume the result can be an improvement in hemodynamics, oxygenation, and lactic acidosis.

(Myburgh & Mythen, 2013; Tinawi, 2021)

Linking Knowledge to Practice

✓ *It is possible for a patient to develop either hypokalemia or hyperkalemia because of 0.9% NS administration.*
  - *0.9% NS does not contain any electrolytes other than sodium and chloride and thus the risk for hypokalemia. This is why potassium is sometimes added to 0.9% NS maintenance IV fluid.*
  - *However, the administration of large volumes of 0.9% NS can lead to a hyperchloremic metabolic acidosis. In the setting of metabolic acidosis potassium shifts from the intracellular space to the extracellular space causing hyperkalemia.*

✓ *The chloride content in 0.9% NS is higher than plasma chloride content and patients can develop elevated serum chloride levels which produces hyperchloremic metabolic acidosis. Hyperchloremia secondary to* 0.9% NS *administration is associated with potential adverse effects including renal and immune dysfunction (Myburgh & Mythen, 2013).*

Balanced Solutions

◆ LR and Plasma-Lyte A are referred to as balanced solutions, as compared to 0.9% NS, although no IV fluid is truly physiologically balanced.

◆ Balanced solutions contain additional electrolytes other than sodium and chloride and thus they more closely mimic the electrolyte content of plasma compared to normal saline.

◆ Balanced electrolyte solutions are designed to be more physiologically normal with the goal of having fewer adverse effects on acid base balance compared to normal saline.

- Balanced solutions are considered relatively hypotonic because they contain a lower sodium concentration compared to extracellular fluid. Hypotonicity can also occur with LR because of its lower osmolarity.
- Potential adverse effects of balanced solutions include hyperkalemia and metabolic alkalosis because these solutions contain potassium and either lactate or acetate, both of which act like a base.
  - While balanced solutions do contain potassium, they also contain buffers (lactate or acetate) which may prevent potassium shifts (intracellular to extracellular) that occur in metabolic acidosis (Toporek et al., 2021). An intracellular to extracellular shift of potassium causes hyperkalemia.
  - The acid base effects of a balanced solution may be more important than the small amount of potassium within the fluid because a normal acid base balance may be more effective in preventing hyperkalemia than the small amount of potassium in the IV fluid in causing hyperkalemia (Potura et al., 2015).
    - In a secondary analysis of the SMART trial (see below) the use of balanced solutions was not associated with more severe hyperkalemia compared to saline (Toporek et al., 2021).
    - Also, in clinical studies involving patients with ESKD undergoing renal transplant, there was no significant difference in rates of hyperkalemia between balanced solutions and 0.9% NS (Potura et al., 2015).
  - LR contains sodium lactate. The liver converts sodium lactate into bicarbonate and water. It does not contain lactic acid, so it does not cause lactic acidosis.
  - LR must be used very cautiously in patients with liver failure because they may not be able to metabolize the lactate to bicarbonate.

(Myburgh & Mythen, 2013; Tinawi, 2021)

Comparison of 0.9% NS and Balanced IV Solutions

- Several research studies have tested balanced solutions against 0.9% NS and found potential benefits with the use of balanced solutions. The use of balanced solutions for fluid resuscitation, especially in patients with sepsis may prevent or reduce the risk of AKI (Tinawi, 2021).
- In an observational study of surgical patients Plasma-Lyte A was associated with lower in-hospital mortality and fewer major complications (AKI requiring RRT, postoperative infection, need for transfusion, and acidosis) compared to 0.9% NS (Shaw et al., 2012). And in another observational study there was a lower incidence of AKI and need for RRT in patients who received Plasma-Lyte A compared to 0.9% NS (Bellomo et al., 2012).
- In a systematic review and meta-analysis IV fluids with a chloride content of > 111 mEq/L were associated with statistically significant higher rates of AKI, blood transfusion rates, and longer mechanical ventilation times (Krajewski et al., 2015).
- In a single center study (SMART) of more than 15,000 patients in 5 ICUs 0.9% NS administration was compared to the administration of either LR or Plasma-Lyte A. Balanced crystalloids compared to saline had a favorable effect on the composite outcome of death, need for new RRT, or persistent renal dysfunction (Semler et al., 2018).
- In another single center study (SALT-ED), comparing 0.9% NS to balanced solutions in more than 13,000 non-critically ill patients, the number of hospital free days did not differ between patients who received 0.9% NS in the emergency department from those who received a balanced solution in the emergency department. However, the patients who received a balanced solution had fewer major adverse kidney events over the following 30-day period (Self et al., 2018).
- The BaSICS double blind randomized clinical trial enrolled more 10,000 ICU patients across 75 ICUs in Brazil and evaluated the impact of 0.9% NS versus Plasma-Lyte 148 on 90-day mortality.

The result was no significant difference in 90-day mortality between patients who received 0.9% NS and patients who received a balanced IV solution. The authors concluded that the findings do not support the use of a balanced solution (Zampieri et al., 2021).

- It is unclear if balanced solutions are harmful in patients with traumatic brain injury. Balanced solutions have a lower osmolarity compared to 0.9% NS making them relatively more hypotonic compared to saline. LR has an osmolarity of 279 mOsm/L compared to 0.9% NS which has an osmolarity of 308 mOsm/L. In an observational study, LR was associated with a higher mortality rate compared to 0.9% NS in patients with traumatic brain injury (Rowell et al., 2016). In the above BaSICS trial, there was a signal for possible harm with the use of Plasma-Lyte 148 in patients with traumatic brain injury (Zampieri et al., 2021).
- Some experts recommend the use of balanced solutions over 0.9% NS unless there is a clear indication for the use of 0.9% NS such as the presence of hyponatremia or chloride sensitive metabolic alkalosis. Other experts promote the use of 0.9% NS over LR in 1) patients with abnormal renal function and concurrent hyperkalemia, 2) patients with intracranial trauma at high risk for cerebral edema and thus the need to avoid relative hypotonicity, and 3) patients with cirrhosis who have a reduced ability to metabolize lactate (Mikhael et al., 2022).

Table 15

Isotonic Crystalloids

0.9% NS	**LR**	**Plasma-Lyte A (Plasma-Lyte 148)**
Osmolarity 308 mOsm/L	Osmolarity 279 mOsm/L	Osmolarity 295 mOsm/L
Content: Sodium 154 mEq/L Chloride 154 mEq/L <u>Note</u>: No potassium or other electrolytes.	**Content:** Sodium 130 mEq/L Chloride 109 mEq/L Potassium 4 mEq/L Calcium 2.7 mEq/L Lactate 28 mEq/L	**Content:** Sodium 140 mEq/L Chloride 98 mEq/L Potassium 5 mEq/L Acetate 27 mEq/L Gluconate 23 mEq/L

(Baxter, 2007; Baxter, 2019; Tinawi, 2021)

Linking Knowledge to Practice

- ✓ *Chloride sensitive metabolic alkalosis is one of the clinical conditions where 0.9% NS is preferred over LR.*
- ✓ *Chloride sensitive or chloride responsive alkalosis occurs when there is a loss of hydrogen ions. This occurs with gastrointestinal loss from vomiting or nasogastric suctioning. There can also be a renal loss of hydrogen ions which occurs in the setting of excess aldosterone. Aldosterone is released in the setting of dehydration. Aldosterone tells the body to hold on to salt and water. Alkalosis is resistant to chloride if it develops due to the retention of too many bicarbonate ions or if there is a shift of hydrogen ions from the extracellular space to the intracellular space. This occurs in the setting of hypokalemia.*

Advanced Concept Focus:
IV Fluids and Hyperkalemia Risk

- Historically it has been recommended to avoid LR in patients with hyperkalemia because it contains 4 mEq/L of potassium. However, 4 mEq/L of potassium is less than the serum concentration of potassium in patients who are hyperkalemic.

- In a small study testing 0.9% NS to LR in patients undergoing renal transplant there was more acidosis and hyperkalemia in the patients who received saline compared to those who received LR. In this study patients received an expected large volume of fluid in the immediate post-transplant period (Khajavi et al., 2008).
- It is important to remember that large amounts of 0.9% NS are associated with metabolic acidosis.
- Hyperkalemia can occur in the setting of metabolic acidosis because potassium shifts from the intracellular space to the extracellular space. The reason for this shift of potassium in the setting of metabolic acidosis is because the body moves hydrogen ions out of the plasma and into the cells which happens in exchange for potassium. When hyperkalemia occurs due to an intracellular to extracellular shift in the setting of acidosis the treatment is to correct the acidosis.
- Another important factor in the development of hyperkalemia is the urinary excretion of potassium.
  - Urinary excretion of potassium is directly related to the sodium delivery to the distal tubule in the kidney.
  - In patients with a high degree of sodium delivery to the distal tubule and thus strong urine output, there will be an increase in urinary potassium excretion and hyperkalemia is less likely to develop.
  - However, in a patient who is oliguric and is very dependent on sodium delivery to the distal tubule to maximize urinary potassium excretion, the administration of a relatively more hypotonic solution such as LR will result in less sodium delivery to the distal tubule and therefore less potassium excretion. This increases the risk of development of hyperkalemia.
  - Optimization of sodium delivery to the distal tubule plays an important role in maximizing potassium excretion. LR delivers less sodium to the distal tubule compared to 0.9% NS.
  - Some experts recommend 0.9% NS over LR in patients with hyperkalemia and renal impairment, especially those patients who are oliguric, to enhance sodium delivery to the distal tubule and thus promote potassium excretion.
  - Maximizing sodium delivery to the distal tubule for the purpose of optimizing potassium excretion may be more important in preventing hyperkalemia than avoiding the risk of intracellular to extracellular potassium shift than can develop from metabolic acidosis caused by 0.9% NS.

(Mikhael et al., 2022)

Linking Knowledge to Practice

✓ *The administration of both LR and Plasma-Lyte A will have an alkalizing effect because they contain substances such as lactate and acetate.*

✓ *The administration of LR to a patient with cirrhosis can result in increased levels of lactate in the blood and these increased levels can interfere with the ability to assess the effectiveness of fluid resuscitation because serum lactate levels are often used as an indicator of hypoxia.*

✓ *Elevated lactate levels can also block ATP production. ATP is important because it captures the energy from the breakdown of molecules and then serves as a major energy source for our cells.*

Hypotonic Crystalloids

- A hypotonic solution has a lower concentration of salt (solute) than the blood and cells in the body.
- A hypotonic solution can also be seen as a solution with excess free water compared to what is in the blood and cells in the body.
  - As a result, when given to a patient with a normal serum sodium, water in the solution will move into the cells by osmosis and cell volume will increase.
  - 0.45% NS and dextrose in water are examples of hypotonic solutions. One liter of 0.45% NS is the equivalent of adding 500 mL of free water to 500 mL of 0.9% NS.

- See Table 16 for comparison of 0.45% NS and D5W.

♦ Hypotonic solutions are used to treat hypernatremia because these solutions contain free water.
  - In hypernatremia there is excess sodium in relation to water within the extracellular space.
  - Thus, when a hypotonic solution is added the result is a dilutional effect in the extracellular space and a lower serum sodium.

♦ In hemodynamically stable patients who are volume depleted and have hypernatremia a hypotonic solution such 0.45% NS is used to treat the volume deficit and correct the hypernatremia.

♦ However, if a patient is both hypernatremic and hypotensive from volume depletion the priority is to give isotonic fluids to restore circulating volume.
  - Giving 0.9% NS to a patient who is hypernatremic will have some impact on lowering serum sodium because the 0.9% NS is more dilute compared to hypernatremic extracellular space.
  - However, once the patient is hemodynamically stable, the patient can receive a hypotonic solution such as 0.45% NS which will more efficiently treat hyponatremia.

♦ Hypotonic solutions are not used initially in patients who need fluid resuscitation. However, after successful resuscitation they can be used if indicated in the optimization and stabilization phases.

♦ When administering dextrose in water solutions such as D5W it is important to know that the solution acts as a hypotonic solution although it has an osmolarity of 278 mOsm/L which is like the osmolarity of LR. See the Advanced Concept Focus section below on osmolarity versus tonicity.
  - All solutions containing any amount of dextrose in water act as hypotonic solutions regardless of the osmolarity inside the IV bag. This is because once administered the dextrose is taken up intracellularly by insulin leaving only free water behind.
  - D5W is used to correct hypernatremia or hypoglycemia.
  - D5W provides 170kcal/L. D10W is used for more severe hypoglycemia.
  - While D5W is used as a treatment for hypernatremia it frequently causes hyponatremia in hospitalized patients when given to patients with normal or low normal sodium levels at baseline.

(Tinawi, 2021)

Linking Knowledge to Practice

✓ *Hypotonic IV solutions cause water to enter cells. This can have the therapeutic effect of correcting cellular dehydration.*

✓ *However, if too much fluid enters the cells this results in cellular swelling that can be harmful.*
  - *If too much water enters brain cells they can swell and cause cerebral edema.*
  - *If too much water enters red blood cells they can rupture resulting in hemolysis.*

✓ *When D5W is used as an IV fluid remember that the dextrose is rapidly metabolized leaving only free water behind.*

✓ *Sodium levels should be monitored in all patients receiving D5W.*

✓ *D5W may be used in the treatment of hypernatremia. However, D5W may also be used for calories in patients who are NP0.*

✓ *When D5W is given in patients with a normal or low normal serum sodium level the D5W can cause hyponatremia. It is important to remember that hyponatremia is not benign.*

Hypertonic Crystalloids

♦ A hypertonic solution has a higher concentration of salt (solute) than the blood and cells in the body.

♦ Water will leave cells and enter the extracellular space when a hypertonic solution is administered.

♦ 3% NS is an example of a hypertonic solution. See Table 16.

- 3% saline is used to treat moderate to severe hyponatremia.
- Hyponatremia can cause cerebral edema and neurological symptoms.
- 3% NS is indicated in patients with acute hyponatremia who have any symptoms.
- The goal in acute symptomatic hyponatremia is to correct the serum sodium by 4 to 6 mEq/L over a few hours to prevent brain herniation and then maintain the level over the next 24 hours.
- 3% NS is also used to treat chronic hyponatremia in patients with severe symptoms or in patients with known intracranial pathology.
- The goal in chronic hyponatremia is to correct the serum sodium by 4 to 6 mEq/L over a few hours while not raising the sodium by more than 10 mEq/L in 24 hours.
- Osmotic demyelinating syndrome is a potential complication of the administration of hypertonic saline if the sodium is corrected too quickly.

(Sterns, 2024; UptoDate®,Lexidrug™, 2026)

◆ 23.4% NS (30 to 60 mL) can be given over 10 minutes to temporarily reverse impending cerebral herniation.

- The rapid administration of 23.4% NS can cause transient hypotension. While the administration of the hypertonic saline increases preload, the hypertonicity relaxes vascular smooth muscle and causes vasodilation of the arterioles with a decrease in SV (Strandvik, 2009).
- In one small study on the safety and tolerability of 23.4% NS 13% of the patients had a drop in systolic BP of at least 20 mmHg and 16% of the patients experienced a BP of < 90 mmHg (O'Brien et al., 2023).

Table 16

Hypotonic and Hypertonic Crystalloids

Hypotonic Crystalloids		Hypertonic Crystalloids
0.45% NS	**D5W**	**3% NS**
Osmolarity 154 mOsm/L	Osmolarity 278 mOsm/L	Osmolarity 1026 mOsm/L
Content: Sodium 77 mEq/L Chloride 77 mEq/L Note: No potassium or other electrolytes.	**Content:** Glucose 50g (50 mg/mL) Note: No potassium or other electrolytes.	**Content:** Sodium 513 mEq/L Chloride 513 mEq/L

Note: Tonicity is not the same as osmolarity. 0.45% NS and D5W have very different osmolarities, however, they are both hypotonic. See Advanced Concept Focus section below on osmolarity versus tonicity.
(Tinawi, 2021)

Linking Knowledge to Practice

✓ *When a patient has either hypernatremia or hyponatremia, 0.9% NS will assist in improving either disorder.*
  - *This is because the 0.9% NS is isotonic and will mix with circulating volume that is either too concentrated or too dilute.*
  - *When the 0.9% NS is added, it will help create a normal or a more normal salt to water ratio.*

✓ *However, hypotonic solutions will treat hypernatremia more efficiently and hypertonic solutions will treat hyponatremia more efficiently.*

✓ *The decision on how to treat hypernatremia or hyponatremia is based on the severity of the disorder and whether the sodium imbalance is acute or chronic.*

Sodium Bicarbonate in IV Fluids

Composition of IV Fluids Containing Sodium Bicarbonate

- $NaHCO_3$ can be added to 1 liter 0.45% NS or D5W for use in patients with metabolic acidosis.
- $NaHCO_3$ is not added to 0.9% NS solution because the total sodium content in 1 liter would be too high making the solution hypertonic.
- 150 mEq of $NaHCO_3$ in 1 liter of D5W is essentially the equivalent of 0.9% NS in terms of sodium content. The difference is that bicarb replaces chloride as the anion. However, 150 mEq of $NaHCO_3$ is typically more bicarbonate than needed for maintenance IV fluid.
- When $NaHCO_3$ is added to 1 liter of 0.45% NS the total sodium content is determined by a combination of the sodium in $NaHCO_3$ and the sodium in 0.45% NS.
  - For example, if 75 mEq of $NaHCO_3$ is added to 1 liter 0.45% NS the total sodium content will be 150 mEq because 1 liter of 0.45% NS contains approximately 75 mEq of sodium.
  - The total sodium content of 150 mEq/L makes this solution isotonic. Remember, this sodium content is like the 154 mEq/L of 0.9% NS.
  - However, when $NaHCO_3$ is added to 0.45% NS only half the anion is chloride while the other half is bicarb. With NS all the anions are chloride.
- When $NaHCO_3$ is added to 0.45% NS it will help correct metabolic acidosis even though the patient is still receiving some chloride. The excess bicarbonate dilutes the impact of serum chloride.
- If more than 75 mEq $NaHCO_3$ were added to 1 liter 0.45% NS the sodium content would be higher making it a hypertonic solution. Less than 75 mEq $NaHCO_3$ can be added to 1 liter 0.45% NS if a hypotonic solution is indicated.

Physiologic Effect of Sodium Bicarbonate

- Despite the known adverse effects of metabolic acidosis including impaired cardiac contractility, reduced response to catecholamines, reduced uptake of lactate by the liver, and increased mortality, most studies have shown that treating metabolic acidosis with $NaHCO_3$ does not improve clinical outcomes.
  - It is thought that bicarbonate solutions do not improve clinical outcomes in the setting of metabolic acidosis because the buffering process increases the production and retention of CO_2.
    - This adverse effect occurs more often in patients with inadequate alveolar ventilation and in those with circulatory failure.
    - These conditions promote the accumulation of CO_2 in the tissues, and this facilitates the development of intracellular acidosis.
  - Hypocalcemia, including a reduction in ionized calcium is another adverse effect seen with $NaHCO_3$.

  (Kraut & Madias, 2019)
- However, in one study of patients with severe metabolic acidemia, although $NaHCO_3$ had no effect on the primary composite outcome of death from any cause by day 28 and the presence any organ failure at day 7, $NaHCO_3$ did decrease the primary composite outcome and decreased 28-day mortality in the predefined subgroup of patients with AKI.
  - In this study 4.2% $NaHCO_3$ was used.
  - The results of this study show that there may be a role for the use of $NaHCO_3$ in patients with lactic acidosis from sepsis or shock who also have AKI.

  (Jaber et al., 2018; Kraut & Madias, 2019; Senewiratne et al., 2024; Tinawi, 2021)
- Bicarbonate containing solutions can be used to replace bicarbonate in patients with low levels.
  - Low levels of bicarbonate can occur in the setting of AKI which is a bicarbonate losing state.

- Bicarbonate containing solutions should only be ordered by providers with specialized knowledge regarding the management of acid base imbalances.

Prescribing Pearls for IV Fluids

- When choosing an IV fluid you must consider the patient's serum sodium level, potassium level, and acid base status.
- It is important to monitor body weight and cumulative fluid balance in a patient who is receiving IV fluids or has recently received IV fluids. The cumulative dose of resuscitation and maintenance IV fluids is associated with the development of interstitial edema which is considered pathologic and results in organ dysfunction. There is an association between a positive fluid balance and adverse outcomes in patients with sepsis.
- Oliguria is a normal response to hypovolemia. However, it should not be used as the only trigger or end point for determining the need for continued IV fluids. Multiple parameters should be considered together when evaluating for the presence of volume depletion or the patient's response to fluid resuscitation.
- A balanced IV solution is indicated in most patients requiring a large volume of IV fluids. 0.9% NS should be considered in patients who have hypovolemia and alkalosis. 0.9% NS should also be used in patients who have hypotension and hyponatremia.
- Albumin can be considered in early resuscitation in patients with severe sepsis. Albumin should never be used in a patient with traumatic brain injury.

(Myburgh & Mythen 2013)

Colloids

- Colloids contain large molecules which increase the plasma oncotic (pulling) pressure. The molecular weight of the molecules in colloids will not allow the molecules to cross a healthy semi-permeable capillary membrane. Colloids will remain in the intravascular space unless there is a break in the capillary barrier that holds fluid in the vascular space. This break in the capillary barrier can occur in severe critical illness.
- Colloids are typically hypertonic solutions except for 5% albumin which is approximately isotonic compared to human plasma (Octapharma, 2006).
- There are different types of colloids including human albumin solutions, semisynthetic colloids such as hydroxyethyl starch (HES or hetastarch), dextran, and gelatins. Gelatin based colloids are currently not available in the United States.
- Colloids are more expensive than crystalloids.
- When using colloids in resuscitation less volume is required compared to crystalloids.
  - However, despite the potential perceived benefit of using colloids instead of crystalloids, colloids have not been proven to be superior to crystalloids in treating critically ill patients (Myburgh & Mythen, 2013; Tinawi, 2021).
  - In the CRISTAL study a variety of colloids were tested against crystalloids including isotonic LR and 0.9% NS as well as hypertonic saline.
    - In ICU patients with hypovolemia there was no significant difference in 28-day mortality between those treated with crystalloids and those treated with colloids.
    - At 90 days there was a lower mortality in those treated with colloids, however, it was concluded that more research is needed to confirm this benefit (Annane et al., 2013).

(Ismail & Elbaih, 2020)

Albumin

- Albumin solutions are the most used colloids. Albumin increases the oncotic pressure in the plasma. Each 1 g of albumin attracts 18 mL of water.
- A 100 mL vial of 25% albumin will expand intravascular volume by about 450 mL which is the equivalent of about 1.8 liters of 0.9% NS or LR.
- 12.5 to 25 g (250 or 500 mL) of 5% albumin is given over 30 minutes.
- 25 g (100 mL) of 25% albumin is given over 2 hours.
- Albumin ½ life is approximately 16 to 24 hours.
- It is important to monitor for an allergic reaction when giving albumin.

(Tinawi, 2021)

- Albumin is commonly available as 5% or 25% solutions.
  - 5% solutions are available in 50 mL, 100 mL 250 ml or 500 mL.
    - A 5% 50 mL solution contains 2.5 g of albumin.
    - A 5% 100 mL solution contains 5 g of albumin.
    - A 5% 250 mL solution contains 12.5 g of albumin.
    - A 5% 500 mL solution contains 25 g of albumin.
  - 25% solutions are available in 20 mL, 50 mL or 100 mL.
    - A 25% 20 mL solution contains 5 g of albumin.
    - A 25% 50 mL solution contains 12.5 g of albumin.
    - A 25% 100 mL solution contains 25 g of albumin.

(UptoDate, Lexidrug™, 2024)

- The SAFE study (Saline versus Albumin Fluid Evaluation) included almost 7,000 critically ill patients in medical and surgical ICUs and demonstrated the safety of albumin in critically ill patients but also showed no difference in the rate of death or development of new organ failure between isotonic saline and 4% albumin.
  - The SAFE study did show a potential benefit in the use of albumin in patients with severe sepsis. In a predetermined subgroup analysis of patients with severe sepsis, albumin demonstrated a lower adjusted risk of death compared to 0.9% NS.
  - The SAFE study also showed that resuscitation with albumin was associated with an increase in the rate of death at 2 years in patients who had traumatic brain injury, likely due to increased intracranial pressure

(SAFE Study Investigators, 2004)

- In the ALBIOS trial that studied patients with severe sepsis, albumin replacement in addition to crystalloids, as compared with crystalloids alone, was not associated with improved survival at either 28 or 90 days despite improvement in some hemodynamic variables. These results did not confirm the results of the subgroup analysis in the SAFE study above. However, there were differences in the amount and concentration of albumin used between the 2 studies. In the ALBIOS trial a post-hoc analysis did show benefit in the subgroup of patients who had septic shock (Caironi, et al., 2014).
- A meta-analysis of 55 research studies involving critically ill patients showed no beneficial effect of albumin on mortality compared to crystalloids (Wilkes & Navickis, 2001).
- Due to its anti-inflammatory effects, albumin is recommended for use in patients with hepatorenal syndrome, patients who are status post large volume paracentesis, and patients with spontaneous bacterial peritonitis (Tinawi, 2021).
- Unfortunately, in a randomized clinical trial, albumin was not effective in increasing serum albumin to 3 g/dL in patients with decompensated liver cirrhosis (China at al., 2021).

- Some observational studies raised concern about an increased risk of AKI with the use of hypertonic albumin. However, a meta-analysis of ten studies in patients with sepsis showed no increased need for RRT in patients receiving albumin compared to those receiving crystalloids only (Rochwerg et al., 2015).
- Albumin is commonly used for the prevention and treatment of hypotension associated with dialysis (Tinawi, 2021).

HES (Hydroxyethyl Starch)

- HES is a synthetic colloid that can successfully expand intravascular volume. It has a long half-life of 50 hours.
- HES has been associated with adverse events in several clinical trials.
    - In one randomized trial comparing HES to LR in patients with severe sepsis, HES was associated with higher risk for AKI and RRT compared to LR (Brunkhorst et al., 2008).
    - In another trial of 7000 ICU patients, HES was compared to 0.9% NS. There was no difference in mortality at 90 days. However, the incidence of AKI and need for RRT was higher in the patients who were treated with HES compared to those treated with 0.9% NS. HES was also associated with overall more adverse events compared to normal saline. The most common adverse effects were rash and pruritis (Myburgh et al., 2012).
    - In the FLASH randomized trial patients undergoing major abdominal surgery were randomized to receive either HES or 0.9% NS at the time of surgery and for up to 24 hours postoperatively. Patients who received HES had a significantly higher rate of AKI (Futier et al., 2020).
    - In a meta-analysis of 38 trials, HES, when used for acute volume resuscitation in critically ill patients, was associated with an increased risk of AKI and mortality compared to other fluids (Zarychanski et al., 2013).
- The FDA has warned against the use of HES in critically ill patients due to the increased risk of AKI and death (FDA, 2013, June 24). The FDA has also warned about excess bleeding, increased AKI with need for RRT, and increased mortality in surgical patients treated with HES; as well as increased AKI and morality in blunt trauma patients who received HES (FDA, 2021, July 7).
- HES is also associated with anaphylactic reactions (Tinawi, 2021).
- HES solutions have the potential to accumulate in the tissues and therefore there is a recommended maximum dose of 33 to 50 mL/kg/day (Myburgh & Mythen, 2013).

Dextran 40

- Dextran 40, a linear glucose polysaccharide, is considered an artificial colloid and is classified as a volume expander.
- Dextran 40 is a preparation of low molecular weight dextran in either D5W or 0.9% NS. Dextran 40 is also described as low viscous or low viscosity dextran.
- In addition to the indication for volume expansion in shock, Dextran can also be used to prime a cardiopulmonary bypass circuit.
- Several hemodynamic parameters are impacted by Dextran 40. When used in the treatment of shock it increases blood volume with a subsequent increase in CVP, CO, SV, BP and urinary output.
- Dextran 40 enhances blood flow specifically in microcirculation because the primary effect of Dextran 40 is volume expansion resulting in hemodilution. Other effects of Dextran 40 include coating red blood cells and platelets and decreasing the viscosity of blood. All the effects of Dextran work together to enhance blood flow. Dextran 40 also improves peripheral blood flow with the release of sequestered blood cells and as a result there is a subsequent increase in venous return.

(Hospira, 2018a; UptoDate, Lexidrug™, 2024)

Table 17 compares common colloidal solutions.

Table 17

Colloids

Albumin 5%	Albumin 25%	HES 6%	Dextran 40
Osmolarity 308 mOsm/L	Osmolarity 308 mOsm/L	Osmolarity 310 mOsm/L	Osmolarity 255 mOsm/L (if in D5W); or 310 mOsm/L if in 0.9% NS
Content: Sodium 154 mEq/L Chloride 154 mEq/L Albumin 50 g/L	**Content:** Sodium 154 mEq/L Chloride 154 mEq/L Albumin 250 g/L	**Content:** Sodium 154 mEq/L Chloride 154 mEq/L HES 60 g/L	**Content:** 10 g dextran 40 and 5 g dextrose hydrous in water per 100 mL OR 10 g dextran 40 and 0.9 g sodium chloride per 100 mL = Sodium 154 mEq/L Chloride 154 mEq/L
(Hospira, 2018a; Tinawi, 2021; UptoDate, Lexidrug™, 2024)			

Linking Knowledge to Practice

✓ *Colloids should normally remain in the vascular space more readily than crystalloids because of their oncotic pressure.*

✓ *Conditions like sepsis can cause capillaries to become leaky and if this occurs colloids can leak into the interstitial space. This is called 3rd spacing.*

✓ *3rd spacing will worsen interstitial edema.*

Advanced Concept Focus:
Osmolarity versus Tonicity

◆ Hyperosmotic, normal osmotic, and hypoosmotic are not the same as hypertonic, isotonic, and hypotonic.

◆ Osmolality is the number of solute particles per kilogram of solvent, and osmolarity is the number of solute particles per liter of solvent. Osmolality and osmolarity are assessments of the solution and can be measured by an osmometer. Often these terms are used interchangeably.

◆ Tonicity describes the behavior of the solution in terms of what it will do to the cell's volume when exposed to the solution. Will cell volume remain constant, or will water leave or enter the cells?

◆ An isotonic solution has the same concentration of salt (solute) as the blood and cells in the body.
- A hypotonic solution has a lower concentration of salt than the blood and cells in the body.
- A hypertonic solution has a higher concentration of salt than the blood and cells in the body.

◆ An isotonic solution will keep the cell volume constant.
- A hypotonic solution will cause water to enter the cells and results in cellular swelling.
- A hypertonic solution will cause water to leave the cells and results in cellular dehydration.

◆ Important point:
Hypoosmolar solutions are always hypotonic. But normal osmolar solutions are not always isotonic, and hyper osmolar solutions are not always hypertonic.

- For example: D5W and 0.9% NS have similar measured osmolarities when they are in IV bags. However, they have different effects on the volume of cells.
- Any solution of pure glucose will be hypotonic regardless of the osmolarity.
- For example, if a patient receives a hyperosmolar yet hypotonic IV solution of D10W, initially water will leave the cell via osmosis because the solution is hyperosmolar.
  - Water always crosses cell membranes before solutes cross cell membranes.
  - However, after glucose is transported into the cell water will follow via osmosis so the net result is water entering into the cell. The cell will have a net increase in water and thus the solution is considered hypotonic.

(Silverthorn, 2016)

VASOACTIVE DRUGS OVERVIEW

- The term "vasoactive" technically refers to drugs that affect (constrict or dilate) blood vessels; however, clinically the term is expanded to incorporate drugs that affect myocardial function as well as blood vessel vasodilation or vasoconstriction.
- In this book, the term vasoactive is used to include drugs that increase myocardial contractility or cause peripheral vasoconstriction or vasodilation.
- Vasoactive drugs are used to improve overall CV performance to achieve hemodynamic stability in patients with HF or shock states.
- Vasoactive drugs include positive inotropes that increase myocardial contractility, vasodilators that cause peripheral arterial or venous vasodilation or both, pulmonary arterial specific vasodilators, and vasoconstrictors that cause peripheral arterial or venous vasoconstriction or both.
- Several drugs have more than one effect on the CV system and some medications have different effects at different doses. For these reasons, nurses must understand the effect of each individual medication at the dose the patient is receiving.

Inotropes

Inotropes increase myocardial contractility by a variety of mechanisms.

- Dobutamine is a sympathomimetic drug that stimulates SNS receptors, most importantly $\beta1$ receptors.
- Milrinone is a PDE-3 inhibitor in both cardiac and vascular tissue that results in increased contractility and vasodilation.
- Digoxin increases contractility by one of its mechanisms resulting in calcium influx via the sodium-calcium exchange pump. The calcium influx leads to increased contractility.

Vasopressors

Vasopressors cause constriction of peripheral arteries and increase SVR and afterload.

- Norepinephrine, epinephrine (high dose), dopamine (high dose), and phenylephrine are vasopressors that stimulate $\alpha1$ receptors in peripheral blood vessels to cause arterial vasoconstriction.
  - Dopamine and epinephrine depending on the dose can also be used for an inotropic effect because of their $\beta1$stimulation.
  - Norepinephrine is not used as an inotrope but there will be some $\beta1$ stimulation when it is used as a vasopressor although $\alpha1$ stimulation is greater than $\beta1$ stimulation.
  - Phenylephrine has virtually no $\beta1$ stimulation.

- Vasopressin, also known as arginine vasopressin, is a vasopressor used only in refractory shock and its mechanism of vasoconstriction is through the activation of V1a receptors.

Vasodilators

Vasodilators are drugs that dilate blood vessels, either veins, arteries, or both. Venous vasodilation reduces preload; arterial vasodilation reduces afterload. Many drugs can cause vasodilation:

- ACEIs and ARBs are vasodilators that reduce both preload and afterload by inhibition of the RAAS.
- CCBs (especially the dihydropyridines) inhibit calcium entry into the muscle layer of arterial blood vessels and result in arterial vasodilation and afterload reduction.
- Drugs that block postsynaptic α_1 receptors in peripheral arteries result in arterial vasodilation. Examples: prazosin, terazosin, and doxazosin.
- Drugs that stimulate central or pre-synaptic α_2 receptors cause peripheral vasodilation. Examples: clonidine, guanfacine, and methyldopa.
- Drugs that directly dilate peripheral arteries (the mechanism of this action is not well understood) include hydralazine and minoxidil.
- Drugs that increase nitric oxide in vascular tissue cause vasodilation. IV NTG, a nitrate, is used predominantly as a venous vasodilator, although at higher doses it dilates both veins and arteries. Nitroprusside is a more balanced dilator, however with more arterial than venous effect.
- The PDE-3 inhibitor, milrinone, causes peripheral arterial and venous vasodilation as well as increased myocardial contractility.

SYMPATHOMIMETIC VASOACTIVE DRUGS

Sympathomimetics mimic the actions of the SNS and exert their therapeutic effects by stimulating one or more of the following receptors: α1, β1, β2, or dopaminergic receptors. See Table 18 for a comparison of receptor affinity for sympathomimetic vasoactive medications.

- When stimulated, β1receptors located in the heart will increase sinus node firing, conduction through the AV node, and ventricular muscle firing resulting in an increase in HR (chronotropic response) and increase in contractility (inotropic response).
- Beta-1 receptors are also located in the kidney and in fat cells.
  - When β1 receptors in the kidney are stimulated renin is released and the RAAS system is activated.
  - When β1 receptors are stimulated in fat cells there is an increase in the breakdown of fats and other lipids to release fatty acids.

  (Alhayek & Preuss, 2023)
- $Beta_2$ receptors are predominantly located in the smooth muscle of the airways.
  - They are also located in cardiac, uterine and skeletal muscles and exist in various types of cells.
  - When stimulated the clinical effect includes bronchodilation and peripheral vasodilation.

  (Abosamak & Shahin, 2023)
- $Alpha_1$ receptors are in the vascular smooth muscle and affect the tone of the small arterioles responsible for determining SVR.
  - When α1 receptors are stimulated there is ultimately an increase in intracellular calcium that results in the contraction of smooth muscle, peripheral vasoconstriction, and an increase in SVR.
  - $Alpha_1$ receptors are also found in myocardial tissue so stimulation will also produce some inotropic effect.

  (Dean & Reddivari, 2023)

- ♦ $Alpha_1$ and β2 stimulation oppose each other in the periphery and have opposite impact on SVR. The net result of SNS stimulation on α and β receptors depends on the degree to which each receptor is stimulated.
- ♦ The renal, mesenteric, and coronary blood vessels also contain dopaminergic receptors.
  - $Dopaminergic_1$ receptors (D1) receptors are in coronary, cerebral, renal, and mesenteric beds while $Dopaminergic_2$ (D2) receptors are in renal tissues and the vasculature.
  - Stimulation of dopaminergic receptors results in vasodilation and increased blood flow to these tissues.

  (Overgaard & Dzavík, 2008)
- ♦ Commercially prepared solutions of vasoactive medications (epinephrine, dobutamine, dopamine, norepinephrine and phenylephrine) contain sodium metabisulfite which can cause allergic type reactions including anaphylaxis and can trigger life-threatening asthmatic episodes in patients with asthma.

> ***Linking Knowledge to Practice***
>
> ✓ *Each sympathomimetic medication will have unique effects based on the receptors stimulated and the degree of stimulation of each receptor.*
>
> ✓ *Example 1: Dobutamine is a medication that predominantly stimulates β1 receptors and this results in dobutamine being a potent inotrope.*
> - *However, dobutamine also stimulates α1 and β2 receptors but does not stimulate these receptors equally.*
> - *There is more β2 stimulation than α1 stimulation that results in modest vasodilation.*
>
> ✓ *Example 2: Phenylephrine strictly stimulates α1 resulting in only vasopressor effects.*

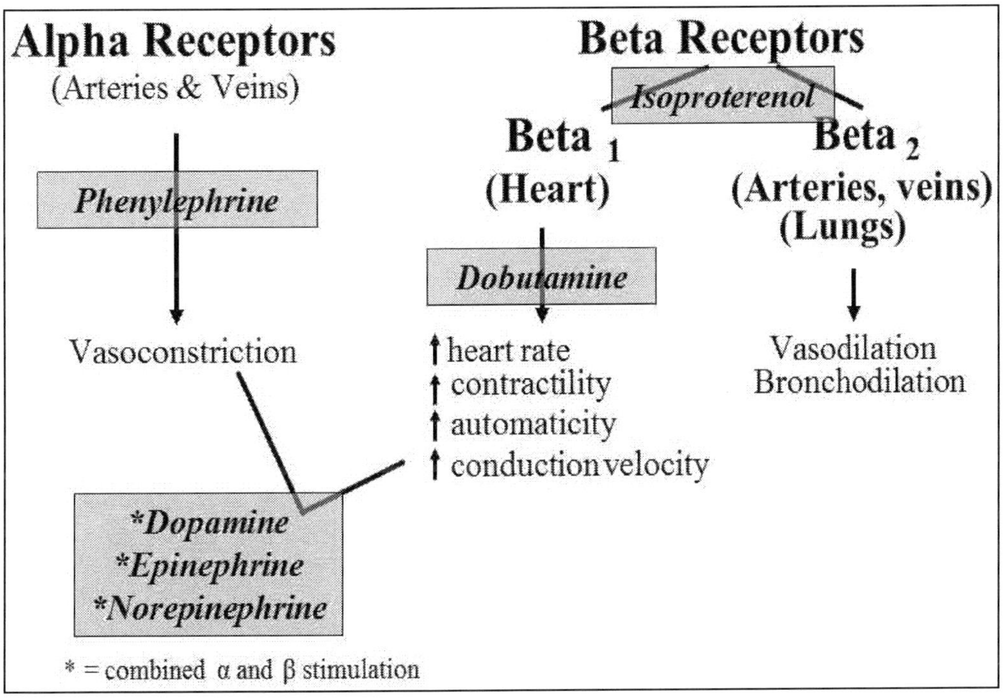

Figure 9: Sympathomimetic Drugs

Figure 9 illustrates where these drugs work in relation to the SNS.

Appendix 10 provides additional details regarding individual sympathomimetics.

Table 18

Comparison of Sympathomimetic Medications and Receptor Stimulation

	β1	β2	α1	Dopaminergic
Isoproterenol	Nonselective beta agonist with maximal affinity for β1 and β2 receptors.		Zero	N/A
Epinephrine	At lower doses great affinity for β1 and β2 receptors. Slightly greater affinity for β1 receptors (++++) compared to β2 receptors (+++).		At higher doses maximal affinity (+++++) for α1 receptors.	N/A
Dobutamine	Predominant β1 stimulator with maximal affinity for β1receptors.	β2 affinity (+++) > α1 affinity (+) = modest vasodilation.	α1affinity (+) < β2 affinity (+++) therefore no vasoconstriction.	N/A
Dopamine	A moderate doses β1 affinity (++++) > β2 affinity (++).		At high doses affinity for α1recptors (+++).	Maximal affinity (+++++) at low doses.
Norepinephrine	Less β1(+++) compared to Dopamine β1 affinity (+++) > β2 affinity (++).		Maximal affinity (+++++) for α1 receptors.	N/A
Phenylephrine	Zero	Zero	Maximal affinity (+++++) for α1 receptors.	N/A

(Overgaard & Dzavík, 2008)

Isoproterenol

Mechanism of Action of Isoproterenol

- Isoproterenol stimulates both β1and β2 receptors.
  - Beta-1 stimulation results in a powerful increase in HR and contractility.
  - Beta-2 stimulation results in potent peripheral vasodilation and mild pulmonary vasodilation.
- The stimulation of β1 receptors leads to an increase in SV.
- However, the simultaneous reduction in SVR from β2 stimulation leads to an overall neutral effect on CO.
- There is also relaxation of the bronchial, gastrointestinal, and uterine smooth muscle.
- Isoproterenol has very little affinity for α1 receptors.

(Overgaard & Dzavík, 2008; UptoDate®, Lexidrug™, 2024)

Indications for Isoproterenol

- Symptomatic bradycardia or AV block that is unresponsive to atropine.
- Cardiogenic shock caused by bradycardia [off label].
- Torsade de pointes: to reduce recurrence [off label].
- Tilt table testing: to diagnose syncope [off label].

(UptoDate®, Lexidrug™, 2024)

Special Dosing Information for Isoproterenol

- There are no manufacturer recommendations for dose adjustment in the setting of renal or hepatic dysfunction.
- When using isoproterenol to treat bradycardia the dose range is 1 to 2 mcg/min. The medication should be started at a low dose and titrated to achieve an increase in HR.

(UptoDate®, Lexidrug™, 2024)

Select Adverse Effects of Isoproterenol

- Coronary vasospasm has been reported as a potential complication when isoproterenol is used during title table testing or cardiac ablation (Duong et al., 2020; Okuya et al., 2021).
- Unexpected adverse effects have also occurred including AV block and a vasovagal response with the patient in a supine position (Barold et al., 2015; Suwa et al., 2004).
- Isoproterenol may cause Adams-Stokes syndrome (also referred to as cardiac syncope) which is a drop in CO that leads to a brief loss of consciousness.

(UptoDate®, Lexidrug™, 2024)

- See Table 19 for additional potential adverse effects of sympathomimetic medications.

Contraindication Highlights for Isoproterenol

- Consult manufacturer recommendations for use in children, pregnant women, and nursing women.
- Isoproterenol is contraindicated in conditions where β1 stimulation would aggravate the patient's baseline clinical status. These conditions include angina, tachycardia, and history of ventricular arrhythmias.
- Isoproterenol is also contraindicated in the setting of digoxin toxicity because it will exacerbate arrhythmias caused by the increased digoxin level.
- Isoproterenol should not be used in any type of vasodilatory shock because SVR can be further reduced through β2 stimulation.

(UptoDate®, Lexidrug™, 2024)

Special Considerations & Monitoring with Isoproterenol

- Isoproterenol, like epinephrine but to a lesser degree, can cause hyperglycemia (Hospira Inc., 2018b). Monitor blood glucose levels carefully especially in patients with DMT1 due to reported cases of DKA (Hoff & Koh 2018).
- See Table 20 for recommended monitoring in patients receiving sympathomimetic vasoactive medications.

Key Pharmacokinetic & Pharmacodynamic Information for Isoproterenol

- The onset of action is immediate, and the duration is 10 to 15 minutes when given IV.
- Half-life elimination is 2.5 to 5 minutes

(UptoDate®, Lexidrug™, 2024)

Important Medication Interactions with Isoproterenol

Epinephrine and isoproterenol are structurally related and therefore should not be used in combination with each other (Hospira Inc, 2018b; UptoDate®, Lexidrug™, 2024).

> ***Linking Knowledge to Practice***
>
> ✓ *All medications that stimulate β1 receptors will increase HR. Doses of isoproterenol that result in a HR of more than 130 may increase the risk of ventricular arrhythmias.*
>
> *(Hospira Inc., 2018b)*

Dobutamine

Mechanism of Action of Dobutamine

- Dobutamine is a synthetic catecholamine that has a strong affinity for both β1 and β2 receptors but binds them at a 3:1 ratio favoring β1.
- As a predominant β1stimulator, dobutamine increases contractility which results in a decrease in LV preload. SV is usually increased with dobutamine. β1 stimulation also results in increased HR, automaticity, and conduction velocity yet the inotropic effect is greater than the chronotropic effect.
- Dobutamine also stimulates α1 receptors but β2 stimulation is greater than α1 stimulation resulting in mild vasodilation. The modest vasodilation results in some reduction of LV afterload particularly at doses < 5mcg/kg/min.
- At higher doses there is not a substantial effect on SVR because β2 vasodilation is counterbalanced by α1 vasoconstriction. The higher the dose the more dominant the α1 vasoconstrictive effects. Dobutamine has little effect on PVR.

(Hospira Inc, 2016; Overgaard & Dzavík, 2008)

Indications for Dobutamine

- Dobutamine is used as an inotrope in the setting of acute decompensated HF in patients with a low cardiac index who have either end organ hypoperfusion or hypotension.
- Dobutamine can be used off label in shock (e.g., septic shock) when hemodynamic goals are not achieved with fluid resuscitation and vasopressor therapy.
- Dobutamine can also be used off label in routine stress echocardiography or with stress echocardiography done for the purpose of myocardial viability assessment.

(UptoDate, Lexidrug™, 2024)

> ***Linking Knowledge to Practice***
>
> ✓ *At low to medium doses dobutamine causes a substantial increase in MVO_2 and that is why it can be used for chemical stress testing. However, when used in other clinical settings this increase in MVO_2 can lead to the adverse effect of ischemia.*
>
> *(Overgaard & Dzavík, 2008)*

Special Dosing Information for Dobutamine

- In the setting of acute decompensated HF, the initial dose is between 2 and 5 mcg/kg/minute and may be adjusted based on systemic or end organ perfusion. The typical dose in acute decompensated HF does not exceed 10 mcg/kg/min. Much higher doses of dobutamine are used during stress echocardiography.
- In the setting of obesity, it is recommended to use the ideal body weight for continuous infusions and the actual body weight for stress testing.
- The manufacturer does not recommend any dose adjustments for renal or hepatic impairment.

(UptoDate, Lexidrug™, 2024)

Select Adverse Effects of Dobutamine

- ♦ BP response can be variable ranging from an increase in systolic BP to hypotension. The clinical rationale for the variable BP response is explained in the ***Linking Knowledge to Practice*** box below. Hypotension secondary to vasodilation usually occurs at higher doses (UptoDate, Lexidrug™, 2024).
- ♦ Life threatening ventricular arrhythmias can occur at any dose (Overgaard & Dzavík, 2008).
- ♦ See Table 19 for additional potential adverse effects of sympathomimetic medications.

> ***Linking Knowledge to Practice***
>
> - ✓ *Adrenergic receptors can be desensitized or downregulated in the setting of chronic heart failure.*
> - ✓ *The ability of an inotrope or a vasopressor to bind to adrenergic receptors can be altered by some clinical conditions.*
>   - *Acidosis and hypoxia can interfere with the ability of sympathomimetics to bind to receptors.*
>   - *As a result, the clinical effect of the medication can be reduced.*
>
>   *(Overgaard & Dzavík, 2008)*
> - ✓ *Patients who are taking beta blockers may not get an adequate response from drugs stimulating beta receptors because the beta blocker interferes with the beta stimulating effects of those drugs.*
>   - *In such patients, a better response may be obtained by using a drug that is not a sympathomimetic agent, such as milrinone, for inotropic support.*
>   - *Milrinone is discussed below.*

Contraindication Highlights for Dobutamine

- ♦ Consult manufacturer recommendations for use in children, pregnant women, and nursing women.
- ♦ Dobutamine should not be used in the setting of volume depletion.
- ♦ HOCM is a contraindication to dobutamine.
- ♦ Dobutamine should not be used for chemical stress testing when clinical conditions exist that prohibit exercise stress testing (e.g. unstable angina).
- ♦ Pheochromocytoma is also a contraindication according to Canadian labeling.

(UptoDate, Lexidrug™, 2024)

Special Considerations & Monitoring with Dobutamine

- ♦ Tolerance can develop after a few days on the medication (Overgaard & Dzavík, 2008).
- ♦ See Table 20 for recommended monitoring in patients receiving sympathomimetic vasoactive medications.

Key Pharmacokinetic & Pharmacodynamic Information for Dobutamine

- ♦ The onset of action is 1 to 10 minutes.
- ♦ The peak effect is 10 to 20 minutes.
- ♦ Half-life elimination is 2 minutes.

(UptoDate, Lexidrug™, 2024)

Important Medication Interactions with Dobutamine

- ♦ Beta blockers will block the effects of dobutamine and can be used as an antidote if needed.
- ♦ The following medications should be avoided with dobutamine:

- A medication change should be considered if the patient is receiving topical cocaine or linezolid. These agents may enhance the hypertensive effects of sympathomimetics.
- Kratom should be avoided with dobutamine because it may enhance the toxic effects of sympathomimetics.

(UptoDate, Lexidrug™, 2024)

> ***Linking Knowledge to Practice***
>
> ✓ *Dobutamine will result in increased forward blood flow and consequently a decrease in LV preload. For both these reasons, it is important that dobutamine or any other inotrope only used when there is adequate LV volume. Adequate LV volume is a prerequisite for an increase in forward flow. A reduction in LV preload would be detrimental in the setting of inadequate baseline preload.*
>
> ✓ *In older adults the initial dose should be started at the lower end of the dose range.*
>
> ✓ *Dobutamine is <u>not</u> a vasopressor and should not be independently titrated up in the event of hypotension. Dose increases for dobutamine are usually ordered by the provider compared to doses for vasopressors which are often titrated based on BP.*
>
> ✓ *Dobutamine can have a variable effect on BP. If the patient has adequate LV volume and the ordered dose is effective in increasing SV, the systolic BP will likely increase. However, if the ordered dose does not effectively increase SV there can be hypotension because of the modest vasodilation.*
>
> ✓ *If the patient is in atrial fibrillation or atrial flutter it is very important that the ventricular rate is controlled before starting dobutamine.*
>
> ✓ *Hypokalemia and hypomagnesemia should be corrected before starting therapy to help minimize the risk of arrhythmias.*

Epinephrine

Mechanism of Action of Epinephrine

- Epinephrine, also referred to as adrenaline, is an endogenous catecholamine produced by the adrenal glands. Epinephrine has an affinity for β1, β2, and α1 receptors and can cause increased cardiac inotropy, bronchial smooth muscle relaxation, and dilation of skeletal muscle vasculature. At lower doses epinephrine has great affinity for β receptors and at higher doses there is more affinity for α1 receptors.
- When epinephrine stimulates β1receptors there is an increase in HR and contractility and a release of renin. Epinephrine is a more potent β1 stimulator compared to norepinephrine.
- The primary clinical effect of β2 stimulation is bronchodilation. There is also a decrease in both SVR and diastolic BP because of vasodilation in response to β2 stimulation.
- At higher doses there is peripheral vasoconstriction in response to α1 stimulation and there is a subsequent increase in BP. There is an increase in both systolic and diastolic BP but the increase in systolic BP is more substantial because the vasodilation from β2 stimulation offsets the vasoconstriction from α1stimulation limiting the rise in diastolic BP. As a result, the MAP increase is less with epinephrine compared to norepinephrine.
- Pulmonary pressures (both arterial and venous) are increased. This is due to an increase in pulmonary blood flow and by direct pulmonary vasoconstriction.
- Epinephrine constricts most all vascular beds including renal, splanchnic, mucosal, and skin.
- When epinephrine stimulates α1 receptors the result also includes pupillary dilator muscle contraction and intestinal sphincter muscle contraction.

(Hospira, Inc. 2019; Overgaard & Dzavík, 2008; UptoDate, Lexidrug™, 2024)

Indications for Epinephrine

- Anaphylaxis / severe hypersensitivity reactions.
  - Early administration, ideally prior to hospital arrival, is essential.
  - IM administration in anterolateral aspect of the middle $^1/_3$ of the thigh is preferred. IV and intraosseous are alternate routes.
  - Patients can self-treat with an autoinjector. IM is the preferred route and SQ administration is an alternative.
- Hypotension / shock except for hemorrhagic shock.
  - Administration is via a continuous IV infusion.
  - It is indicated as an adjunctive agent in septic or other vasodilatory shock states. Epinephrine is not a first-line agent in septic shock.
  - It may also be used off label in cardiogenic or post-cardiac arrest shock although not as a first-line agent.
- Sudden cardiac death due to asystole, pulseless electrical activity (PEA), ventricular fibrillation, or pulseless VT [off label]. IV or intraosseous is the preferred route and endotracheal is an alternative route for administration.
- Inotropic support via continuous IV infusion [off label].
- Symptomatic bradycardia or AV block via continuous IV infusion [off label].
- Acute severe asthma [off label].
  - Epinephrine can be used in patients who cannot be treated with inhaled beta-agonists. It can also be considered in patients who are not responding to standard therapy and who are facing an impending respiratory arrest.
  - IM is the preferred route of administration and SQ is an alternative.
- Mydriasis during intraocular surgery. Consult an evidence-based drug reference for details regarding the use of epinephrine for this indication.

(UptoDate, Lexidrug™, 2024)

Special Dosing Information for Epinephrine

- When given IM epinephrine is dosed in mg (e.g., 0.3 mg or 0.5 mg IM) using a 1 mg/mL concentration.
- When given as a continuous infusion epinephrine is dosed either weight based in mcg/kg/min (e.g., 0.01 to 0.5 mg/kg/min) or non-weight based in mcg/min (e.g., 1 mcg/min to 80 mcg/min). The specific dose will vary based on the indication.
- A continuous infusion of epinephrine at lower doses will produce more inotropic effects and higher doses will produce more vasoconstrictive effects.
- When given IV, intraosseous, or endotracheal for asystole or pulseless arrest the dose is 0.01 mg/kg (0.1 mL/kg of a 0.1 mg/mL solution). IV or intraosseous is preferred over endotracheal administration.
- There are no recommended renal or hepatic dose adjustments per manufacturer labeling.
- The following are dosing recommendations in obesity:
  - Ideal body weight should be used for IV continuous infusion weight-based dosing. The drip should be titrated based on clinical effect.
  - Do not make changes between using ideal body weight and actual body weight during therapy. Do not make changes between weight-based dosing and non-weight-based dosing during therapy.
  - Use non-weight-base dosing for IM, SQ, intraosseous, and endotracheal administration.

(UptoDate, Lexidrug™, 2024)

> ***Linking Knowledge to Practice***
>
> ✓ *Endotracheal administration of epinephrine is not preferred during asystole or pulseless arrest because the concentrations delivered via this route may produce transient β2 effects resulting in peripheral vasodilation and subsequent hypotension. The IV or intraosseous routes are preferred.*
>
> *(American Heart Association, 2025; Manisterski et al., 2002)*

Select Adverse Effects of Epinephrine

- Hyperglycemia can occur with epinephrine administration.
  - Epinephrine is an exogenous stress hormone.
  - It inhibits the release of insulin by the pancreas, decreases glucose uptake by the tissues, and increases glycogenolysis resulting in hyperglycemia.
- There can be an increase in lactic acid because epinephrine causes glycolysis and thus the production of pyruvate which is an acid. This can result in the development of lactic acidosis.
- Epinephrine inhibits gastric motility and decreases gastric mucosa perfusion.
- Prolonged use and high doses can lead to direct cardiac toxicity. Mechanisms include:
  - Direct stimulation of myocyte apoptosis.
  - Damage of arterial walls leading to focal areas of myocyte cells death and myocardial contraction band necrosis.
- See Table 19 for additional potential adverse effects of sympathomimetic medications.

(Becker et al., 2020; Dalal & Grujic, 2023; Hospira, Inc. 2019; Jozwiak et al., 2022; Overgaard & Dzavík, 2008; UpToDate, Lexidrug™, 2024)

Contraindication Highlights for Epinephrine

- Consult manufacturer recommendations for use in children, pregnant women, and nursing women.
- There are no absolute contraindications to using injectable epinephrine in the setting of a life-threatening emergency (UpToDate®, Lexidrug™, 2024). Consult a pharmacist, package insert, or drug reference for contraindications to epinephrine when used for other indications.
- Hypovolemia should be corrected before the use of any inotrope or vasopressor.

> ***Linking Knowledge to Practice***
>
> ✓ *The development of lactic acidosis associated with epinephrine use is thought to be independent of the lactic acidosis that develops secondary to tissue hypoxia in the setting of shock.*
>
> *(Jozwiak, 2022)*

Special Considerations & Monitoring with Epinephrine

- Monitor blood glucose levels with a goal keeping the blood glucose level at < 180 mg/dl.
- Use with caution in patients with the following diagnoses:
  - Parkinson's disease: Patients can experience psychomotor agitation or temporary worsening of symptoms.
  - Thyroid disease: A patient in a hyperthyroid state is more prone to tachycardia, atrial fibrillation, and increased cardiac contractility. Epinephrine will potentiate these CV effects of hyperthyroidism (Ross, 2024).

  (UptoDate, Lexidrug™, 2024)
- See Table 20 for recommended monitoring in patients receiving sympathomimetic vasoactive medications.

> ***Linking Knowledge to Practice***
>
> ✓ *Diligent glucose monitoring is vital with epinephrine due to the risk of hyperglycemia.*
>
> ✓ *An average daily blood glucose level of < 180 mg/dl in a medically critically ill patient decreases the odds of subsequent in hospital mortality.*
>
> *(Becker et al., 2020)*

Key Pharmacokinetic & Pharmacodynamic Information for Epinephrine

- With IV administration a BP increase will occur in < 5 minutes. The offset of BP response occurs within 20 minutes.
- With IV injection the effective half-life of < 5 minutes.
- With continuous IV infusion a steady state is achieved in 10 to 15 minutes.
- Epinephrine is extensively metabolized.
  - Epinephrine is rapidly degraded to vanillylmandelic acid, an inactive metabolite.
  - The liver, kidneys, and skeletal muscle contribute the most to the removal of exogenous epinephrine.
- Higher body weight has been associated with a higher plasma epinephrine clearance and a lower concentration plateau.
- One small study demonstrated there was prolonged elimination of epinephrine when given IV for cardiac arrest thus potentially leading to increased plasma levels (Heradstveit, et al., 2023).

(Hospira, Inc. 2019)

Important Medication Interactions with Epinephrine

See Table 21 for important medication interactions with sympathomimetic vasopressors.

> ***Linking Knowledge to Practice***
>
> ✓ *Older patients have reduced drug clearance due to decreased renal or hepatic function and need to be monitored for signs of drug accumulation and toxicity.*
>
> ✓ *Many cardiac patients are older and have multiple comorbid conditions requiring polypharmacy and thus are at higher risk for medication interactions.*

Dopamine

Mechanism of Action of Dopamine

Dopamine is an immediate precursor to norepinephrine and epinephrine. Dopamine stimulates dopaminergic, α1, and β1 receptors depending on the dose.

- At lower doses (≈ 0.5 to 2 to 3 mcg/kg/min [maybe up to 5 mcg/kg/min]) dopamine stimulates dopaminergic receptors (D_1 and D_2) resulting in coronary, cerebral, renal and mesenteric vasodilation and increased blood flow to these tissues. There is no effect on BP at low doses.
- Dopamine also has a direct natriuretic effect related to action at the level of the renal tubules.
- At moderate doses (≈ 2 or 3 to 10 mcg/kg/min [some sources say 5 to 10 mcg/kg/min]) dopamine stimulates β_1 receptors and α1 receptors. Dopamine weakly binds to β_1 receptors and promotes the release of norepinephrine. At these doses there is an increase in contractility and HR and a mild increase in SVR.
- At higher doses (≈ 10 to 20 mcg/kg/min) there is dominant α1 stimulation and arterial and venous vasoconstriction. There is an increase in venous return and LV afterload.

(Jozwiak et al., 2022; Overgaard & Dzavík, 2008; UptoDate ®, Lexidrug™, 2024)

> ***Linking Knowledge to Practice***
>
> ✓ *Although dopamine stimulates the dopaminergic receptors causing renal vasodilation and increased renal blood flow, there is no evidence that this results in an increase in the glomerular filtration rate. There is also no proven renal protection with the use of low dose dopamine.*
>
> *(Overgaard & Dzavík, 2008)*

Indications for Dopamine

- Hypotension or shock: Dopamine can be used as an alternative vasopressor in cardiogenic or septic or other vasodilatory shock.
  - Dopamine is not the preferred first-line vasopressor in cardiogenic shock due to increased risk of arrhythmia and potential increased risk of mortality in this patient population (DeBacker et al., 2010).
  - Dopamine is only used in septic shock as an alternative to norepinephrine in patients with bradycardia and a low risk for developing tachyarrhythmias. Compared to norepinephrine there is the potential for worse outcomes with the use of dopamine (Evans et al., 2021).
- Bradycardia or AV block: Dopamine can be used off label when bradycardia or AV block is not responsive to atropine.
- Inotropic support: May be used as an inotrope in patients with severely reduced EF and evidence of decreased end organ perfusion.

(UptoDate, Lexidrug™, 2026)

Special Dosing Information for Dopamine

- Dopamine is dose dependent as discussed above under mechanism of action.
- The initial dose should be calculated based on ideal body weight and then titrated to achieve the goals of therapy.
- The weight that is used during therapy should not change based on the patient's actual weight.
- There are no recommendations for dose changes based on renal or hepatic function.

(UptoDate®, Lexidrug™, 2024)

> ***Linking Knowledge to Practice***
>
> ✓ *Because dopamine has different effects at different doses, it is very important to know the reason the patient is on a dopamine drip. For example, if the patient is receiving dopamine for the purpose of inotropic support, titrating to higher doses may be harmful rather than helpful.*

Select Adverse Effects of Dopamine

See Table 19 for potential adverse effects of sympathomimetic medications.

Contraindication Highlights for Dopamine

- Consult manufacturer recommendations for use in children, pregnant women, and nursing women.
- Dopamine is contraindicated in the presence of pheochromocytoma, a rare type of tumor of the adrenal gland that secretes catecholamines.
- Dopamine is not the preferred vasopressor in septic shock. A meta-analysis showed that in patients with septic shock there was higher mortality with the use of dopamine compared to norepinephrine. In the same population there was also a higher rate of arrhythmic events (De Backer et al., 2012).

- ♦ Dopamine at doses with β_1 stimulation should be used with caution in patients with CV disease due to risk of ischemia and infarction.
  - Dopamine should also be used cautiously in patients with cardiogenic shock.
  - In a randomized controlled trial evaluating dopamine and norepinephrine, the rate of death was higher in predefined subgroup analysis for patients with cardiogenic shock treated with dopamine (De Backer et al., 2010).
- ♦ Hypovolemia should be corrected before the use of any inotrope or vasopressor.

(UptoDate, Lexidrug™, 2024)

Special Considerations & Monitoring with Dopamine

See Table 20 for recommended monitoring in patients receiving sympathomimetic vasoactive medications.

Key Pharmacokinetic & Pharmacodynamic Information for Dopamine

- ♦ The onset of action is within 5 minutes.
- ♦ The duration of action is less than 10 minutes.
- ♦ Half-life elimination is approximately 2 minutes.

(UptoDate, Lexidrug™, 2024)

Important Medication Interactions with Dopamine

See Table 21 for important medication interactions with sympathomimetic vasopressors.

<u>Advanced Concept Focus:</u>
Extravasation

- ♦ Extravasation is the leakage of an IV vesicant (substance that produces blistering) or IV irritant (substance that produces local inflammation and phlebitis) medication / solution from the blood vessel into surrounding tissues resulting in tissue damage.
- ♦ This is different from an IV infiltration which is the leakage of a non-vesicant / non-irritant substance into the surrounding tissues.
- ♦ The most common vesicants are cytotoxic chemotherapy agents, however there are many other non-cytotoxic medications that have the potential to cause tissue damage.
- ♦ Injury from extravasation can damage surrounding tissues and involve nerves, tendons, and joints.
  - The solution or medication that extravasates moves out from the initial site of extravasation.
  - This movement leads to damage and is the reason that the total damage is often much larger than what is seen at the time of extravasation.
- ♦ If treatment is delayed, the patient may require surgical debridement and skin grafting. The need for amputation is a devastating outcome.
- ♦ Extravasation injuries occur more commonly in areas where there is less soft tissue to protect nerves, tendons, and joints. These areas include the dorsum of the hand and foot, the antecubital fossa, and in an area in proximity to a joint or joint spaces.
- ♦ Patient factors can also increase the risk of extravasation. Examples include:
  - A local vascular problem such as lymphedema, presence of peripheral vascular disease, Raynaud's phenomenon, or the presence of superior vena cava syndrome results in reduced venous flow and promotes IV fluid pooling and leaking.

- Fragile veins in older patients that are difficult to canulate or thrombosed veins in patients with a history of IV drug use increases the risk of extravasation.
- The presence of peripheral neuropathy can result in a delay in reporting pain and delay intervention in early extravasation.

◆ Several factors determine the degree of injury from extravasation including the volume of solution and the chemical properties of the solution.
- Many solutions and medications given IV can cause tissue necrosis including total parental nutrition fluids, antibiotics, and electrolyte solutions.
- A vasopressor causes vasoconstriction and ischemia at the site of extravasation. However, a vasodilator has the potential to enhance the effects of extravasation by enhancing blood flow to the area and expanding the amount of injury.
- Osmotic pressure can contribute to cell death.
  - Osmotic pressure is driven by the osmolality of a solution.
  - Tissue damage has been associated with solutions with high osmolality.
  - Hypertonic and hypotonic solutions both affect osmotic pressure.
  - A hypertonic solution given IV will draw fluid out of cells and can cause cell death by dehydration.
    - For example, the administration of hypertonic saline can cause the potential complication of osmotic demyelinating syndrome.
    - X-ray contrast media is hyperosmolar and can also cause cellular dehydration and cell death.
  - Hypotonic solutions given IV can cause cellular swelling and complications such as cerebral edema in high-risk patients.
- A concentrated solution with less volume reduces the risk for extravasation but a concentrated solution also has the potential for more tissue injury if there is leakage into the tissues.

◆ The severity of the reaction in an extravasation depends on the qualities of the medications that are extravasated and the total dose of the medication that was extravasated.

◆ The extent of the injury caused by extravasation might not be known immediately. The injury can evolve over days and even weeks.
- Early after extravasation the local S&S can be similar for a vesicant and an irritant. These include pain, burning, pruritis, mild erythema, and swelling. However, the initial presentation of S&S can be delayed.
- There can be a progression of S&S over the next 2 to 3 days. Pain and erythema can increase along with additional discoloration and blistering. The skin can also thicken (induration) and peel (desquamation).
- S&S of small volume extravasations can disappear over several weeks.
- Large volume extravasations can result in necrosis with the formation of eschar.
- An ulcer can also develop.
  - The edge of the ulcer is often red, raised, and painful.
  - A necrotic ulcer base with yellow slough can develop over days to weeks.
  - Ulcers caused by a vesicant do not have granulation tissue and lack adequate epithelial growth.

◆ The escape of an irritant medication from the vein will not cause tissue sloughing or necrosis. However, the escape of a vesicant from the vein can cause full thickness loss of the skin and damage underlying structures.

◆ Complications of untreated vesicant ulcers include nerve compression syndromes, neurological injury and dysfunction, permanent stiffness of joints, and contractures.

(Buter et al., 2024)

Advanced Concept Focus:
Inotropes & Vasopressors and Coronary Blood Flow

- In a study of 14 healthy people, it was shown that coronary blood flow increases when β-adrenergic receptors are stimulated both during exercise and with infusions of the medications isoproterenol and epinephrine (Vargas et al., 2016).
- Epinephrine and norepinephrine produce physiological responses that enhance coronary blood flow.
  - One of the mechanisms is the stimulation of cardiomyocytes to release local vasodilators. This process helps counterbalance the effects of α1 mediated coronary vasoconstriction.
  - Epinephrine causes an increase in the relative duration of diastole at higher HRs.
  - Norepinephrine increases coronary blood flow due to increased diastolic BP. However, prolonged infusions of norepinephrine have a toxic effect on cardiomyocytes by causing apoptosis (Overgaard & Dzavík, 2008).
  - Dopamine at low doses stimulates dopaminergic receptors D1 and D2. D1 receptors are in the coronary, cerebral, renal, and mesenteric beds and when stimulated there is vasodilation and increase blood flow to these tissues (Overgaard & Dzavík, 2008).

Norepinephrine

Mechanism of Action of Norepinephrine

- Norepinephrine potently stimulates α1 receptors resulting in arterial vasoconstriction and an increase in systolic and diastolic BP as the predominant therapeutic effect. Norepinephrine also produces venous vasoconstriction with an increase in venous return and an increase in preload.
- Norepinephrine modestly stimulates β1 receptors resulting in a positive inotropic effect and increase in SV.
  - The increase in LV afterload from α1 stimulation has the potential to negate the increased SV from β1stimulation. However, in the setting of septic shock there is some evidence that norepinephrine improved systolic function and CO even with the concurrent increased SVR.
  - Beta-1 stimulation resulting in potential increased chronotropy is offset by the baroreflex stimulation that occurs in response to vasoconstriction. Baroreflex stimulation results in bradycardia.
- It has little affinity for β2 receptors.
- Microcirculation may be improved when it is used in the treatment of septic shock.

(Jozwiak et al., 2022; Overgaard & Dzavík, 2008)

Indications for Norepinephrine

Norepinephrine is indicated in the following clinical circumstances:

- Cardiogenic shock.
- Post-cardiac arrest shock.
- Septic shock and other types of vasodilatory shock: Norepinephrine is the preferred first-line agent in septic shock.
- AKI or hepatorenal syndrome type 1 [off label].

(UptoDate, Lexidrug™, 2024)

Special Dosing Information for Norepinephrine

- In cardiogenic shock norepinephrine can be given with or without weight-based dosing. Regardless of dosing strategy, the medication is titrated to achieve end organ perfusion.

- Initial weight-based dosing is 0.05 mcg/kg/min. The typical dose range is 0.05 to 0.4 mcg/kg/min.
- Initial non-weight-based dosing starts at 5 mcg/min. The usual dose range for an 80 kg person ranges from 3 to 30 mcg/min.

◆ The ideal body weight should be used for initial weight-based dosing when the BMI is $\geq$ 30 kg/m^2.
- Continue titrating for clinical effectiveness.
- During therapy there should not be a change to/from weight based or non-weight based.
- Nor should there be a change from one type of weight (actual or ideal) to another.

◆ Dosing recommendations vary to some degree for other indications.

◆ No dose adjustment is necessary based on renal impairment or with any form of RRT since the medication is titrated to clinical effect.

◆ The medication is likely to be dialyzable with intermittent hemodialysis but not significantly dialyzable with continuous RRT.

◆ There is no recommended dose adjustment in hepatic dysfunction.

(UptoDate, Lexidrug™, 2024)

Linking Knowledge to Practice

✓ *When titrating any vasoactive drug that is being used as a vasopressor, the systolic, diastolic, and mean BP as well as the pulse pressure needs to be considered.*
- *The systolic BP provides information regarding the patient's LV SV.*
- *The pulse pressure and diastolic BP provide information about LV afterload.*
- *The mean BP is the pressure that is important for the kidneys and brain to autoregulate blood flow.*

Select Adverse Effects of Norepinephrine

◆ Post-marketing there have been reports of peripheral ischemia and gangrene.

◆ See Table 19 for additional potential adverse effects of sympathomimetic medications.

(UptoDate, Lexidrug™, 2024)

Contraindication Highlights for Norepinephrine

◆ Consult manufacturer recommendations for use in children, pregnant women, and nursing women.

◆ There are no contraindications in the manufacturer labeling in the United States.

◆ Hypovolemia should be corrected before the use of any vasopressor.

◆ Extreme caution should be used in patients who are hypoxemic or who have hypercapnia due to an increased risk of VT or ventricular fibrillation (VF).

(UptoDate, Lexidrug™, 2024)

Special Considerations & Monitoring with Norepinephrine

See Table 20 for recommended monitoring in patients receiving sympathomimetic vasoactive medications.

Key Pharmacokinetic & Pharmacodynamic Information for Norepinephrine

◆ Norepinephrine has a very rapid onset of action.

◆ The duration of action is only 1 to 2 minutes.

- ♦ The medication reaches a steady state in 5 minutes.
- ♦ The mean half-life elimination is 2.4 minutes.

(UptoDate, Lexidrug™, 2024)

> ***Linking Knowledge to Practice***
>
> - ✓ *When up titrating a vasopressor for hypotension both the onset of action and the peak action of the medication should be considered.*
> - ✓ *For example:*
>   - *If the onset is 1 to 2 minutes you want to wait 2 minutes to observe the impact of the initial dose of the medication.*
>   - *If the peak action is 10 minutes, and if the clinical condition allows, you want to wait 10 minutes to see the full effect of that dose before deciding if the patient needs up titration.*
> - ✓ *If hypotension occurs because of drug initiation it can be discontinued immediately.*

Important Medication Interactions with Norepinephrine

See Table 21 for important medication interactions with sympathomimetic vasopressors.

Advanced Concept Focus:
Weight Based versus Non-Weight Based Vasopressor Titration in Obese and Nonobese Patients

- ♦ In one retrospective study of 200 patients in septic shock the dose requirements of norepinephrine were compared in obese and nonobese patients. The primary outcome was the dose requirement of norepinephrine at 60 minutes after the start of the infusion.
    - At 60 minutes the mean infusion rate for weight-based dosing was 0.09 mcg/kg/min in the obese group and 0.13 mcg/kg/min in the nonobese group which was statistically significant ($P = .006$).
    - At 60 minutes the non–weight-based dose was 9 mcg/min in obese patients and 8 mcg/min in nonobese patients showing no statistical difference. ($P = .72$).
    - The conclusion was that compared to nonobese patients, obese patients with septic shock require lower weight-based doses of norepinephrine yet similar total norepinephrine doses (Radosevich et. al., 2016).
- ♦ In a multicenter retrospective study of 308 patients with septic shock who required vasopressor therapy, all patients received non-weight-based dosing. Patients were divided into 2 groups, obese and non-obese. The primary outcome was the requirement of a second hemodynamic support drug to obtain a MAP of ≥ 65 mmHg.
    - In the obese group 27% of patients required secondary medication to achieve a mean BP of > 65 mmHg compared to 19% in the non-obese group. The results were statistically significant.
    - It took 5.3 hours to achieve hemodynamic stability in the obese group compared to 3.5 hours in the nonobese group (P=.006) (Adams et al., 2017).
- ♦ In another multicenter retrospective study obese patients were studied to determine if weight-based dosing of norepinephrine leads to earlier time to goal MAP compared with non- weight-based dosing in obese patients with septic shock.
    - The primary outcome was time to goal MAP. Researchers concluded that weight-based dosing of norepinephrine does not achieve an earlier time to the goal MAP.
    - However, weight-based dosing may lead to higher norepinephrine cumulative dose requirements and prolonged time until norepinephrine discontinuation.

(Vadiei et al., 2017)

Linking Knowledge to Practice

- ✓ *Most IV drugs with cardiac and vascular effects need to be titrated down prior to discontinuation as opposed to being terminated abruptly.*
- ✓ *When weaning a patient off a vasopressor you need to consider the duration of action and the half-life of the medication being titrated. Drugs with a short half-life need to be titrated more slowly than drugs with a longer half-life.*
- ✓ *For example:*
  - *If the half-life of a medication is very short and the duration of the medication is only 1 to 2 minutes, then the patient's BP should be checked 2 minutes after a decrease in dose to assure the patient is tolerating the reduced dose.*
  - *Many vasoactive drugs like dopamine, dobutamine, and nitroprusside have a half-life of about 2 minutes, and they should be weaned over a period of 2 to 3 hours while monitoring the patient's response each time the infusion rate is decreased.*
  - *It is important to know if you are weaning a medication with a very short half-life and duration of action to ensure that you stay in the room to evaluate the patient's response after each downward titration.*
  - *Drugs like lidocaine and milrinone, with a longer half-life of about 2 hours are typically stopped rather than weaned. Patients don't require the same frequent vital sign assessment as patients who are being weaned from a vasoactive medication with a very short half-life, and they do not require the same frequent vital sign assessment after discontinuation. After discontinuation the body essentially "weans" the drug over the next few hours.*

Phenylephrine

Mechanism of Action of Phenylephrine

- ♦ Phenylephrine, a potent systemic arterial vasoconstrictor, acts by directly stimulating α1 receptors. The clinical result is an increase in SVR with increases in systolic and diastolic BP.
- ♦ In addition to increasing LV afterload there is also evidence that phenylephrine may increase cardiac filling in preload dependent patients by increasing systemic venous return. However, the mechanism of action is complex because phenylephrine also increases the resistance to venous return which can decrease systemic venous return. This makes the effects on CO hard to predict.
- ♦ There is essentially zero beta effect and thus no direct HR effects.

(Jozwiak et al., 2022; Kalmar et al., 2018; Overgaard & Dzavík, 2008; UptoDate, Lexidrug™, 2024)

Indications for Phenylephrine

Only the indications for IV phenylephrine are discussed below. Phenylephrine is also available OTC for nasal decongestion, and intracavernous injection of phenylephrine can be used off label to treat acute ischemic priapism.

Indications for IV phenylephrine include:

- ♦ Cardiogenic shock: Phenylephrine is the first-line vasoactive medication in treating cardiogenic shock in patients with HOCM, aortic stenosis, or mitral stenosis.
- ♦ Septic or other vasodilatory shock:
  - Phenylephrine is no longer recommended in critically ill patients with septic shock.
  - It is only used in septic shock in specific circumstances: 1) when norepinephrine (the preferred agent) causes serious arrhythmias, 2) when CO is known to be high, but BP remain low, or 3) as part of salvage therapy in combination with other vasopressor / inotropic agents.
- ♦ Hypotension that is associated with anesthesia.

- Additional clinical uses:
  - To treat severe hypotension in patients with aortic stenosis.
  - To decrease the outflow tract gradient in patients with HOCM.
  - To correct hypotension caused by the combination of nitrates and PDE-5 inhibitors.
  - To correct vagally mediated hypotension that can occur during percutaneous procedures.

(UptoDate, Lexidrug™, 2024)

> ***Linking Knowledge to Practice***
>
> ✓ *A preload dependent patient is a patient who has an increase in SV in response to an increase in end diastolic volume in either the RV or the LV.*
>
> ✓ *While there are no direct HR effects with phenylephrine, patients can have a significant baroreceptor mediated reflex bradycardia in response to a rapid increase in MAP.*
>
> ✓ *In a patient with reduced EF the increase in SVR produced by phenylephrine may result in a decrease in CO.*

Special Dosing Information for Phenylephrine

- When used in cardiogenic shock a continuous infusion is used, and the medication is titrated to clinical effect. The dose range is 0.1 to 10 mcg/kg/min.
- Phenylephrine may be used as a bolus to rapidly raise the BP in patients with septic shock.
  - In a retrospective study of patients with septic shock who were started on norepinephrine but remained hypotensive, those who received a phenylephrine bolus were compared to those who did not.
  - Patients who received a phenylephrine bolus had a higher rate of achieving hemodynamic stability, but this was not sustained.
  - Phenylephrine boluses were also associated with a higher ICU mortality, and thus the use of phenylephrine boluses should be done with caution.

  (Hawn et al., 2021)
- The manufacturer does not recommend any dose adjustments based on kidney or liver function.
- In the setting of renal dysfunction there may be increased responsiveness, and lower initial doses may be indicated.
- In the setting of hepatic dysfunction there may be decreased responsiveness and higher initial doses may be indicated.

(Hawn et al., 2021; UptoDate, Lexidrug™, 2024)

> ***Linking Knowledge to Practice***
>
> ✓ *In patients with aortic stenosis the LV afterload is essentially fixed due to the stenosis of the aortic valve. Thus, the rise in diastolic BP caused by phenylephrine may increase coronary perfusion without any detrimental effect of increasing afterload.*
>
> ✓ *Phenylephrine is effective in HOCM because it supports keeping the LV outflow tract open by its sustained increase in preload.*

Select Adverse Effects of Phenylephrine

See Table 19 for potential adverse effects of sympathomimetic medications.

Linking Knowledge to Practice

- ✓ *Mesenteric ischemia is an uncommon but potentially fatal complication of vasopressor therapy. Any new abdominal pain could represent mesenteric ischemia and should be reported immediately.*
- ✓ *When administering a vasopressor that stimulates α1 receptors resulting in vasoconstriction, anticipate that the patient may have a reflex response resulting in a profound bradycardia.*

Management of Peripheral Extravasation of Dobutamine, Dopamine, Epinephrine, Norepinephrine, Phenylephrine and Vasopressin

- Stop infusion immediately.
- Leave cannula or needle in place temporarily.
- Do NOT flush the line.
- Do NOT apply pressure to the site.
- Gently aspirate the infiltrated solution.
- Remove the needle or cannula after aspiration and administration of any antidote that is ordered.
- Elevate the extremity and apply dry warm compresses.
  - Dry warm compresses should be applied to the affected area for 20 minutes every 4 to 6 hours for 1 to 2 days after removal of the IV catheter.
  - If the dry warm compress provides comfort the frequency can be up to 20 minutes per hour.
  - Warm compresses are not recommended if topical NTG is initiated.
- Initiate an antidote (phentolamine, topical NTG, or terbutaline) in severe cases.
- Surgical consultation is indicated if there is skin compromise or a mass effect from the infiltrate.
- Phentolamine is a non-selective alpha blocker, blocking both α1 and α2 receptors. It is the preferred antidote for vasopressors that are stimulating α1 receptors.
  - Dilute 5 to 10 mg in 10 mL NS.
  - Divide the above dose into multiple SQ injections along the area of infiltration.
  - If the IV catheter is still in place, administer the first dose of phentolamine through the IV catheter.
  - The initial dose can be repeated in 60 minutes if the patient remains symptomatic.
  - Phentolamine should be administered as soon as possible and within 12 hours of the infiltrate.
- Terbutaline, a β2 agonist is an alternative antidote.
  - Terbutaline is injected SQ in a similar manner as phentolamine.
  - 1 mg of terbutaline is diluted in 10 mL NS.
  - For small extravasations 0.5 mg can be given by using 1 mg of terbutaline diluted in 1 mL NS.
  - The dose can be repeated if needed after 15 minutes.
- Topical NTG 2% ointment is also an alternative antidote. NTG does not act directly on the α1 or β2 receptors. It is a vasodilator through smooth muscle relaxation.
  - NOTE: Topical NTG is preferred antidote for vasopressin extravasation.
  - Topical NTG should be applied within 1 hour of the infiltration.
  - Warm compresses are not recommended when topical NTG is used.
  - A 1-inch strip of NTG should be applied to the site and the area should be covered.
  - The dose may be repeated every 8 hours as needed.
  - Topical NTG may be used in conjunction with phentolamine and terbutaline.
  - Longer term therapy may be needed if NTG is used as the sole treatment.
- Phentolamine is the preferred agent when α1receptors are being stimulated by the vasoactive medications such as with norepinephrine and higher doses of dopamine. However, with dobutamine topical NTG or terbutaline may be preferred because dobutamine is not a predominant α1stimulator.

(Buter, et al., 2024; UptoDate, Lexidrug™, 2024)

Contraindication Highlights for Phenylephrine

- Consult manufacturer recommendations for use in children, pregnant women, and nursing women.
- Hypovolemia should be corrected before the use of any vasopressor.
- Phenylephrine should not be used if the SVR is more than 1200 dynes x sec/cm^5.
- Do not use phenylephrine in patients with HF or cardiogenic shock because increased LV afterload will result in a decrease in CO.

(UptoDate, Lexidrug™, 2024)

Special Considerations & Monitoring with Phenylephrine

See Table 20 for recommended monitoring in patients receiving sympathomimetic vasoactive medications.

Key Pharmacokinetic & Pharmacodynamic Information for Phenylephrine

- IV onset of action is immediate.
- IV duration is 15 to 20 minutes.

(UptoDate, Lexidrug™, 2024)

Linking Knowledge to Practice

- ✓ *The half-life of a drug is the amount of time that it takes for the plasma concentration of the drug to fall to half its original level.*
- ✓ *Drugs with a long half-life stay in the body longer than those with a short half-life. It takes about 5 half-lives for 95% of a drug to be eliminated, and about 7 half-lives for 99% of a drug to be eliminated.*
- ✓ *Clinically, most drugs are considered "gone" in about 5 half- lives. For example, amiodarone has a very long half-life (average of 53 days), so it takes approximately 265 days for 95% of the drug to disappear; while adenosine has a half-life of 9 seconds, so 95% of it is gone in 45 seconds.*

Important Medication Interactions with Phenylephrine

See Table 21 for important medication interactions with sympathomimetic vasopressors.

Advanced Concept Focus:
Vasopressors and Acute Mesenteric Ischemia

- Acute mesenteric ischemia is a rare complication of vasopressor therapy.
- However, if it occurs it is frequently fatal with a mortality rate of approximately 28% in patients who require surgical intervention (Gupta et al., 2011).
- All vasopressors have been associated with the development of mesenteric ischemia. However, patients requiring vasopressor therapy also have hypoperfusion which is also a contributing factor.
- Even when vasopressors are effective in increasing perfusion pressure, the restored microcirculatory blood flow is not distributed evenly, particularly in the abdominal organs.
- Vasopressors may divert blood away from mesenteric circulation.
- Vasopressor therapy may decrease gastrointestinal (GI) motility but critical illness itself and the use of sedatives in critical care also reduce GI motility. Compared to other vasopressors, epinephrine has the greatest effect on inhibiting gut motility.

- A reduction in splanchnic blood flow plays a role in the development of mesenteric ischemia and vasopressors can cause splanchnic vasoconstriction. The effect of vasopressors on splanchnic circulation is unpredictable.
- Non-occlusive acute mesenteric ischemia (GI ischemia in the setting of normal vessels) may result from vasopressor induced splanchnic vasoconstriction. Phenylephrine's $\alpha 1$ stimulation produces a more substantial splanchnic vasoconstriction than norepinephrine.
- Microcirculation of the GI tract is also affected by vasopressors. Epinephrine and norepinephrine might have a greater adverse effect on GI microcirculation than phenylephrine. In a study of patients on mechanical ventilation low dose dopamine at 4 mcg/kg/min had an adverse effect on gastroduodenal motility (Dive et al., 2000).
- Although there is an association between vasopressors and acute mesenteric ischemia there has been no proven causation in randomized controlled studies.
- In the setting of metabolic acidosis, patients with abdominal pain out of proportion of the physical abdominal exam, should be considered to have intestinal ischemia until proven otherwise.

(Gilani, 2024; Jozwiak et al., 2022)

Prescribing Pearls for Norepinephrine

- Throughout the world there are different preparations of norepinephrine. All preparations are formulated to a salt solution to make the solution stable and safe for IV use. There is no pure norepinephrine base available.
- However, in some publications the recommendations for norepinephrine dosing are made based on base equivalents.
- Norepinephrine is available as norepinephrine tartrate, norepinephrine bitartrate, and norepinephrine hydrochloride. The equivalents are as follows:
  - noradrenaline base: 1 mg/mL.
  - noradrenaline tartrate: 2 mg/mL.
  - noradrenaline bitartrate: 1.89 mg/mL.
  - noradrenaline hydrochloride: 1.22 mg/mL.
- Until recently there has not been standards regarding labeling. The labeling of some preparations of IV norepinephrine listed the base equivalency followed by the concentration of the conjugated salt. For example: noradrenaline base = 1 mg/mL and noradrenaline tartrate = 2 mg/mL. Other commercial products only listed the conjugated salt equivalent with no base equivalent.
- The implications are important when reading studies, recommendations, or guidelines regarding norepinephrine dosing. For example, if a recommendation is made based on base equivalent dosing and an organization is using a tartrate formulation there could be a twofold dosing discrepancy during implementation.
- In an international study regarding adherence to sepsis guidelines, 50% of those responding did not know the preparation of norepinephrine in their hospital (Mongardon et al., 2023).
- There are ongoing discussions worldwide on steps needed to improve communication regarding norepinephrine dosing.
- It is recommended that the labeling of all norepinephrine products include the base equivalent.
- Also, all recommendations regarding norepinephrine dosing should be expressed in the base equivalent.
- There is a recommendation for all research studies involving norepinephrine to clearly state the formulation of norepinephrine that is used in the study.

(Goyer et al., 2024; Kotani et al., 2023)

Table 19 **Potential Adverse Effects of Sympathomimetic Medications**
▪ Inotropic effects from β1stimulation can result in tachycardia, premature atrial and ventricular beats, atrial and ventricular arrhythmias, and palpitations.
▪ Beta-1 stimulation will also cause an increase in MVO_2 and cause chest pain and ischemia in patients with CAD.
▪ Vasoconstrictive effects from α1stimulation can increase BP, LV afterload, and can also decrease blood flow to limbs resulting in distal ischemia. ▪ Tissue necrosis can also occur at local injection sites.
▪ The combination of cardiac stimulation and peripheral vasoconstriction can result in pulmonary edema.
▪ If a medication produces a predominant α1stimulation a severe reflex bradycardia can occur in response to the increase in LV afterload and rise in BP.
▪ HTN or hypertensive emergencies may occur in response to vasopressor therapy, particularly phenylephrine.
▪ Visceral vasoconstriction can lead to decreased blood flow and potential ischemia to the intestines, liver, and spleen. ▪ See Advanced Concept Focus section above on acute mesenteric ischemia.
▪ Renal vasoconstriction can also occur with some sympathomimetic medications.
▪ Many sympathomimetic medications are vesicants and capable of causing extravasation. Management of extravasation is outlined in the box above. ▪ See Advanced Concept Focus section above on extravasation.
(Jozwiak et al., 2022; UptoDate, Lexidrug™, 2024)

Table 20 Part 1 **Patient Monitoring for Sympathomimetic Vasoactive Medications**
Monitor volume status: Adequate volume status is a prerequisite for the administration of an inotrope or vasopressor. ▪ Volume is always the first-line treatment for hypotension unless it is certain that the patient has adequate or excess intravascular volume. ▪ An inotrope will not be effective in increasing SV if there is not adequate ventricular filling.
Monitor the patient's hemodynamic status as an indicator of clinical improvement: The following parameters should be monitored: ▪ BP, HR, and cardiac rhythm. ▪ Invasive or non-invasive hemodynamic parameters of CO, SV, preload, and afterload should be closely monitored.
Monitor urine output: Renal vasoconstriction and a subsequent reduction in urine output can occur depending on the medication and the dose. ▪ Dopamine at low doses can cause renal vasodilation. ▪ If an inotrope or vasopressor is effective at improving end organ perfusion in the setting of shock, there can be an improvement in urine output.
Monitor for ischemia and arrhythmias (atrial or ventricular): Patients with underlying cardiac disease are at high risk of experiencing complications of ischemia or arrhythmias with sympathomimetic medications. ▪ These medications result in an increase in myocardial O_2 demand. ▪ There is an increase in myocardial O_2 demand with any increase in HR, contractility, or afterload.

Table 20 Part 2 Patient Monitoring for Sympathomimetic Vasoactive Medications
Monitor for pulmonary edema: Patients are at risk for pulmonary edema when a medication produces simultaneous cardiac stimulation with an increase in SVR. This may be seen with epinephrine.
Monitor for exaggerated response in patients with autonomic dysfunction: There are several causes of autonomic dysfunction including autoimmune disorders, degenerative neurological diseases, drug toxicity, chronic liver disease, diabetes mellitus, and infectious processes.
Monitor for signs of mesenteric or peripheral vascular ischemia: This is particularly important in patients with any history of mesenteric or peripheral vascular thrombosis. ▪ Vasopressors at therapeutic doses cause peripheral vasoconstriction and can increase the risk of peripheral vascular ischemia. ▪ Vasopressors, depending on the medication and dose, also have the potential to cause mesenteric vasoconstriction and increase the risk for mesenteric ischemia. ▪ Assess for adequate peripheral perfusion including skin temperature and color and the presence of peripheral pulses. ▪ Also assess for and report any new onset abdominal pain in a patient receiving vasopressor therapy. See Advanced Concept Focus section on acute mesenteric ischemia.
Monitor for extravasation: Many vasoactive medications are vesicants. ▪ See Advanced Concept Focus section above section on extravasation. ▪ The steps for the management of extravasation are outlined in the box above.
Monitor for tolerance when weaning: As a vasopressor is weaned and vasoconstriction is reduced the intravascular space will get bigger. ▪ The patient will usually require additional volume to fill the expanded vascular space. ▪ If the patient's volume status is not adequate, profound hypotension can develop when the medication is weaned.

Table 21 Part 1

Important Medication Interactions with Sympathomimetic Vasopressors

Medication	Potential Effect	Epinephrine	Dopamine	Norepinephrine	Phenylephrine
Blonanserin	↓ therapeutic effect	Avoid	Not listed	Not listed	Not listed
Bromocriptine	↑ HTN effect	Consider med change	Consider med change	Consider med change	Consider med change
Bromperidol	↓ therapeutic effect	Avoid	Not listed	Not listed	Not listed
Ergot derivatives*	↑ vasoconstrictive effect	Avoid	Avoid	Avoid	Avoid
Haloperidol	↓ vasoconstrictive effect	Consider med change	Not listed	Not listed	Not listed
Hyaluronidase	↑ vasoconstrictive effect	Consider med change	Consider med change	Consider med change	Consider med change
Linezolid	↑ HTN effect	Consider med change	Consider med change	Consider med change	Consider med change
Lisuride	↑ HTN effect	Avoid	Avoid	Avoid	Avoid

Table 21 Part 2 Important Medication Interactions with Sympathomimetic Vasopressors					
MAO inhibitors	↑ HTN effect	Monitor	Consider med change	Monitor	Avoid
Promethazine	↓ vasoconstrictive effect	Consider med change	Not listed	Not listed	Not listed
SNRIs	↑ vasopressor & tachycardiac effect	Consider med change	Consider med change	Consider med change	Not listed
Topical cocaine	↑ HTN effect	Consider med change	Consider med change	Consider med change	Consider med change
Tricyclic anti-depressants	↑ vasopressor effect	Consider med change	Consider med change	Consider med change	Monitor
(UptoDate, Lexidrug™, 2024) MAO: monoamine oxidase					

NON-SYMPATHOMIMETIC VASOACTIVE DRUGS

Non-sympathomimetic vasoactive medications exert their therapeutic action on arteries and veins through mechanisms outside the receptors of the SNS. Each drug or class of drug impacts a unique receptor or system outside the SNS to either stimulate or oppose to gain the desired effect.

Milrinone

Milrinone is a non-sympathomimetic inotrope meaning its mechanism of action is not through activation of the SNS. In addition to exerting an inotropic effect, milrinone also improves cardiac lusitropy (diastolic function or rate of myocardial relaxation). Milrinone also has the additional hemodynamic effects of preload and afterload reduction.

Appendix 11 provides additional details regarding Milrinone.

Mechanism of Action of Milrinone

- Milrinone is a selective PDE-3 inhibitor at low doses. PDE-3 is present in cardiac sarcoplasmic reticulum and in the smooth muscle of arteries and veins.
- In the myocardium the drug slows the hydrolysis of cyclic adenosine monophosphate (cAMP) buildup.
  - The increased concentration of cAMP results in increased availability of calcium in the cardiac sarcomere (contractile unit of the muscle) resulting in increased inotropy.
  - There is also a subsequent increase in calcium reuptake into the sarcoplasmic reticulum resulting in cardiac relaxation and improved diastolic function.
  - The effect of improved relaxation and diastolic function is called lusitropy.
- The clinical effects of milrinone also include both venous and arterial vasodilation.
  - Milrinone prevents cyclic guanosine monophosphate (cGMP) metabolism and the increased cGMP levels lead to vasodilation.
  - Systemic BP and cardiac filling pressures are lowered due to venous and arterial vasodilation.
- Milrinone is also a pulmonary vasodilator causing a reduction in PVR. This reduction in RV afterload can be beneficial in patients with RV dysfunction.
- Some increase in HR is expected but unlike dobutamine, there is no strong chronotropic effect. (Chong et al., 2018; Mathew et al., 2021; UptoDate®, Lexidrug™, 2025).

Linking Knowledge to Practice

✓ *Milrinone and dobutamine are both inotropic medications that may also be referred to as inodilators. An inodilator is an inotropic medication that also has vasodilator effects. Milrinone results in both venous and arterial vasodilation by preventing cGMP metabolism. Increased cGMP results in vasodilation. Dobutamine has more modest vasodilation resulting from greater ß2 stimulation than α1 stimulation.*

Advanced Concept Focus:
Physiological Effects of Milrinone Compared to Clinical Outcomes

- Patients with HFrEF have reduced contractility which can lead to hypoperfusion of end organs.
  - Patients with HFrEF also typically have an increased SVR which occurs to compensate for low SV. Unfortunately, this increased SVR results in an increased workload for the failing LV.
  - Patients with HFrEF are also at risk for backwards failure which results in increased volume in the LV after ejection. This increased volume can be transmitted backwards to the LA and then to the pulmonary veins. From the pulmonary veins fluid can be pushed into the interstitial space and then ultimately into the alveoli resulting in pulmonary edema.
- Milrinone is an inotropic medication that increases SV and reduces both preload and afterload. These hemodynamic effects seem favorable in a patient with HFrEF. Milrinone has the effects of increasing contractility, decreasing SVR, and decreasing cardiac filling pressures without a substantial increase in HR and without an increase in MVO_2. These effects are hemodynamically desirable in a patient with decompensated HFrEF.
- Other positive effects of milrinone includes lusitropy which is improvement in cardiac relaxation or diastolic function.
- Milrinone improves the interaction between LV contraction and the elasticity and resistance of the arterial vascular system. This benefit is referred to as improved LV-arterial coupling.
- However, with all medications it is important to know whether the perceived beneficial physiological effects produce an improvement in one or more patient clinical outcomes.
- The Optime trial evaluated 951 patients from 78 different hospitals in the United States. Patients were admitted with an exacerbation of HFrEF (mean LVEF 23%) who required hospitalization but in whom there was not an urgent need for inotropic support.
  - In this study patients were randomized to receive either a milrinone drip starting at 0.5 mcg/kg/min or a placebo infusion of saline.
  - The study outcome was the cumulative days of hospitalization for any CV cause within 60 days of being randomized into the clinical trial.
  - There was no statistical difference in the cumulative days of hospitalization between the groups. There was also no statistical difference in in-hospital mortality or 60-day mortality between the groups.
  - In the patients who received milrinone there was more hypotension that required treatment and there were also more new onset atrial arrhythmias in the milrinone group.
- The conclusion of the study was that the regular use of milrinone in patients with an exacerbation of HFrEF is not indicated to reduce hospital length of stay (LOS) or prevent a readmission.
- Remember, in the Optime trial the patients enrolled did not have an urgent clinical need for inotropic support. Milrinone or dobutamine, however, will be used in clinical practice when a patient's clinical and hemodynamic status requires inotropic support.

(Ayres & Maani, 2023; Cuffe et al., 2002)

Comparison of Milrinone and Dobutamine

- Milrinone (a non-sympathomimetic) and dobutamine (a sympathomimetic) are both inotropic medications that may be used in acute decompensated HF or cardiogenic shock.
- However, in addition to its inotropic action milrinone also results in both venous and arterial vasodilation.
- In contrast dobutamine only results in a modest vasodilation of the arterial bed because the stimulation of ß2 receptors is somewhat greater than the stimulation of α1 receptors. The vasodilatory effects of ß2 stimulation are not as potent as the vasodilatory effects of milrinone (Ayres & Maani, 2023).
- The net effects of dobutamine result in an increase in MVO_2 while the net effect of milrinone does not result in the same increase in MVO_2.
- The vasodilation effects of milrinone decrease preload and afterload which offset any increase in MVO_2 from increased contractility.
- In one study milrinone and dobutamine were found to be comparable in the treatment of low CO in patients after cardiac surgery. In this study dobutamine was associated with a higher incidence of atrial fibrillation and milrinone was associated with a higher incidence of sinus bradycardia (Feneck et al., 2001).
- In a randomized study comparing dobutamine and milrinone there was no difference in the primary outcomes between these medications. The primary outcome was a composite of in hospital death from any cause, resuscitated cardiac arrest, treatment with cardiac transplant or mechanical circulatory support, non-fatal MI, stroke or transient ischemic attack (TIA), or need for RRT (Mathew et al., 2021).

Linking Knowledge to Practice

✓ *Milrinone may be preferred to dobutamine in patients with pulmonary HTN because milrinone reduces pulmonary pressures and may help improve RV function.*

(Mathew et al., 2021)

Indications for Milrinone

- Acute decompensated HF.
  - In patients with low cardiac index and either hypotension or end organ hypoperfusion.
  - Short-term use only.
- Inotropic support pre or post-heart transplant [off label].
- Weaning post-cardiac surgery in patients with preexisting LV dysfunction [off label].
- There is also interest in the use of milrinone to treat pulmonary HTN in neonates (James et al., 2016; Matsushita et al., 2024; Qasim & Jain, 2020).

(Ayres & Maani, 2023; UptoDate®, Lexidrug™, 2025)

Special Dosing Information for Milrinone

- IV bolus dose is not recommended due to risk of hypotension.
- A continuous infusion is used for all indications.
- Initial dose in acute decompensated HF is 0.125 to 0.25 mcg/kg/min.
  - Titration should occur to achieve the desired clinical endpoint.
  - Usual dose range does not exceed 0.75 mcg/kg/min.
- Usual dose range for inotropic support post-heart transplant is 0.375 to 0.75 mcg/kg/min.

- The lowest effective dose should be used.
- The medication should be weaned within 3 to 5 days after surgery.

♦ Lower initial doses should be used with renal impairment because clearance is dependent on kidney function.
  - For CrCl 10 to 50 mL/min start at 0.0625 to 0.125 mcg/kg/min.
  - Doses > 0.375 mcg/kg/min are not recommended if there is substantial renal impairment because the of the risk of drug accumulation. Some experts recommend milrinone be avoided in patients with AKI or ESKD.
  - In obesity the initial dose should be based on ideal body weight followed by titration to clinical effect. However, once therapy has been started the weight parameter should not be changed but rather the drug should be titrated based on clinical effect.

♦ There are no manufacturer recommendations for dose adjustment in patients with hepatic dysfunction.
(Ayres & Maani, 2023; Chong et al., 2018; UptoDate®, Lexidrug™, 2025)

> ***Linking Knowledge to Practice***
>
> ✓ *If milrinone is used in a patient with renal dysfunction the patient should be monitored closely for hypotension and cardiac arrhythmias.*
>
> ✓ *Complications of milrinone occur more frequently in patients with abnormal kidney function.*
>
> *(UptoDate®,Lexidrug™, 2025)*

Select Adverse Effects of Milrinone

♦ Ventricular ectopy is the most common adverse effect. Nonsustained VT and other ventricular arrhythmia can also occur. The adverse effect of ventricular arrhythmias does not seem to be related to dose.

♦ Supraventricular arrhythmias may also occur including atrial fibrillation. One small study showed that milrinone was an independent risk factor for the development of atrial fibrillation in patients undergoing elective cardiac surgery (Fleming et al., 2008).

♦ Milrinone can cause hypotension due to its impact on reducing preload.
  - This can occur especially if the patient has received aggressive diuresis for heart failure.
  - The risk of hypotension increases at higher doses.

♦ HA, secondary to a reduction in preload has also been reported in approximately 3% of patients.
(UptoDate®, Lexidrug™, 2025)

> ***Linking Knowledge to Practice***
>
> ✓ *Milrinone has a much longer half-life compared to the inotrope dobutamine.*
>
> ✓ *In patients with renal dysfunction the half-life of milrinone is longer. For this reason, the risk for ventricular or atrial arrhythmias may continue even after the medication is stopped. In addition, any hypotension from the medication will be prolonged in the setting of renal dysfunction.*
>
> *(UptoDate®,Lexidrug™, 2025)*

Contraindication Highlights for Milrinone

♦ Consult manufacturer recommendations for use in children, pregnant women, and nursing women.

♦ Hypersensitivity is the only listed absolute contraindication.

♦ However, inotropes should be avoided in patients with HCOM and in patients with severe pulmonic or aortic valve stenosis causing obstruction.

- ♦ Milrinone should also be used with caution and under the direction of an expert clinician when treating patients with severe HF or severe pulmonary HTN due to the risk of hemodynamic changes in highly complex patients.
- ♦ Based on the manufacturer's recommendation milrinone should not be used for more than 48 hours. There is no evidence for safety or efficacy beyond 48 hours of use.

(Ayres & Maani, 2023; UptoDate®, Lexidrug™, 2025)

Special Considerations and Monitoring with Milrinone

- ♦ Continuous cardiac monitoring is required due to the risk of ventricular and atrial arrhythmias.
- ♦ Electrolyte abnormalities, particularly hypokalemia and hypomagnesemia, should be corrected to minimize the risk of cardiac arrhythmias.
- ♦ A right heart catheterization may be performed before starting therapy to obtain baseline hemodynamic status; however, invasive hemodynamic monitoring is not routinely recommended.
- ♦ The following parameters should be carefully monitored:
  - BP, HR, cardiac rhythm, and jugular vein assessment to determine intravascular volume.
  - Hemodynamic parameters if available from a pulmonary artery catheter or central venous catheter.
  - Urine output and kidney function.
  - Electrolytes, especially potassium and magnesium.
  - Platelets: Thrombocytopenia is a rare potential adverse reaction.

(Ayres & Maani, 2023; UptoDate®, Lexidrug™, 2025)

> ***Linking Knowledge to Practice***
>
> ✓ *Potassium should be closely monitored in patients receiving milrinone therapy because enhanced diuresis is an anticipated outcome of therapy.*
>
> ✓ *When increased diuresis occurs because of an improvement in CO the dose of diuretics may need to be decreased.*
>
> *(Ayres & Maani, 2023)*

Key Pharmacokinetic and Pharmacodynamics Information for Milrinone

- ♦ IV onset of action is 5 to 15 minutes.
- ♦ Half-life elimination in patients with HF is between 2 and 2.5 hours.
- ♦ If the patient has any kidney impairment the half-life elimination will be prolonged.
- ♦ The half-life will also prolong as the length of infusion time increases because tissue stores become saturated.

(Ayres & Maani, 2023; Heidenreich et al., 2022; Chong et al., 2018; UptoDate®, Lexidrug™, 2025)

> ***Linking Knowledge to Practice***
>
> ✓ *In a patient who is in atrial fibrillation prior to starting milrinone it is important that the ventricular rate is controlled. Although milrinone does not exert a strong chronotropic effect there can still be an increase in ventricular rate in the setting of atrial fibrillation.*

Important Medication Interactions with Milrinone

- ♦ Anagrelide, a medication used to treat thrombocythemia, can increase the adverse effects of milrinone.
  - Anagrelide also inhibits PDE-3.
  - Anagrelide should not be given in patients receiving milrinone.

(Ayres & Maani, 2023; UptoDate®, Lexidrug™, 2025)

Vasopressin Agonists

Mechanism of Action & Types of Vasopressin Agonists

- Vasopressin is a non-catecholamine hormone that is produced in the hypothalamus and released by the posterior pituitary gland. This hormone plays an important role in overall homeostasis. The term vasopressin will be used in this section, and it is synonymous with arginine vasopressin.
  - Vasopressin is known as ADH and is responsible for osmoregulation through water conservation. It regulates the permeability of the renal collecting ducts to water.
  - Vasopressin is also secreted based on the baroreflex and causes constriction of smooth muscle and thus participates in regulating homeostasis of the CV system.
- Vasopressin stimulates a group of receptors named vasopressin receptors. It also can stimulate oxytocin and purinergic receptors that work together to regulate physiological responses.
- The V1 receptor (also known as the AVPR1a receptor and previously known as the V1a receptor) is mainly vascular. When the V1 receptor is stimulated the following effects occur:
  - Vasoconstriction of vascular smooth muscle.
  - Efferent arteriole constriction.
  - Platelet aggregation.
  - Glycogenolysis (the process of stored glycogen being broken down into glucose).
  - Endothelial release of nitric oxide leading to vasodilation of coronary and pulmonary vessels.
  - Note: When vasopressin is used at pressor doses the V1 receptors also cause contraction of the smooth muscle in the GI tract.
- The V2 receptors (also known as AVPR2 receptors) are in the distal tubule, connecting tubule, and collecting ducts. These receptors regulate the antidiuretic effect of vasopressin. V2 receptors are also found on vascular endothelium. When V2 receptors are stimulated the following effects occur:
  - Antidiuretic effect:
    - cAMP increases resulting in increased water permeability at the renal tubule which increases water reabsorption and decreases urine volume.
    - Vasopressin keeps plasma osmolality between 275 and 290 mOsm/kg.
    - An increase in osmolarity or a decrease in blood volume will stimulate the release of vasopressin.
  - Release of clotting factor VIII and von Willebrand factor.
- V3 receptors (previously known as V1b receptors) are mainly central. When V3 receptors are stimulated the following effects occur:
  - Secretion of ACTH, also called corticotropin.
  - Possible involvement in the secretion of other hormones including insulin and prolactin.

(Burnstock, 2018; García-Álvarez & Arboleda-Salazar, 2023; Landry & Oliver, 2001; Robben et al., 2004; UptoDate®, Lexidrug™, 2025)

- Table 21 lists the types of vasopressin agonists. In addition to AVP, two analogs were created by altering the sequence of one or more amino acids. The purpose of vasopressin analogs is to offer a longer half-life and receptor selectivity. The remainder of this section will focus on AVP.

The Baroreceptor Reflex

Baroreceptors in the aortic arch and carotid sinus, sense arterial wall tension and respond (baroreceptor reflex). Decreased arterial wall tension activates the SNS and RAAS, and releases vasopressin to raise BP by vasoconstriction and water retention. When HTN is sensed, the SNS, RAAS, and vasopressin response decrease, and the parasympathetic system is activated to lower BP by decreasing HR and vasodilating vessels (Palma & Kaufman, 2025).

Table 21 Types of Vasopressin Agonists			
Name of Medication	**Drug Specifics**	**Receptors**	**Use**
Vasopressin or Arginine Vasopressin	Synonymous with ADH.	V1, V2, V3.	Sepsis, other vasodilatory shocks, cardiac arrest.
Desmopressin Acetate	Synthetic analog of vasopressin.	V2.	Central DI, bleeding disorders.
Terlipressin	Synthetic analog of vasopressin.	Selectivity highest for V1 (also some V2 & V3).	Portal HTN, hepatorenal syndrome, bleeding gastric or esophageal varices, septic shock.
(García-Álvarez & Arboleda-Salazar, 2023)			

Linking Knowledge to Practice

✓ *ACTH is a hormone produced by the anterior pituitary gland. One of its important functions is to stimulate the adrenal glands to release cortisol (a glucocorticoid), aldosterone (a mineralocorticoid), and epinephrine and norepinephrine (medullary hormones). ACTH also affects attention, learning, and memory.*

Indications for Vasopressin

- Septic shock and other vasodilatory shock states
  - Vasopressin should be considered as an adjunctive medication when MAP goal is not achieved with a sympathomimetic vasopressor such as norepinephrine.
  - Vasopressin can also be used as an adjunctive agent to decrease the dose requirement of a sympathomimetic agent.
- DI (central, acute) [off label]. Vasopressin may be considered short term in the early postoperative period after transsphenoidal surgery.
- Deceased organ management [off label]. Vasopressin can be used in deceased organ donors, particularly those who are declared brain dead, to stabilize BP or to treat DI.

(UptoDate®, Lexidrug™, 2025)

Linking Knowledge to Practice

✓ *DI is caused by a vasopressin deficiency or an abnormal response to vasopressin. There are two types of DI.*
- *In central DI there is a decreased production of vasopressin by the hypothalamus or a decreased release of vasopressin from the pituitary. Central DI can be idiopathic, or it can occur secondary to a brain tumor or head injury.*
- *In nephrogenic DI the problem is the kidneys do not appropriately respond to vasopressin due to a mutation of the V2 receptor.*

(García-Álvare & Arboleda-Salazar, 2023)

Linking Knowledge to Practice

✓ *When vasopressin is used to treat DI the minimum effective dose is used to prevent the development of hyponatremia. Vasopressin will cause the kidneys to reabsorb water. If too much water is reabsorbed the amount of sodium in the bloodstream will be diluted and the patient will develop hyponatremia.*

Advanced Concept Focus:
Rationale for Vasopressin in Septic Shock

- Vasodilation, caused by prostacyclin synthesis and increased nitric oxide production triggered by inflammatory cytokines, is the primary driver of hypotension in sepsis.
- Fluid resuscitation to fill a dilated vascular bed is the first-line treatment followed by vasopressor therapy.
- In septic shock there are appropriate and substantial increased levels of catecholamines such as norepinephrine and appropriate activation of the RAAS resulting in increased levels of angiotensin II.
  - However, there is failure to respond appropriately to these vasoconstrictors thus vasodilation and hypotension persist.
  - The underlying pathophysiology is failure of the smooth vascular muscle to constrict.
- Adequate vasoconstriction requires norepinephrine and angiotensin II to bind to and activate receptors on the surface of smooth muscle cells initiating a process that results in increased intracellular calcium.
  - Increased intracellular calcium occurs because calcium is both released from intracellular stores and extracellular calcium enters the cell through calcium channels.
  - The high concentration of intracellular calcium triggers subsequent activity that results in muscle contraction.
  - If intracellular calcium is not adequate vasoconstriction will not occur even though there are increased circulating levels of norepinephrine and angiotensin II.
- There are several pathological processes that occur in sepsis that hinder appropriate muscle contraction, and this contributes to hypotension.
  - Desensitization of $\alpha 1$ receptors due to the inflammatory response and metabolic acidosis.
  - Adrenergic receptors are less responsive in the setting of high circulating levels of catecholamines.
  - The cell membrane potential is altered. The mechanisms at work are discussed below:
    - The resting action potential of vascular smooth muscle cells is negative.
    - When the membrane potential becomes positive a depolarization occurs, and calcium channels are opened and the concentration of intracellular calcium increases.
    - However, when the membrane potential becomes more negative (referred to as hyperpolarization) calcium channels are closed and relaxation occurs due to decreased intracellular calcium.
    - Several factors impact the cell membrane actional potential including potassium channels. While circulating levels of norepinephrine and angiotensin II are high in septic shock there is not an appropriate vascular response to these levels likely because of the activation of potassium channels in the vascular smooth muscle.
    - When a specific type of potassium channel (K_{ATP}) is opened potassium leaves the cell resulting in hyperpolarization of the membrane potential which prevents calcium from entering the cell. K_{ATP} channels are activated when there is a decrease of intracellular ATP and when there is an increase in cellular concentrations of hydrogen ions and lactate as seen in metabolic acidosis.
  - There are also known activators of the K_{ATP} channels including atrial natriuretic peptide and adenosine. Levels of atrial natriuretic peptide and adenosine are elevated in sepsis. Potassium channels can also be activated by increased nitric oxide discussed below.

- Vasopressin can block K_{ATP} channels and interfere with nitric oxide signaling (discussed below) resulting in an increased impact of adrenergic drugs on vascular smooth muscle. This enhances the effects of catecholamines on vascular smooth muscle.

♦ Increased synthesis of nitric oxide contributes to hypotension:
- Increased nitric oxide synthesis contributes to both hypotension and resistance to vasopressor therapy that is seen in septic shock.
- In septic shock there is increased production of nitric oxide in different types of cells including smooth muscle cells. Pro-inflammatory cytokines and endotoxin contribute to increased inducible nitric oxide synthase and thus increased nitric oxide.
- In addition to the direct effect of nitric oxide on vasodilation and vasopressor resistance, nitric oxide also contributes to the activation of potassium channels in the vascular smooth muscle.
- Even though nitric oxide is a primary driver of hypotension in septic shock, complete inhibition of nitric oxide is not desirable because nitric oxide plays a valuable role in the immune response to infection. For this reason, selective inhibitors of nitric oxide are thought to be preferred in the treatment of refractory septic shock.
- Harm has been shown with the use of a non-selective nitric oxide inhibitor (López et al., 2004).

♦ Vasopressin deficiency contributes to hypotension:
- Under normal physiological conditions, vasopressin does not play a major role in the maintenance of arterial BP because its most important action is water conservation.
- The water conservation effect of vasopressin occurs at low plasma levels of vasopressin, but the vasoconstrictive effects only occur at much higher plasma levels.
- Vasopressin is secreted in response to the baroreflex and when this occurs vasopressin participates in vasoconstriction.
- Vasopressin is released early from the posterior lobe of the pituitary in response to hypotension in sepsis. When vasopressin is released, it has several effects including:
  - Potentiation of the effects of elevated plasma norepinephrine levels.
  - Inactivation of potassium channels in vascular smooth muscle.
  - Blunting of the increase in cGMP that is induced by nitric oxide and decreasing the synthesis of inducible nitric oxide synthase.
- As septic shock worsens the initial high levels of vasopressin fall to an inadequate level over a period of 72 hours.
  - Possible reasons include: 1) depletion of pituitary stores of vasopressin following a full-scale release of vasopressin in the early stage of septic shock, 2) impaired synthesis of vasopressin, and 3) autonomic dysfunction in the setting of septic shock.
  - Autonomic dysfunction can interfere with the normal baroreflex that regulates the release of vasopressin in response to a decrease in BP.
- Vasopressin levels remain remarkably low for up to 7 days from the onset of septic shock and this contributes to the vasodilatation and hypotension seen in septic shock.
- A greater vasopressin deficiency is seen with more severe infections.
- Even though there is not adequate vasopressin to produce a vasoconstrictor effect, the level of vasopressin remains adequate for appropriate antidiuretic effect.

♦ Vasopressin administration can reduce the catecholamine requirements and thus potentially reduce complications associated with high doses of catecholamine vasopressors.

♦ Vasopressin also improves the vascular responsiveness to catecholamines.

♦ Vasopressin receptors may be better preserved than adrenergic receptors in an environment where there is a high level of circulating catecholamines and in the environment of metabolic acidosis.

(Arias-Ortiz & Vincent, 2024; García-Álvarez & Arboleda-Salazar, 2023; Holmes et al., 2021; Landry & Oliver, 2001)

Linking Knowledge to Practice

- ✓ *Maintenance of BP involves the interaction of three systems: SNS, RAAS, and AVP system. Under normal circumstances the role of vasopressin in BP maintenance is minimal.*
- ✓ *However, when the RAAS or SNS is compromised, vasopressin becomes more important. This is the case in sepsis where patients may not respond appropriately to medications that stimulate the SNS or RAAS.*

Linking Knowledge to Practice

- ✓ *At a therapeutic dose for the treatment of vasodilatory shock vasopressin stimulates V1 receptors resulting in an increase in SVR and a rise in MAP. In response to the rise in MAP there may be a decrease in CO and HR.*
- ✓ *The goal is for vasopressin to restore vascular tone and decrease the need for catecholamine vasopressors that are associated with undesirable adverse effects. High doses of catecholamines are associated with arrhythmias and end organ/tissue ischemia.*
- ✓ *However, vasopressin is also associated with undesirable effects related to potential reduced blood flow to the heart, kidneys, and intestines. Vasopressin has been associated with mesenteric ischemia, skin necrosis, digital ischemia, and decreased cardiac output. Vasopressin is not recommended at a dose of more than 0.04 units/minute to reduce the risk of ischemic complications.*

(Russell et al., 2008; UptoDate®, Lexidrug™, 2025)

Terlipressin: A Vasopressin Analog

- Terlipressin, a synthetic analog of vasopressin, is a predominantly V1 receptor agonist with high vascular selectivity. It is a prodrug that has a longer half-life than vasopressin.
- Terlipressin has been studied as an alternative to norepinephrine in the setting of septic shock.
- In a randomized double blind clinical trial of more than 500 patients there was no difference in 28-day mortality between norepinephrine and terlipressin. However, there were more serious adverse events in the terlipressin group (Liu et al., 2018).
- In a meta-analysis of six research studies, terlipressin did not add survival benefit compared to norepinephrine in patients with septic shock (Huang et al., 2019).
- In a small, randomized controlled trial norepinephrine was compared to norepinephrine plus terlipressin in patients with septic shock. At 12 hours patients treated with norepinephrine and terlipressin had 1) lower norepinephrine dose requirements, 2) shorter duration of vasopressor administration during the ICU stay, 3) lower lactate levels, 4) increased urine output, and 5) greater reduction in the sequential organ failure assessment (SOFA) score. These results pointed to the conclusion that norepinephrine plus terlipressin might be helpful in achieving early resuscitation goals in septic shock. However, there was no difference in ICU mortality between the groups (Sahoo et al., 2022).

Linking Knowledge to Practice

- ✓ *Desmopressin acetate, a vasopressin analog, is more commonly used in the treatment of bleeding disorders due to fewer adverse effects compared to vasopressin.*

(García-Álvare & Arboleda-Salazar, 2023)

Advanced Concept Focus:

Vasopressors and Outcomes in Septic Shock

- Vasopressin was tested against norepinephrine in the treatment of septic shock in a multi-center, randomized, double-blind trial, the Vasopressin in Septic Shock Trial (VASST study).
  - The primary endpoint was 28-day mortality after the start of either vasopressin or norepinephrine. There was no difference in 28-day mortality between the medications.
  - The conclusion of the study was that vasopressin did not reduce mortality compared to norepinephrine in the treatment of septic shock.

(Russell et al., 2008)

- In an analysis of the VASST study data the major hemodynamic difference in patients initially treated with vasopressin compared to norepinephrine was a reduction in HR in those receiving vasopressin.
  - There was no difference in cardiac index or SV index between the groups although more inotropic agents were used in the vasopressin group in patients with more severe shock.
  - Any reduction in CO with vasopressin seemed due to a reduction in HR as opposed to a reduction in SV index.

(Gordon et al., 2012)

- In a double-blind randomized study including 409 patients, four initial interventions were tested in patients with septic shock: 1) vasopressin plus hydrocortisone, 2) vasopressin plus placebo, 3) norepinephrine plus hydrocortisone, and 4) norepinephrine plus placebo.
  - The hypothesis was the potential early use of vasopressin in improving renal outcomes. The primary outcome was the number of AKI free days.
  - The percentage of patients who developed AKI was not statistically different between those receiving vasopressin and those receiving norepinephrine. There was less use of RRT in the vasopressin group but no statistically significant difference in mortality between the patients who were treated with vasopressin compared to those treated with norepinephrine.
  - This study did not provide evidence that vasopressin should be the first-line agent over norepinephrine in the treatment of septic shock, although there were some findings pointing to potential benefit with the use of vasopressin.

(Gordon et al., 2016)

- In a small retrospective study, the early addition of vasopressin within 4 hours was evaluated against treatment with norepinephrine alone. The study outcome was the time to goal MAP.
  - Patients started on early vasopressin achieved and maintained the goal MAP sooner.
  - These findings generated the hypothesis that the early addition of vasopressin in septic shock may result in achieving the goal MAP sooner and contribute to the resolution of end organ dysfunction at the 72-hour mark compared to later or no addition of vasopressin.

(Hammond, Cullen et al., 2019).

- In a review of the safety and efficacy of vasopressors in the treatment of shock, norepinephrine was ranked the first choice followed by either vasopressin or epinephrine. Angiotensin II and dopamine were found to have limited indications in shock (Russell, 2019).
- In a systematic review and meta-analysis of 23 trials, authors found that new onset atrial fibrillation occurred 23% less frequently when vasopressin was used in conjunction with a catecholamine (McIntyre et al., 2018).
- In a subsequent analysis comparing norepinephrine alone to norepinephrine in combination in vasopressin, there was a lower risk of cardiac arrhythmia when norepinephrine was used in combination with vasopressin but there was also a higher risk of digital ischemia. The risk of digital ischemia was higher when vasopressin was used without optimization of fluid status and CO (García-Álvarez & Arboleda-Salazar, 2023; Nagendran et al., 2019).

- In a systematic review and meta-analysis of 23 randomized trials involving patients in septic shock, the use of vasopressin or vasopressin analogs showed no significant improvement in reducing 28-day or 30-day mortality compared to catecholamines alone.
  - However, in a subgroup analysis the use of terlipressin was shown to have possible survival benefit compared to the use of catecholamines alone.
  - This analysis also showed that vasopressin or its analogs increased the risk of digital ischemia compared to the use of catecholamines.

(Yao et al., 2020).

- In a small, randomized trial of patients with septic shock, norepinephrine alone versus norepinephrine in combination with vasopressin was tested.
  - The primary outcome was lactate levels.
  - Lactate levels were significantly higher in the norepinephrine group at 6, 12, 18, and 48 hours compared to the group who received norepinephrine in combination with vasopressin.
  - There was also improvement in the secondary outcomes of renal function and earlier recovery of septic shock in patients who received a combination of norepinephrine and vasopressin compared to patients who received only norepinephrine.

(Hussien et al., 2021)

- In a systematic review and meta-analysis of 5 studies the authors evaluated the impact of starting vasopressin within 6 hours of the diagnosis of septic shock compared to starting vasopressin later or not at all.
  - In this analysis starting vasopressin within 6 hours of diagnosis did not result in decreased short term mortality or shorter ICU LOS.
  - However, starting vasopressin within the first 6 hours of septic shock diagnosis was associated with less need for RRT.

(Huang et al., 2021)

- A retrospective study of patients with septic shock who received vasopressin demonstrated the following:
  - When vasopressin was started in patients with higher norepinephrine doses, or in patients with higher lactate levels, there was an associated higher in-hospital mortality.
  - This raised the question regarding the potential benefit of vasopressin use earlier in septic shock.

(Sacha et al., 2022).

- In a systematic review and meta-analysis of 11 trials involving 4,803 patients, the authors compared outcomes of norepinephrine in septic shock compared to other vasopressors.
  - Other vasopressors included dopamine, phenylephrine, epinephrine, vasopressin, and terlipressin.
  - The results of this analysis did not show the superiority of norepinephrine in terms of the achievement of the goal MAP or a reduction in mortality.
  - However, the results did show norepinephrine to be superior in terms of preventing cardiac arrhythmias, thus making it a safe vasopressor option in the treatment of septic shock.

(Ruslan et al., 2021)

- In a review of 8 multicenter randomized trials of vasopressors in septic shock, norepinephrine remained the first-line vasopressor in the treatment of septic shock.
  - Second-line vasopressors included vasopressin, epinephrine, and angiotensin II.
  - More research is needed to determine the optimal dose of angiotensin II and the types of patients who would most benefit from its use.
  - Two synthetic analogs of vasopressin, (terlipressin and selepressin), are not recommended in the treatment of septic shock due to their potential risk of ischemic complications.
  - The use of methylene blue remains controversial due to limited clinical evidence.

(Jozwiak, 2022)

- In a multi treatment meta-analysis of randomized controlled trials involving septic shock the authors evaluated 8 different treatment options involving either a single vasoactive medication treatment or combination treatment. Treatment options included epinephrine, norepinephrine, dopamine, dobutamine, vasopressin, terlipressin, norepinephrine in combination with dobutamine, and norepinephrine in combination with vasopressin.
  - The results of this analysis suggest that norepinephrine in combination with dobutamine may result in lower 28-day mortality.
  - Also in this study, dopamine was associated with a higher 28-day mortality compared to norepinephrine, vasopressin, and terlipressin.

(Jia et al., 2023)

- In an updated meta-analysis of 14 randomized controlled trials norepinephrine was found to be favorable over other vasopressors in improving outcomes in septic shock.
  - Eight of the 14 studies evaluated 28-day mortality and norepinephrine was associated with lower 28-day mortality compared to other vasopressors.
  - Seven studies evaluated ICU LOS, and norepinephrine was associated with fewer ICU days.
  - Norepinephrine is also associated with less cardiac arrhythmias compared to other vasopressors.
  - Interestingly, norepinephrine did not have an advantage over other vasopressors in achieving the goal MAP. This is why vasopressin has been studied as an agent to add to norepinephrine in the treatment of septic shock.
  - Larger randomized, blinded, controlled trials are needed to confirm the efficacy of norepinephrine compared to other vasopressors.

(Xu et al., 2025).

- In a systematic review and meta-analysis of eight studies comparing norepinephrine and vasopressin as first-line agents in septic shock, there was less need for RRT in the patients treated initially with vasopressin.
  - There was no difference in mortality, other adverse outcomes, or LOS between the use of vasopressin or norepinephrine as a first-line agent.
  - The authors concluded that vasopressin can be considered as a first-line agent in septic shock in patients with risk factors for kidney injury that may lead to the need for RRT.

(Sedhai et al., 2022)

- In a multicenter retrospective study of 385 patients, investigators evaluated whether or not the administration of vasopressin earlier in septic shock would reduce end organ damage and all-cause mortality.
  - The primary outcome was a composite of a change in the SOFA score of >3 from baseline at 72 hours and / or in-hospital mortality.
  - All patients received vasopressin within 48 hours of shock onset with a mean time of initiation of 7.3 hours after the start of norepinephrine.
  - The primary outcome was driven by in-hospital mortality. For every hour delay in initiating vasopressin, the odds of experiencing one of the components of the primary outcome increased.
  - The conclusion of the study is that the earlier administration of vasopressin in septic shock may decrease organ dysfunction and all-cause mortality.

(Rydz et al., 2022)

- In a single center multi-site retrospective study patients who had vasopressin started within 3 hours of norepinephrine had a shorter time to shock resolution compared to patients who had vasopressin added more than 3 hours after the start of norepinephrine. The authors concluded that there may be an opportunity to improve clinical outcomes with the early addition of vasopressin to norepinephrine in patients with septic shock (Brask et al., 2023).
- In a retrospective study of 938 patients who received vasopressin as adjunctive therapy to catecholamines, patients were determined to be either a vasopressin responder or a non-responder.

A vasopressin responder was a patient who required a lower catecholamine dose 6 hours after the start of vasopressin. Vasopressin responders were found to have a better clinical trajectory than vasopressin non-responders and thus vasopressin responsiveness may be a prognostic marker for the patient's short term clinical trajectory.

(Bauer et al., 2023)

- ♦ A recent multicenter observational study evaluated responsiveness to vasopressin when added to norepinephrine in patients with septic shock.
  - There was a positive hemodynamic response rate of 79% 2 hours after the initiation of vasopressin.
  - This positive hemodynamic response resulted in a significant reduction in norepinephrine requirements or other equivalent vasopressor requirements.
  - Factors that negatively affected vasopressin responsiveness included high lactate levels, obesity, and baseline norepinephrine dose of < 0.3 mcg/kg/min.

(Melchers et al., 2025)

> ***Linking Knowledge to Practice***
>
> ✓ *It is important to understand that there are several limitations to single center retrospective studies.*
> - *The interventions in retrospective studies were not implemented in a randomized fashion, and this can introduce bias in the results.*
> - *Additionally, retrospective studies while they may show an association between interventions and outcomes, they cannot prove causation.*
>
> ✓ *For these reasons randomized controlled clinical trials are preferred when evaluating the impact of an intervention on an outcome.*

Advanced Concept Focus:

Weaning of Vasopressors / Vasopressin in Septic Shock

Discontinuation of Norepinephrine First or Vasopressin First in Shock

- ♦ Several studies have identified an increased risk of hypotension or hemodynamic instability when vasopressin is discontinued prior to norepinephrine (Bauer et al., 2010; Bissell et al., 2019; Musallam et al., 2018).
- ♦ However, another small study was stopped early because of the increased risk of hypotension when norepinephrine was tapered first (Jeon et al., 2018).
- ♦ In a retrospective study of 585 patients there was no difference in the incidence of hypotension between patients who had norepinephrine weaned first and those who had vasopressin weaned first (Sacha et al., 2018).
- ♦ In several of the above clinical studies the method for de-escalating vasopressin (abrupt discontinuation versus down titration or weaning) was not defined.
- ♦ In a systematic review and metanalysis of six studies the discontinuation of norepinephrine prior to vasopressin resulted in less clinically significant hypotension. However, there was no difference in LOS or hospital mortality. Larger studies were recommended to confirm findings (Hammond, Sacha et al., 2019).
- ♦ A Mayo Clinic retrospective cohort study of 2,035 patients who received both norepinephrine and vasopressin for the diagnosis of shock evaluated the differences in outcomes between patients in whom norepinephrine was discontinued first and patients in whom vasopressin was discontinued first.
  - In this study there was a higher incidence of hypotension in patients who had vasopressin discontinued prior to norepinephrine.

Also, there was increased hospital mortality and 28-day mortality in the group where vasopressin was discontinued first, although there was no difference in ICU LOS or mortality between the groups.

- In this study vasopressin was not weaned or down titrated, but rather it was turned on or off based on patient needs. Vasopressin was turned off in this study when the patient's norepinephrine requirements were trending downward. In the group where norepinephrine was stopped first, the medication was titrated down rather than abruptly stopped.

(Song et al., 2021)

- ♦ In a small retrospective study of 78 patients with septic shock who had an LVEF of < 40%, there was no difference in clinically significant hypotension between patients in whom norepinephrine was discontinued first and patients in whom vasopressin was discontinued first (Taylor et al., 2022).
- ♦ In a more recent single center study in Brazil, there was no statistical difference in the incidence of hypotension between patients who had vasopressin discontinued first or those who had norepinephrine discontinued first. In this study vasopressin was titrated off (weaned) rather than simply discontinued (Mallmann et al., 2025).
- ♦ At this time the question of which vasopressor should be discontinued first has not been fully answered (Bhattacharjee & Maitra 2023; Hamzaoui et al., 2023). The marker copeptin is easier to measure than vasopressin and correlates with the plasma vasopressin concentration. It has been suggested that copeptin may be helpful in guiding decision making about which vasopressor to discontinue first (Hamzaoui et al., 2023).

Vasopressin Weaning or Abrupt Discontinuation

- ♦ In a single center retrospective review 46 patients were evaluated to determine the difference between abrupt discontinuation or the gradual weaning of vasopressin. Although not statistically significant, the study found a higher rate of hypotension with abrupt discontinuation of vasopressin. There was no difference in hospital mortality between the methods of vasopressin discontinuation suggesting abrupt discontinuation of vasopressin may be safe. A larger study was recommended (Garimella et al., 2020).
- ♦ A multicenter retrospective study evaluated the abrupt discontinuation of vasopressin compared to the down titration of vasopressin. The outcome was time to ICU discharge. In this study there was no difference in time to ICU discharge between abrupt discontinuation of vasopressin compared to down titration (Lam et al., 2021).
- ♦ In another single center retrospective study of patients with septic shock, the abrupt discontinuation of vasopressin was compared to the incremental weaning of vasopressin. In this study there was no difference in the primary endpoint of clinically significant hypotension between the discontinuation strategies. The authors' conclusion was that either discontinuation strategy is acceptable (Murata et al., 2023).

Linking Knowledge to Practice

- ✓ *Vasopressors are classified as either pure vasopressors or inopressors.*
- ✓ *Pure vasopressors (phenylephrine, vasopressin, and angiotensin II) result in arterial vasoconstriction while having no to minimal impact on HR or contractility.*
- ✓ *Inopressors (epinephrine, dopamine, and norepinephrine) can produce arterial vasoconstriction but also impacts cardiac contractility and HR.*

Special Dosing Information for Vasopressin

- ♦ In septic or other vasodilatory shock, vasopressin is given in a fixed dose as opposed to being titrated. The typical dose range is 0.01 to 0.04 units/min. Doses higher than this recommended range are only used as a salvage strategy because these higher doses are associated with ischemic complications.

- The discontinuation strategy for vasopressin has been the subject of recent research. See the Advanced Concept Focus section above on research comparing abrupt discontinuation to incremental weaning. According to UptoDate®, Lexidrug™, vasopressin should be tapered slowly by 0.01 units/min every 30 to 60 minutes because weaning more quickly can result in hypotension.
- In the treatment of DI (central, acute) a continuous infusion may be used. Infusion rates vary based on hospital protocols, but doses are adjusted based on urine output. SQ administration 2 to 3 times daily is another dosing option.
- There is no dose adjustment required for any degree of renal impairment.
  - The medication is unlikely to be significantly dialyzable for patients receiving either peritoneal dialysis or 3 times weekly hemodialysis.
  - Although there is some removal by continuous RRT, the clinical significance is not known.
- The manufacturer labeling has no recommendations regarding hepatic dysfunction.
- Consult drug reference for special dosing information when vasopressin is used for deceased organ donor management or treatment of DI.

Select Adverse Effects of Vasopressin

- Ischemic complications: Stimulation of the V1 receptor results in vasoconstriction. This can potentially result in cardiac, limb, digit, and mesenteric ischemia as well as ischemic skin lesions.
- Decreased platelet count and intractable hemorrhage: Stimulation of the V1 receptor results in platelet activation and this may reduce the overall platelet count.
- Decreased CO / Bradycardia: The vasoconstrictive effects of vasopressin can affect the heart leading to myocardial depression. Additionally, an increase in BP from vasopressin can result in the triggering of a vagal reflex. Vasopressin has CNS effects that can contribute to lowering of HR.
- Renal insufficiency: Renal blood flow can be reduced due to the vasoconstrictive effects of vasopressin.
- Hyponatremia: Hyponatremia can occur due to stimulation of the V2 receptors resulting in an antidiuretic response.

Contraindication Highlights for Vasopressin

- Consult manufacturer recommendations for use in children, pregnant women, and nursing women.
- Hypersensitivity is the only listed absolute contraindication in the United States labeling.
- Vasopressin should be used with caution in patients with atherosclerosis and other forms of CV disease because the medication can potentially worsen cardiac output. The primary mechanism for potential worsening of cardiac out is the increase in SVR from vasoconstriction.
- Also, because of the vasoconstrictive effects of the vasopressin it should be used with caution in patients with renal impairment or other forms of vascular disease.
- The vasoconstrictive effects of vasopressin may trigger a migraine or worsen H/A pain in patients with a history of migraines and therefore should be used with caution in patients with a history of migraines.

Linking Knowledge to Practice

✓ *Adequate fluid resuscitation is vital in any vasodilatory shock. Adequate fluid administration with the use of vasopressin has been shown to prevent the potential complication of mesenteric and splanchnic ischemia.*

(García-Álvarez & Arboleda-Salazar, 2023)

Vasopressin In Cardiac Surgical Patients

- Vasoplegia, a form of vasodilatory shock can be seen in cardiac surgical patients after they are separated from cardiopulmonary bypass.
- In vasoplegia there is hypotension and low SVR in the setting of normal to high CO and adequate fluid resuscitation. Vasoplegia is associated with a poor prognosis.
- Vasoplegia has been associated with certain clinical factors such as LVEF < 35%, the need for a LV assist device (LVAD), thyroid disease, and the preoperative use of certain medications including ACEIs, beta blockers, and IV heparin.
- There are multiple pathways that are activated during major cardiac surgery that results in a systemic inflammatory response syndrome (SIRS).
  - In response to SIRS there is a release of multiple cytokines and proinflammatory and prothrombotic substances.
  - There is also endothelial cell activation and the release of nitric oxide and prostacyclin. Nitric oxide and prostacyclin cause vasodilation.
  - Additionally, retrieved blood from the surgical field that is filtered and reinfused also contains proinflammatory substances.
- Patients with vasoplegia after cardiac surgery have lower levels of vasopressin compared to patients who do not have vasoplegia.
  - Perioperative vasopressin deficiency is particularly prominent in patients undergoing surgery for LVAD placement.
  - Autonomic failure has been proposed as the reason for a more severe vasopressin deficiency in patients who undergo surgery for LVAD placement.
  - There is evidence that those with the greatest vasopressin deficiency will have the most substantial response to vasopressin administration.
- In a randomized double-blind trial 330 patients with vasoplegic shock were randomized to receive vasopressin or norepinephrine as the first-line vasopressor.
  - The primary endpoint was a composite of mortality or severe complications within 30 days. The primary endpoint occurred in 32% of the patients who received vasopressin and in 49% of the patients who received norepinephrine.
  - There was no difference between the groups in the rates of digital or mesenteric ischemia. The authors suggest that vasopressin can be used as the first-line agent in vasoplegic shock post-cardiac surgery to improve outcomes.

  (Hajjar et al., 2017).
- A meta-analysis of randomized studies involving patients undergoing elective and emergency cardiac surgery suggested that vasopressin may reduce complications (Duenser et al., 2018).
- The following recommendations are made in Vasopressor Therapy in Cardiac Surgery-An Experts' Consensus Statement (Guarracino et al., 2021).
  - Norepinephrine, vasopressin, or both drugs in combination is strongly recommended to maintain or restore systemic perfusion pressure in patients undergoing cardiac surgery.
  - There is no recommendation for either medication regarding the risk of ischemic complications.
  - There is a strong recommendation against the use of dopamine in treating vasoplegic shock and there is a recommendation against the use of methylene blue except as a salvage therapy.
  - There is a weak recommendation to add a second vasopressor (either norepinephrine or vasopressin) depending on the initial vasopressor of choice.
  - There is an additional recommendation to consider vasopressin as a first-line agent or to add it to norepinephrine in cardiac surgical patients who have pulmonary HTN or right sided heart failure.

(Levin et al., 2009; García-Álvarez & Arboleda-Salazar, 2023)

Linking Knowledge to Practice

✓ *Patients with HFrEF have chronically elevated levels of vasopressin and copeptin (a precursor). These chronically elevated levels may result in vasopressin depletion and place the patient at risk for vasoplegia when undergoing cardiac surgery.*

(García-Álvarez & Arboleda-Salazar, 2023)

Vasopressin and Renal Function

- AVP may play a role in protecting renal perfusion. There is a higher concentration of V1 receptors in the efferent arterioles than in the afferent arterioles.
  - Afferent arteriole vasoconstriction results in decreased blood flow entering the glomerulus.
  - Constriction of the efferent arteriole (the exiting arteriole) increases intraglomerular pressure and maintains GFR.
  - In a meta-analysis and systematic review of 17 studies of patients with distributive shock, the use of vasopressin (or analog) was associated with a lower incidence of AKI and a reduced need for RRT compared to those treated with catecholamines alone (Nedel et al., 2019).

Society of Critical Care Medicine Recommendations for Vasopressors in Septic Shock in Adult Patients

- For patients on vasopressors the recommended initial target MAP is 65 mmHg rather than a higher MAP target.
- Norepinephrine is the recommended first-line vasopressor over other vasopressors.
- When there is an inadequate MAP on norepinephrine, the addition of vasopressin is recommended over escalating the dose of norepinephrine.
- When there is an inadequate MAP on norepinephrine and vasopressin, the addition of epinephrine is recommended.
- The addition of dobutamine to norepinephrine or the use of epinephrine alone is recommended when there is cardiac dysfunction and persistent hypoperfusion in the setting adequate BP and volume status.
- When central venous access is not already available it is recommended to start vasopressors via peripheral access rather than delaying their start until central venous access is achieved.
- The use of terlipressin is not recommended in septic shock.
- IV corticosteroids are suggested for patients who have an ongoing vasopressor requirement. The typical corticosteroid is IV hydrocortisone. The suggestion is to start IV hydrocortisone when the norepinephrine or epinephrine dose is $\geq$ 0.25 mcg/kg/min at least 4 hours after initiation.
- Note: Refer to full guidelines regarding fluid administration, antimicrobials, and other patient management recommendations.

(Evans et al., 2021)

Advanced Concept Focus:

Why Methylene Blue is Being Investigated in Refractory Septic Shock

♦ Rationale for methylene blue: Methylene blue is an agent that inhibits inducible nitric oxide synthase (Mayer et al., 1993) and has been used as a rescue agent in refractory shock.

The mechanism of action of methylene blue is the inhibition of the soluble guanylate cyclase enzyme. The activation of this enzyme is important in nitric oxide signaling pathway. The mechanism of action of methylene blue may allow it to block the harmful effects of nitric oxide while allowing it to maintain some of its beneficial effects (Arias-Ortiz & Vincent, 2024).

- In a small single center randomized clinical trial in patients with septic shock methylene blue was tested against placebo. The primary outcome was time to discontinuation of vasopressors. Patients who received methylene blue had a shorter time to the discontinuation of vasopressors. There was no difference in mortality (a secondary outcome) between the groups. The results support the need for a larger randomized controlled trial (Ibarra-Estrada et al., 2023).
- In a systematic review and meta-analysis of 6 randomized controlled trials the authors concluded that methylene blue may reduce the duration of vasopressors, hospital LOS, and short-term mortality. However, there was low certainty of evidence due to study limitations, and a large rigorous clinical trial is needed to evaluate the effect of methylene blue in septic shock on patient outcomes (Fernando et al., 2024). In another systematic review and meta-analysis of 3 randomized controlled trials the authors found that treatment with methylene blue reduced the time to discontinuation of vasopressors, days on mechanical ventilation, and ICU LOS. The authors concluded that methylene blue could be a promising vasopressor sparing agent used in the management of septic shock. Again, low certainty of evidence was a limitation to this analysis (Ballarin et al., 2024).
- In another systematic review and meta-analysis of both randomized controlled trials and prospective observational studies there was a significant reduction in mortality in patients with septic shock who were treated with methylene blue. Additional research is needed to confirm these results (Alkazemi et al., 2024).
- In a pilot randomized study 42 patients were evaluated. Patients with septic shock were randomized to receive either standard treatment or standard treatment plus the early administration of methylene blue. Standard treatment included IV fluid, vasopressors, and antibiotics. Patients in the methylene blue group received both a loading dose of methylene blue and a maintenance infusion.
  - In this study methylene blue was started along with vasopressin at the time a second vasopressor was indicated. Methylene blue was administered for 48 hours.
  - Methylene blue resulted in an immediate reduction in the norepinephrine dose and an earlier reduction in the vasopressin dose. It was concluded that methylene blue when added to standard treatment might reduce vasopressor requirements. The use of methylene blue was considered safe.

  (Luis-Silva et al., 2024)
- The current guidelines from the Society of Critical Care Medicine do not give a recommendation regarding the use of methylene blue in refractory septic shock. Larger randomized trials are needed to determine if methylene blue will become a safe and effective option in the treatment of refractory septic shock.

Special Considerations and Monitoring with Vasopressin

- Vasopressin is an ADH analog. The following monitoring is required during administration.
  - Serum and urine sodium.
  - Serum and urine osmolality.
  - Strict measurement of intake and output.
  - Urine specific gravity.
- Water intoxication can occur with vasopressin administration.
  - Nurses should assess for early S&S including H/A, drowsiness, and listlessness.
  - Recognition of early S&S of water intoxication are important to prevent the development of seizure or potential coma.

- ♦ Reversible DI may occur after vasopressin has been discontinued.
  - Urine output, volume status, and electrolytes need to be carefully monitored after vasopressin is discontinued.
  - If DI develops after discontinuation of vasopressin, the vasopressin may need to be restarted to treat the DI.
  - Desmopressin, a synthetic analogue of AVP (ADH) may also be used in the treatment of reversible DI.
- ♦ Meticulous assessment of the IV site is required to avoid extravasation of the medication. The severe vasoconstrictive effects of the medication can cause tissue necrosis. See the Advanced Concept Focus section above on extravasation located in the section on sympathomimetic vasoactive drugs.
- ♦ Careful monitoring for potential ischemic complications is required. Patients are at risk for ischemic colitis and gangrene of the tongue and extremities.

Key Pharmacokinetic & Pharmacodynamics Information for Vasopressin

- ♦ The vasopressor effect of vasopressin is rapid, and peak effect is within 15 minutes of the start of a continuous IV infusion.
- ♦ The peak anti-diuretic effect occurs in 1 to 2 hours.
- ♦ The duration of the vasopressor effect lasts for less than 20 minutes after discontinuation of IV drip.
- ♦ Half-life elimination is 5 to 10, up to 15 to 20 minutes.
- ♦ There is no absorption from the GI tract so the medication must be administered parentally.
- ♦ The medication is not protein bound.
- ♦ AVP does not cross the blood brain barrier.

(García-Álvarez & Arboleda-Salazar, 2023; Up to Date®, Lexidrug™ 2025)

Important Medication Interactions with Vasopressin

- ♦ Consider therapy modification with the following medications due to risk of bradycardia.
  - Ceritinib (an antineoplastic agent)
  - Fingolimod (medication in treatment of multiple sclerosis)
  - Ponesimod (medication in treatment of multiple sclerosis)
  - Siponimod (medication in treatment of multiple sclerosis)
- ♦ Avoid using with landiolol (new beta blocker approved 11/2024) due to the risk of bradycardia. Vasopressin may increase the bradycardic effects of any medication that results in bradycardia.

(Up to Date®, Lexidrug™ 2025)

Appendix 11 provides additional details regarding vasopressin.

Nitroglycerin

NTG is a non-sympathomimetic medication available in various formulations including IV, sublingual (SL), oral, paste, and transdermal patch.

As a vasoactive agent, NTG exerts different levels of the therapeutic action of vasodilation depending on the dosage administered. It is utilized for multiple CV and other clinical indications. It is used in multiple clinical settings and is prescribed for patient use at home.

Appendix 11 provides additional details regarding NTG.

Mechanism of Action of Nitroglycerin

- NTG donates a free radical nitric oxide to activate guanylate cyclase in vascular smooth muscle. This leads to the dephosphorylation of the myosin light chain and subsequent marked venous vasodilation and modest arterial vasodilation.
- Both NTG and isosorbide dinitrate are powerful dilators of vascular smooth muscle.
- All forms of NTG impact preload and afterload in varying degrees depending on dose.
- Venous vasodilation occurs at very low doses of nitrates and very little increase in venous vasodilation is seen with increased doses.
  - Venous vasodilation results in pooling of blood in the periphery leading to a reduction in preload. There is a decrease in RAP, pulmonary artery pressure, PAOP and LV end diastolic pressure.
  - Nitrates are considered better venous than arterial vasodilators.
- At low to moderate doses, nitrates increase the diameter of larger arteries and lower resistance to arterial flow.
  - Nitrates preferentially dilate large coronary arteries and arterioles that meet a certain size.
  - These larger arteries respond better to NTG because of their increased compliance compared to smaller vessels.
  - Nitrates result in a decrease in LV afterload with a reduction in aortic systolic pressure even though there is not a change in brachial artery pressure. This fall in aortic systolic pressure also results in a decrease in O_2 demand.
  - Nitrates affect coronary circulation in both the normal and the ischemic heart. They redistribute blood flow to the collateral channels and from the epicardial areas to the endocardial areas. This allows O_2 and nutrient rich blood to reach ischemic areas.
  - Nitrates also prevent or relieve coronary spasm, and relieve coronary stenosis caused by exercise. There is also evidence that nitrates dilate areas with atherosclerotic stenoses.
- At high doses, nitrates dilate the arterioles most responsible for SVR.
- One study demonstrated that NTG acted as an afterload reducer in patients who had excessive afterload given their level of LV function (patients with severe congestive HF), and it acted as a preload reducer in patients without an increased level of afterload (Haber et al., 1993).
- The hemodynamic effect of nitrates on an individual patient will depend on the patient's LV function and the degree of SNS stimulation. The dose of the nitrate and the presence or absence of drug tachyphylaxis (sometimes called tolerance) will also impact the hemodynamic effect.
- Nitrates also impact regional circulation in the following ways:
  - There is decreased vascular resistance and increased arterial blood flow to peripheral circulation (arms and legs).
  - Venous vasodilation also occurs in the extremities.
  - There is an initial vasodilation in the splanchnic and mesenteric beds, followed by a reflex vasoconstriction.
  - Under normal conditions there is little change in hepatic blood flow.
  - Renal blood flow either is unchanged or decreases slightly; however, a reflex SNS response may cause secondary vasoconstriction.
  - Pulmonary blood flow is decreased, and pulmonary artery pressures are reduced.

(Abrams, 1985; Katzung, 2024; Opie & Horowitz, 2013)

- Oral and topical (paste and transdermal) nitrate preparations are forms of NTG that provide primarily venous vasodilation. IV NTG at lower doses (< 100 mcg/min as defined by some experts) is also primarily a venous vasodilator.

- ♦ SL nitrate tablets and lingual nitrate sprays are fast acting nitrates that impact both venous and arterial vasodilation. Although these formulations have a relatively balanced effect, they exert a more pronounced impact on veins compared to arteries.
- ♦ IV NTG at higher doses (> 100 mcg/min as defined by some experts) will result in a more pronounced arterial vasodilation and more prominent reductions in BP.

(Kelly et al., 2023; Lopez-Rivera et al., 2019; Opie & Horowitz, 2013; Up to Date®, Lexidrug™ 2024)

Linking Knowledge to Practice

✓ *IV NTG at low doses is effective in relieving angina even with predominant venous vasodilation because venous vasodilation reduces preload which decreases MVO_2.*

Linking Knowledge to Practice

✓ *Topical and transdermal formulations are not recommended in clinical emergencies such as hypertensive pulmonary edema because the patient may be diaphoretic. The diaphoresis can interfere with absorption leading to inconsistent dosing.*

(Lopez-Rivera et al., 2019)

Indications for Nitroglycerin

- ♦ Oral and topical NTG (paste or transdermal patch) are used for:
  - Prevention of angina in patients with established coronary artery disease.
  - Treatment of HFrEF in combination with hydralazine to improve outcomes (isosorbide dinitrate only) (Heidenreich et al., 2022).
- ♦ SL tablets and lingual sprays are used for:
  - Prevention of angina in patients with established CAD and chronic stable angina.
  - Acute relief of an acute anginal attack.
  - Termination of an acute angina attack caused by coronary vasospasm (SL NTG only).
  - Adjunct therapy to IV diuretics in acute decompensated HF to relieve congestion and dyspnea (SL only) (Heidenreich et al., 2022).

(Espero Pharmaceuticals, Inc., 2018; Parke-Davis Division of Pfizer, 2018)

- ♦ IV NTG is used for:
  - Acute severe angina or rest angina not responsive to SL NTG.
  - Perioperative HTN and induction of intraoperative hypotension.
  - Acute decompensated HF secondary to acute hypertensive episode.
- ♦ Off label indications include:
  - Hypertensive emergency.
  - Extravasation management with sympathomimetic vasopressor infiltration (NTG paste only). See the Advanced Concept Focus section above on extravasation located in the section on sympathomimetic vasoactive drugs.
  - A diagnostic aid in tilt table testing (SL NTG most commonly, or IV NTG) to provoke symptoms of vasovagal syncope in a patient who has not demonstrated signs of vasovagal syncope during the passive portion of the tilt table test (≥ 20 minutes of head-up tilt to 60-70 degrees).
- ♦ Non-CV indications for NTG include:
  - Anal fissure (alternative agent) (ointment).
  - Tendinopathy persistent (adjunctive agent) (patch) [off label].
  - Uterine relaxation (IV) [off label].

(Up to Date®, Lexidrug™ 2024)

> ***Linking Knowledge to Practice***
>
> ✓ *Patient education should include the following:*
> - *Store SL NTG tablets at room temperature.*
> - *After the first opening of the bottle, keep SL tablets in the original dark container with the lid tightly in place.*
>
> *(Merck Sharp & Dohme Corp., 2014; Parke-Davis Division of Pfizer, 2018)*

Special Dosing Information for Nitroglycerin

IV NTG

- Nonabsorbable IV tubing is recommended and preferred when administering IV NTG. When using a non-absorbable administration set begin at 5 to 10 mcg/min and titrate at increments of 5 mcg/min every 5 minutes. When using an absorbable polyvinyl chloride IV administration set, begin at a dose 20 to 25 mcg/min and titrate at increments of 10 mcg every 5 minutes (American Regent, Inc., 2021; Baxter Health Corporation, 2016).
- When titrating IV NTG with nonabsorbable tubing, it is recommended to initially only increase the dosage by 5 mcg/min every 3 to 5 minutes. Patients with normal or low LV filling pressure may develop hypotension at doses as low as 5 mcg/min.
- Incremental increases of 10 mcg/min can be used if there is no clinical response after titration up to 20 mcg/min. If patients are not responsive to changes of 10 mcg/min, titrations increments can be increased to 20 mcg/min.
- The dose of IV NTG should not exceed 200 mcg/min.
- IV NTG can be started at a higher dose for acute hypertensive cardiac pulmonary edema since this represents a hypertensive crisis. In this situation it is recommended to begin at approximately 20 mcg/min and increase by 15 to 20 mcg/min every 3 to 5 minutes. The typical dose in this situation is usually 100 mcg/min with a maximum dose of 400 mcg/min. At these higher doses there is a decrease in SVR and a reduction in LV afterload (Lopez-Rivera et al., 2019).
- NTG tachyphylaxis (decrease in drug effectiveness) can occur as soon as 24 hours of IV continuous infusion. This will be evident by the loss of symptom control or loss of BP control. Patients should be transitioned to oral therapy prior to reaching 24 hours of a continuous infusion.

(American Regent, 2021; Pfizer, 2016)

> ***Linking Knowledge to Practice***
>
> ✓ *Many IV administration sets are produced with polyvinyl chloride, a plastic that will absorb NTG. This absorption is enhanced by longer administration sets, lower infusion rates, and higher concentrations of IV NTG* (Espero Pharmaceuticals, Inc., 2018).
>
> ✓ *When caring for a patient receiving IV NTG, changing from a polyvinyl chloride administration set to a nonabsorptive administration set will increase the amount of NTG the patient receives by 20 to 60% if a rate adjustment is not made.*
>
> ✓ *If the concentration of the NTG drip is changed for any reason a new IV administration set should be flushed with the new concentration prior to use to assure the proper dose of the NTG is administered.*

Sublingual NTG

- 0.3 or 0.4 mg tablets are used in the treatment of acute angina. The dose can be repeated every 5 minutes if angina is not relieved, up to a total of 3 doses.

- Patients with chest pain who do not have a diagnosis of chronic stable angina should call 911 if symptoms are not relieved within 3 to 5 minutes of taking the first SL tablet. The additional 2 NTG SL tablets can be taken 5 minutes apart while waiting for EMS arrival.
- Patients with chronic stable angina have predictable exertional angina and their use of SL NTG is different from that of a patient in whom angina is not expected.
  - Patients with chronic stable angina are usually instructed to take up to 3 SL NTG with 5 minutes between each dose.
  - SL NTG may also be used to prevent angina. In this case a SL NTG tablet would be taken 5 to 10 minutes prior to an activity known to provoke angina.

(Merck Sharp & Dohme Corp., 2014; Parke-Davis Division of Pfizer, 2018)

> ***Linking Knowledge to Practice***
>
> ✓ *The rationale for educating patients to call 911 if chest symptoms suspicious of acute angina are not relieved by 1 SL NTG tablet is to shorten the time from symptom onset to reperfusion in the event the patient is experiencing an ACS event.*
>
> ✓ *ACS is caused by an acute plaque rupture followed by thrombus formation resulting in either a stable clot (STEMI) or an unstable clot (NSTE-ACS). Both conditions warrant urgent treatment to disrupt the clot and restore perfusion.*
>
> ✓ *ACS is different from stable angina. Patients with stable angina have predictable angina when performing activities that increase demand and thus MVO_2.*

> ***Linking Knowledge to Practice***
>
> ✓ *The usual anti-anginal SL NTG dose of 0.4 mg every 5 minutes for 3 doses is equivalent to 80 mcg/min as an IV infusion. A SL dose of 0.3 mg rather than 0.4 mg may be preferred in older or more frail patients to minimize the risk of hypotension.*
>
> *(López-Rivera et al., 2019)*

Lingual NTG Spray

- The spray pump needs to be primed with 5 sprays prior to use. Once primed it will then deliver the proper dose. If not used for 6 weeks the spray will need to be primed again prior to use.
- Spray should be aimed towards or under the tongue.
- Spray should not be inhaled.
- The patient should not expectorate the dose, nor should the mouth be rinsed for 5 to 10 minutes after the dose is given.
- One spray should deliver 400 mcg NTG (after priming).
- The spray can be repeated once every 5 minutes for a maximum dose of 3 sprays within 15 minutes.
- As with the use of SL NTG, patients should call 911 if no relief of symptoms within 5 minutes of 1 spray. Patients with stable angina are an exception and should follow provider instructions.

(Espero Pharmaceuticals Inc., 2018)

Topical NTG

- The onset of action of both forms of topical NTG is approximately 15 to 20 minutes. This makes these preparations unsuitable for acute angina.

- ♦ The initial dose of a transdermal NTG patch is 0.2 to 0.4 mg/hr. The dose can be increased to a maximum of 0.8 mg/hr. The NTG patch has a duration of 10 to 12 hours. One-time daily dosing, with removal of the patch after 12 hours, allows for the nitrate free period of 12 hours.
- ♦ The duration of NTG paste is only 6 to 7 hours. This requires 2 doses at 6-hour intervals which provides 12 hours of treatment followed by a 12-hour nitrate free period each day. See the box below for details about dosing and the safe and accurate utilization of NTG paste.

(Merck Sharp & Dohme Corp., 2014; Savage Laboratories, 2021)

NTG Paste: Pearls for Application and NTG Free Period

- The proper application of NTG paste impacts the effectiveness of the paste. Note that ½ inch of paste is equal to 7.5 mgs of NTG with 2 inches equaling 30 mgs.
- Place the measuring paper supplied with tube of NTG paste printed side down on a flat surface.
- Squeeze the prescribed amount of ointment onto the measuring paper.
  - The length of the expelled ointment should be the prescribed dose (½ inch, 1 inch, etc.) as marked on the paper.
  - The width of the ointment should be about the size between the 2 dark lines on the measuring paper.
- Turn the measuring paper over and apply the ointment to the skin on the desired location. Application to the chest wall is often the chosen location but other areas can be used. Hair may interfere with absorption of the medication, so find an area with the least hair.
- Once the paper has been placed on the skin, spread the ointment around to an area about the size of the paper (3½″ by 2 ¼″). Do not try to rub the ointment into the skin.
  After gently applying the ointment to the skin surface tape the paper in place.
  - The ointment can stain clothing, so some prefer to cover the area with plastic wrap to assure any ointment that is beyond the sides of the paper won't stain clothes.
  - Plastic wrap is used because it will not absorb the ointment as a gauze pad will.
- Wash hands after application. The presence of ointment on the fingers may result in a H/A.
- When the next application is due, remove the old paper. The next dose will require a new piece of paper. Wipe off any of the old ointment that has not been absorbed by the body.
- Rotating sites can be helpful in preventing skin irritation.
- It is important to have nitrate free periods of time to prevent nitrate tolerance. This nitrate free period is usually scheduled for during the night when people are sleeping and not experiencing activity induced angina.
- The nitrate free period should be 10 to12 hours.
  - Doses should be administered at equally spaced intervals.
  - For example:
    - If the order is NTG paste ½ inch every 6 hours twice a day the first dose would be applied shorty after rising in the morning.
    - The second dose will be applied 6 hours later.
    - Six hours after the second dose was applied the paper should be removed, and any remaining ointment should be wiped off the skin surface to assure the nitrate free period.

(Savage Laboratories, 2021)

Linking Knowledge to Practice

- ✓ *When applying NTG paste the nurse should not touch the paste because digital contact with the paste can result in the nurse developing a H/A that can be severe in some cases.*
- ✓ *NTG paste and patches should be removed from the chest prior to defibrillation. There are reports of arcing and small explosions (Wrenn, 1990).*

Oral NTG

- Oral NTG includes the ER capsule and the oral medications isosorbide mononitrate and isosorbide dinitrate. The onset of action for these agents range from 30 to 60 minutes and therefore none of these medications can be used for acute angina.
- NTG ER is started at an initial low dose and is titrated up based on an achievement of the desired effect (freedom from angina) and the patient's ability to tolerate the dose. Dosing is 3 to 4 times a day. The nitrate free interval is 10 to 12 hours per day. Timing principles described in the box above for achieving a nitrate free period with NTG paste can be applied to the ER NTG capsule.
- Isosorbide mononitrate is longer acting than isosorbide dinitrate allowing for twice a day (intermediate release) or one-time daily dosing (extended release). Isosorbide mononitrate has an elimination half-life of 5 hours and thus 2 doses, 7 hours apart, during waking hours is recommended to allow for the recommended nitrate free period. Isosorbide mononitrate is also available in an ER form allowing for one-time daily dosing.
- Isosorbide dinitrate has a duration of action of 4 to 6 hours. To allow the appropriate nitrate free period isosorbide dinitrate is usually dosed 2 to 3 times a day during waking hours, with a schedule of 7 am and 1pm or 7am, 12 noon and 5pm. The nitrate free period should be 12 to14 hours.

(Merck & Co, 2010; Pfizer, 2022a; Up to Date®, Lexidrug™ 2024)

> ***Linking Knowledge to Practice***
>
> ✓ *With all nitrate preparations the reduction in preload can reduce blood pressure, most specifically in those that are "dry" or preload dependent.*
>
> ✓ *The impact on systolic BP is often slight with oral nitrates, topical nitrates or low dose IV NTG.*
>
> ✓ *When titrating IV NTG the crossover to the "high" dose NTG can occur resulting in more arterial vasodilation and a more substantial decrease in the systolic BP.*
>
> ✓ *When titrating NTG at higher doses the increases should be in smaller increments with longer intervals of time between dose adjustments.*

Select Adverse Effects of Nitroglycerin

- Most adverse effects are dose related and secondary to the vasodilatory effects of NTG.
  - H/As, which can be from mild to severe in some cases, are the most common side effect and worsen with increased doses. H/A can occur immediately after use.
    - Many patients experience a decrease in H/As over time with chronic use.
    - The dose should be decreased in those experiencing H/As. Starting with a lower dose and using slow incremental increases may help reduce the incidence of H/A.
  - Transient lightheadedness or dizziness may occur. These symptoms are often from orthostatic hypotension. Instruct patients on the importance of sitting for a few moments before standing to help diminish the incidence of orthostasis.
  - Hypotension is the most common serious adverse effect and in some cases this can be profound. Patients who are preload dependent or volume depleted are at high risk for considerable hypotension.
  - Patients can develop a reflex compensatory tachycardia in response to vasodilation. Concurrent use of beta blockers can minimize or blunt this reflex tachycardia.
- Uncommon Select Adverse Effects:
  - Syncope is a less common but significant side effect that can occur resulting in falls and other injuries. The likelihood of syncope is diminished with cautious use of other vasodilating medications, in particular PDE-5 inhibitors such as sildenafil, vardenafil, tadalafil, and avanafil.

- Bradycardia, including severe and symptomatic bradycardia, rather than the expected reflex tachycardia, can occur with NTG (American Regent, Inc., 2021; Baxter Health Corporation, 2016). See the ***Linking Knowledge to Practice*** box below for information regarding bradycardia as an adverse effect.
- Crescendo angina can occur with tachyphylaxis (sometimes referred to as tolerance) or with the sudden cessation of higher dose nitrates. Angina may also occur during nitrate free periods.
- Rebound HTN can occur when nitrate preparations are stopped suddenly.
- Rash or skin irritation may occur with paste or transdermal preparations. This is limited by routine site rotation.

♦ Very Rare Side Effect:
- Methemoglobinemia has occurred in patients receiving IV NTG.
- Cases are very rare (< 1%) and occur with moderate to high doses of NTG. There are case reports of methemoglobinemia occurring with high dose NTG used in stabilizing patients prior to open heart surgery (Bojar et al., 1987).
- Renal or hepatic dysfunction may increase the risk of the development of methemoglobinemia.
- Patients with severe anemia may also be at higher risk.

(Kaplan et al., 1985; Merck Sharp & Dohme Corp., 2014; Opie & Horowitz, 2013; Pfizer, 2016; Up to Date®, Lexidrug™ 2024)

Contraindication Highlights for Nitroglycerin

♦ Consult manufacturer recommendations for use in children, pregnant women, and nursing women.

♦ IV NTG is contraindicated in conditions where CO is preload dependent. Those conditions include HOCM, severe constrictive pericarditis, acute pericardial tamponade. and severe restrictive cardiomyopathy (amyloidosis). See Special Considerations and Monitoring section below.

♦ Avanafil must be held for 12 hours, sildenafil and vardenafil for 24 hours, and tadalafil for 48 hours prior to any NTG use (Rao et al., 2025). Severe hypotension can occur.

♦ NTG is not recommended in patients with severe anemia. Large doses of NTG may cause the oxidation of hemoglobin to methemoglobinemia exacerbating the anemia. When used in patients with severe anemia the signs of cyanosis will be masked if methemoglobinemia develops. See the box below.

♦ NTG is contraindicated in patients with increased intracranial pressure or who are at risk for worsening intracranial pressure. NTG dilates vessels in the brain and leads to an increase of cerebral blood volume which can worsen intracranial pressure. Additionally, NTG reduces BP and leads to a reduction in cerebral perfusion pressure.

(American Regent, Inc. 2021; Espero Pharmaceuticals, Inc., 2018; Omnvium Pharmaceuticals, 2024; Pfizer, 2016; Prchal, 2024; Rangel-Castillo, L., Gopinath, S., & Robertson, C. S., 2008; Savage Laboratories, 2021; Up to Date®, Lexidrug™ 2024)

Why Anemia Can Mask Methemoglobinemia

- The degree of cyanosis observed in a patient with methemoglobinemia is determined by the total amount of methemoglobin which is calculated by multiplying the total hemoglobin by the percent of methemoglobin.
- For a patient with a hemoglobin of 9.0 g/dL and 20% methemoglobin the total methemoglobin would be 9.0 g/dL x .2 = 1.8 g/dL methemoglobin.
- For a patient with a hemoglobin of 15.0 g/dL and 20% methemoglobin the total methemoglobin would be 15.0 g/dL x .2 = 3.0 g/dL methemoglobin.

Clinical Pearl: Signs of cyanosis will be masked in a patient with anemia.

Special Considerations & Monitoring with Nitroglycerin

- Hold if SBP ≤ 90 mmHg or ≥ 30 mmHg below baseline to avoid symptomatic hypotension and shock. Hypotension can occur with even small doses of NTG, and patients should be monitored carefully regardless of the dose.
- Hold if tachycardia is present (HR > 100). As SBP decreases HR increases in a normal compensatory fashion. In an already tachycardic patient this reflex tachycardia can result in significantly elevated HRs and can cause angina and worsen outcomes.
- Hold if severe bradycardia is present (HR < 50).
  - In some patients receiving NTG a severe reflex bradycardia can occur resulting in worsening angina or a syncopal episode if the patient is standing or walking.
  - Reflex bradycardia results in the loss of the normal compensatory tachycardia to increase CO when hypotension develops. The mechanism for this effect remains unclear.

(Amsterdam et al., 2014; O'Gara et al., 2013)

- Cautiously use nitrates in patients who are preload dependent or sensitive.
- Patients with aortic stenosis, constrictive pericarditis, restrictive cardiomyopathy (amyloidosis is most common), severe mitral stenosis and HCM become preload dependent as their condition worsens with time.
  - With diastolic dysfunction there is often a smaller LV chamber due to ventricular hypertrophy. This smaller LV chamber results in reduced LV volume at baseline. The venous vasodilation from NTG further reduces preload and there is a subsequent decrease in SV and cardiac output.
  - Patients with HOCM are further dependent on preload as loss of preload worsens the LV outflow tract obstruction (Braunwald et al., 1964; Ommen et al., 2024).
  - Patients with amyloidosis develop biventricular preload dependence and loss of preload to the RV further worsens CO (Shah et al., 2006).
- Patients with a RV infarct will not tolerate preload reduction.
  - About 1/3 of patients with an inferior wall MI also experience RV infarction.
  - In RV infarction the RV distends and may lose some contractility in the early phases of the MI.
  - Any reduction in preload can result in a reduction in LV filling pressures and hypotension can result.
  - Hypotension, elevated JVD and clear lungs are clinical clues that there is RV involvement in the presence of an inferior wall MI.
  - NTG should be avoided in patients suspected of having an RV infarct as the risk of hypotension is high.

  (Amsterdam et al., 2014).

(American Regent, Inc., 2021; Pfizer, 2016; Up to Date®, Lexidrug™ 2024)

Linking Knowledge to Practice

✓ *Reflex tachycardia is common in response to vasodilator therapy. It is designed to support CO in the setting of vasodilation that can decrease preload and afterload.*

✓ *Therefore, it is important for nurses to recognize bradycardia as an unexpected adverse response to the administration of NTG.*

✓ *Bradycardia can occur at even low doses of IV NTG and this bradycardia has been associated with syncopal episodes resulting in injury.*

✓ *Patients on a NTG drip, even on low doses, and if pain free, should be assisted with any out of bed activity such as using the commode.*

(American Regent, Inc., 2021; Baxter Health Corporation, 2016)

Key Pharmacokinetic & Pharmacodynamic Information for Nitroglycerin

- NTG onset of action, peak effect, and duration of action varies based on the preparation.
- Duration of topical and oral nitrates are discussed in the dosing section above. Duration of these nitrates are important when dosing for a nitrate free period.
- IV NTG, SL tablets, and SL spray are considered fast acting nitrates.
  - SL forms work in 1 to 3 minutes with a peak effect in 5 minutes for the tablets and 4 to 15 minutes for spray.
  - IV NTG provides an immediate peak effect with a duration of 3 to 5 minutes. IV NTG is cleared quickly from the system with a half-life of 3 minutes.
- Topical nitrates include NTG paste and the transdermal NTG patch.
  - NTG paste has an onset of action in approximately 15 minutes with a peak effect in 60 minutes.
  - The transdermal patch begins working in about 30 minutes with a peak effect in 120 minutes.
- Oral NTG preparation includes isosorbide mononitrate, isosorbide dinitrate, and oral NTG ER. The duration of action of these medications is discussed above under dosing because the duration impacts the dosing requirements for a nitrate free period.
  - Isosorbide mononitrate is available in immediate release (IR) and ER formulations.
    - IR onset of action and peak plasma concentrations occur in 30 to 60 minutes. The peak anti-anginal effect is 1 to 4 hours.
    - ER time to peak concentration varies by dose and ranges from 2.9 to 4.5 hours.
  - Isosorbide dinitrate has an onset of action with hemodynamic changes noted in 20 to 60 minutes.
  - NTG ER has an onset of action of approximately 60 minutes. The peak effects is 2.5 to 4 hours.
- Due to IV NTG's short half-life hemodynamic rebound can occur if it is stopped suddenly. To avoid this problem IV NTG should be weaned and discontinued rather than abruptly stopped.
  - Neurohormonal activation occurs in response to vasodilation and decreased BP caused by NTG. This neurohormonal activation results in increased HR and vasoconstriction. With the sudden cessation of IV NTG this neurohormonal activation is left unopposed, and HTN and cardiac ischemia can develop.
  - Down titration of an IV NTG infusion, especially at higher doses, causes the neurohormonal response to downregulate as the dosage of NTG is decreased. This prevents hemodynamic rebound and the development of HTN and angina.
  - Although significant hemodynamic rebound is unusual with the sudden withdrawal of topical or oral therapy, it is wise to withdrawal patients from any nitrate preparation to avoid this potential complication.

  (Bauer & Fung, 1993; Frishman, 1992; Pfizer, 2022; Rehnqvist et al., 1988).
- Dosing recommendations to accomplish a nitrate free period with topical and oral agents are discussed in the dosing section above.
- Tachyphylaxis: See the box below on tachyphylaxis and Advanced Concept Focus section below on tachyphylaxis versus nitrate tolerance.

(American Regent, Inc., 2021; Edenbridge Pharmaceuticals, 2025; Espero Pharmaceuticals, Inc., 2018; Heritage Pharmaceuticals, Inc., 2021; Lopez-Rivera et al., 2019; Merck Sharp & Dohme Corp., 2014; Omnvium Pharmaceuticals, 2024; Opie & Horowitz, 2013; Pfizer, 2022; Savage Laboratories, 2021; Up to Date®, Lexidrug™ 2025)

Linking Knowledge to Practice

✓ *IV NTG should always be weaned rather than abruptly stopped to avoid hemodynamic rebound. Hemodynamic rebound can occur because the vasodilation from the NTG activates the RAAS. If NTG is abruptly stopped there is no opposition to the vasoconstrictive effects of the RASS. Weaning to lower doses will help down regulate the RAAS.*

Linking Knowledge to Practice

✓ *Patients receiving topical or oral nitrates can experience an increase in angina during the 8 to 12 hours of nitrate free time. However, substantial hemodynamic rebound as seen with higher doses of IV NTG is unusual with oral preparations.*

Important Medication Interactions with Nitroglycerin

- Any form of NTG should be used with caution when given with other medications that can reduce BP.
- NTG cannot be given in proximity to PDE-5 inhibitors due to the risk of severe hypotension. Avanafil must be held for 12 hours, sildenafil and vardenafil for 24 hours, and tadalafil for 48 hours prior to any NTG use (Rao et al., 2025).
- Concurrent use with soluble guanylate cyclase stimulators (Riociguat) can result in severe hypotension.
- Medications with strong anticholinergic effects may decrease the absorption of NTG especially through slowing of the rate of dissolution of SL NTG (Sawan et al., 2023; Up to Date®, Lexidrug™ 2024).
- Prescribing literature cautions that the anticoagulant effect of heparin may be diminished in the presence of concomitant use of IV NTG, especially with very high doses of IV NTG (American Regent, Inc, 2021; Opie & Horowitz, 2013; Sawan et al., 2023; Up to Date®, Lexidrug™ 2024). However, several reports evaluating this effect have reported no significant interaction between heparin and IV NTG (Berk et al., 1993; Gonzalez et al., 1992; Koh et al., 1995; Nottestad & Mascette, 1994).
- Nitrates may enhance the adverse/toxic effect of Rosiglitazone. Most importantly there is a higher risk of developing ischemia (Up to Date®, Lexidrug™ 2024).

NTG Tachyphylaxis

- Tachyphylaxis can occur with prolonged or continuous use of NTG.
- The mechanism of tachyphylaxis is complex and includes the neurohormonal mechanisms of vasoconstriction that are in direct opposition to the effects of nitric oxide.
- NTG tachyphylaxis can occur with any preparation but is most often associated with oral or topical agents.
- Tachyphylaxis can develop as soon as 24 hours of use. This includes IV NTG infusions.
- A loss of the hemodynamic effects of the current dose of NTG, such as returning chest pain, decrease in chest pain free activity periods, or an increase in BP provide evidence that the patient has developed tachyphylaxis.
- A daily nitrate free period will decrease the likelihood of nitrate tachyphylaxis.
  - The nitrate free period should occur during the patient's least active time when being treated for chronic stable angina, which is most often during sleep.
  - Guidelines recommend a 10 to12 hour nitrate free period.

(Frishman,1992; Katzung, 2024; Parker & Gori, 2001; Savage Laboratories, 2021; Up to Date®, Lexidrug™ 2024)

<u>Advanced Concept Focus</u>:

Drug Tachyphylaxis Versus Drug Tolerance

- Drug tachyphylaxis and drug tolerance are similar but not synonymous terms. While both imply that drug attenuation (change in drug effect) has occurred, tachyphylaxis is often due to cellular depletion whereas tolerance is thought to be due to cellular adaptation.

♦ The terms tolerance and tachyphylaxis are often used interchangeably because the literature is not always clear in defining these to patterns of attenuation.

♦ Drug tolerance is identified when a medication no longer provides the same benefit that it once did. This usually occurs overtime when the longer a medication is taken the less effective it becomes.

- Tolerance is most often noted when a higher dose of a drug is needed to achieve the same effect that was previously achieved at a lower dose.
- Increasing the dose usually increases the effectiveness of the medication and additional dose increases will be needed overtime as further tolerance develops.
- Opioid medications are often associated with drug tolerance.

♦ Drug tachyphylaxis usually occurs more quickly than drug tolerance and can occur with as few as 1 or 2 doses.

- Tachyphylaxis is recognized when there is a rapid decrease in the response to a drug, or a progressive decreased response to repeated doses over a short period of time.
- This is thought to be a biological response due to a decrease in stores, over time, of the neurotransmitter responsible for producing the drug effect. This is also referred to as drug attenuation secondary to cellular depletion.
- Increasing the dosage of the drug does not increase the drug's effectiveness.
- Tachyphylaxis is reversible with a period of drug cessation. This allows for a period without the drug to "reset" the transmitters which will then elicit a normal response with the next medication administration.
- Nitrates are known for tachyphylaxis or tolerance due to this neurohormonal counter-regulation.

♦ Findings in clinical trials have provided insight into the effect of tachyphylaxis:

- Studies have shown reduced efficacy in BP lowering when NTG is administered at regular intervals within a 24-hour period.
- Research results have also shown that the antianginal effect in chronic angina diminishes without a drug-free period, resulting in more instances of breakthrough angina.
- While these trials refer to this phenomenon as nitrate intolerance, it is noted that increasing the dose of the nitrate did not improve its effectiveness. It is only after a nitrate free period that the initial effectiveness is restored supporting the notion that this phenomenon is indeed tachyphylaxis.

♦ Figure 10 provides a simple schematic of the difference between tachyphylaxis and tolerance.

(Hikma Pharmaceuticals USA Inc., 2025; Münzel et al., 2005; Parker et al., 1983; Svensson, 2022; Valeant Pharmaceuticals North America, 2015)

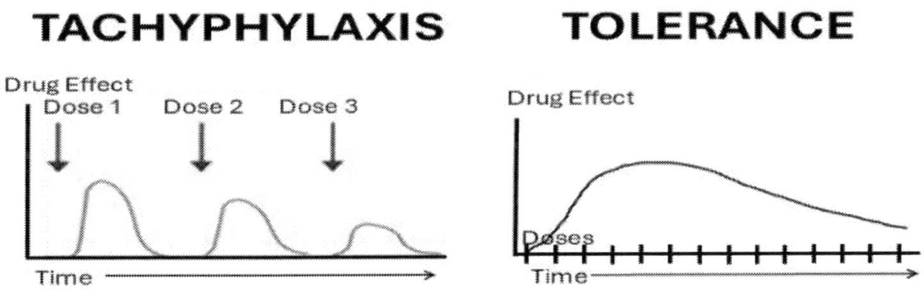

Figure 10: Tachyphylaxis versus Tolerance

> ***Linking Knowledge to Practice***
>
> ✓ *It has been found that in patients with HFrEF who are taking isosorbide dinitrate in combination with hydralazine that hydralazine prevents the nitrate tachyphylaxis. Therefore, in this situation isosorbide dinitrate can be administered 3 or 4 times a day with no nitrate free period.*
>
> *(Gogia et al., 1995)*

Prescribing Pearls for NTG

- The standard dose for SL NTG is 0.4 mg/tablet. In patients at higher risk for hypotension (elderly and frail patients) or in patients who develop hypotension with a dose of 0.4 mg/tablet, the use of a lower dose such as 0.3 mg/tablet might be better tolerated and allow the patient to safely treat or prevent chronic angina.
- Inpatient orders should reflect appropriate monitoring and activity restrictions.
  - Hypotension can occur at even small doses of NTG.
  - Severe paradoxical bradycardia can also occur resulting in syncope.
- H/As from NTG preparations may decrease adherence.
  - Educate patient taking longer acting NTG preparations used in chronic conditions about the possibility of H/As. The patient will usually adjust to the medication over the period of a week or so with the severity of the H/As deceasing.
  - The dose of the medication can also be decreased and slowly up titrated to the recommended dose to help improve tolerance.
  - Acetaminophen may help relieve H/A symptoms.
- Nitrates should not take precedence over beta blocker therapy in the treatment of ACS because nitrates have not demonstrated a mortality benefit in this population and beta blockers do improve mortality (Amsterdam et al., 2014; Byrne et al., 2023; Katzung, 2024; Reeder, 2023). When SBP is considered "soft", choices must be made about which BP lowering medications should be held. BP lowering medications known to improve clinical outcomes in ACS take priority.
- Patients who have critical aortic stenosis present a challenge when presenting with chest pain.
  - NTG will decrease preload in a patient that is preload dependent resulting in a reduced SV leading to hypotension, hemodynamic compromise and a decrease in coronary perfusion.
  - When critical aortic stenosis is present, the impact of the normal sympathetic compensatory mechanism of increased HR to compensate for low CO may not be adequate. In critical AS the volume of blood that can move through the stenosis is fixed. Even with an increase in HR, blood flow through the valve may not be enough to improve cardiac output.
  - There are several small studies demonstrating the benefit of nitrates in patients with AS and acute decompensated pulmonary edema, with both IV and SL NTG without the development of hypotension. However, the studies are small, and providers are encouraged to proceed with caution when using NTG in severe or critical AS (Marquis-Gravel et al., 2016; Otto, 2024).

(American Regent, Inc. 2021; Baxter Health Corporation 2016; Braunwald et al., 1964; Pfizer, Inc. 2016; UptoDate®, Lexidrug™ 2024)

Nitroprusside

Nitroprusside is a powerful venous and arterial vasodilator that can significantly decrease SVR (afterload) as well as decrease ventricular filling (preload) with an overall decrease in BP. When used in the correct population the hemodynamic effects of decreased preload and afterload will improve cardiac output. Nitroprusside is most often used in the treatment of hypertensive crisis and acute decompensated HF. The use of nitroprusside is reserved for a carefully selected group of patients due to its rapid onset of action and potential for life threating adverse effects.

Linking Knowledge to Practice

✓ *Nitroprusside is an effective medication with serious side effects that can become unsafe in the hands of an inexperienced nurse. Therefore, ICU nurses who are caring for a patient with nitroprusside for the first time should seek advice from more experienced ICU nurses or scholarly information to assure patient safety and to prevent avoidable complications.*

(Exela Pharma Sciences, 2017; Namigen, 2016; UptoDate®, Lexidrug™, 2024)

Mechanism of Action of Nitroprusside

- Nitroprusside is comprised of ferrous iron complexes with each ferrous ion binding to 4 cyanide ligands and 1 nitrosyl ligand. Nitroprusside interacts with erythrocytes, albumin and additional proteins to produce nitric oxide. Nitric oxide then reacts with guanylate cyclase in the vascular smooth muscle to produce cGMP which limits the availability of intracellular calcium. Subsequently, vascular smooth muscles relax, and venous and arterial vasodilation occurs.
- Nitroprusside is a powerful arterial vasodilator that can significantly decrease SVR by arterial relaxation. Systolic BP, MAP, and diastolic BP are all decreased. The impact of nitroprusside on diastolic BP is thought to be greater than with NTG because nitroprusside dilates smaller arterioles responsible for SVR while NTG has a stronger effect on larger conductance vessels because they are more compliant. This has been proposed as the reason for the development of coronary steal with nitroprusside (Hottinger et al., 2014). See the box below regarding coronary steal.
- The reduction in LV afterload has been known to improve CO in acute decompensated HFrEF, acute mitral regurgitation, and in patients with severe aortic stenosis with severe LV systolic dysfunction.
- Venous vasodilation results in pooling of venous blood in the periphery and decreases venous return resulting in decreased ventricular filling (reduced preload) with a resultant decrease in LV end diastolic volume and PAOP.

(D'Elia et al., 2024; Hottinger et al., 2014; Khot et al., 2003)

Indications for Nitroprusside

Originally, a first-line agent for the treatment of acute HTN in the mid-1970s, the use of nitroprusside has decreased over the years as newer agents became available. Concerns for the development of significant hypotension and the potential for cyanide toxicity with nitroprusside have resulted in the use of safer medications to treat acute HTN.

In recent years nitroprusside has usually been reserved for the treatment of acute hypertensive emergency and acute decompensated heart failure (Hottinger et al., 2014). Nitroprusside continues to be very effective in select situations due to its rapid onset and short duration of action. It is still used in critical situations, and when HTN is refractory to first-line agents.

See Table 22 for details on the indications for nitroprusside.

Special Dosing Information for Nitroprusside

- Nitroprusside is administered as an IV infusion and is not to be administered as an IV push medication.
- Dosing begins as low as 0.1 to 0.25 mcg/kg/min with titration by 0.5 mcg/kg/min every 5 minutes.
- Typical infusion rates are 0.5 to 4 mcg/kg/min with a maximum dose of 10 mcg/kg/min.
  - Infusions of 8 to 10 mcg/kg/min should not exceed 10 minutes due to cyanide toxicity risk. If BP does not improve, consider an alternative agent.
  - Doses < 2 mcg/kg/min greatly reduce the risk of cyanide toxicity.
- Patients with reduced kidney function are at an increased risk of developing thiocyanate toxicity as serum thiocyanate levels increase with poor renal clearance.
  - Limit infusion rates to < 3 mcg/kg/min if eGFR < 30 mL/min/1.73 m^2.
  - Limit infusion rates of a maximum of 1 mcg/kg/min if the patient is anuric.
- There are no recommendations for adjustments with liver disease. However, patients with hepatic dysfunction are at a higher risk for the development of thiocyanate toxicity.

(Exela Pharma Sciences, 2017; Namigen, 2016; Up to Date®, Lexidrug™, 2024)

Table 22 Indications for Nitroprusside	
Indication	**Key Points**
Hypertensive Emergency	▪ Earliest indication approved by the FDA was for the treatment of HTN due to the drugs profound ability to reduce BP through aggressive arterial vasodilation. ▪ Currently approved for the immediate reduction of BP in hypertensive crisis. ▪ Less toxic medications for the emergent reduction in BP are preferred if effective. ▪ Also indicated for the induction and maintenance of controlled hypotension in the operating room to minimize bleeding (Exela Pharma Sciences, 2017).
Acute Decompensated Heart Failure (adjunctive agent)	▪ Indicated for use in acute decompensated HF with volume overload in those without symptomatic hypotension to reduce LV end diastolic pressure, PAOP, SVR and MAP. With a reduction of MAP and SVR there is a subsequent increase in SV and CO. This results in the unloading of the LV, further decreasing LV end diastolic volume, and is considered an adjunct to diuretic therapy. ▪ Preload is also reduced secondary venous vasodilation. ▪ It is also used in acute HF or cardiogenic shock secondary to acute mitral or aortic regurgitation, when reduction of afterload is critical. By reducing SVR in the presence of acute mitral or aortic regurgitation, the impedance to forward flow decreases and LV output improves (Chatterjee et al., 1973; Harshaw et al., 1975).
Acute Aortic Syndromes / Acute Aortic dissection [off label]	▪ Nitroprusside is not the preferred vasodilator of choice due to its side effect profile but has been used in this population. Vasodilator therapy in an acute aortic dissection is not initiated until therapies to assure adequate HR control (60 to 80 BMP) are implemented as well as therapies to control pain (IV opioids).
Acute Ischemic Stroke [off label]	▪ Nitroprusside may be used for BP management in patients receiving reperfusion therapy in the presence of acute ischemic stroke. Nitroprusside is reserved for the treatment of HTN in this clinical situation when HTN is refractory to other treatment options with first-line agents or the diastolic BP is > 140 mmHg.
Cardiogenic Shock with Elevated SVR [off label]	▪ Nitroprusside lowers SVR which reduces PAOP and LV end diastolic pressure. These changes result in an increase in forward flow with improved SV and subsequently CO with no appreciated change in LVEF or HR.
Critically Ill Patients with Severe Aortic Stenosis and Left Ventricular Dysfunction [off label]	▪ Nitroprusside has been shown to improve cardiac function in patients with non-hypotensive decompensated HF with significant LV dysfunction and severe aortic stenosis. The reduction in afterload allows for better forward flow and improves cardiac function as demonstrated by increased cardiac output. The use of nitroprusside in these critically ill patients can allow time for clinical decision making regarding next steps. (Ikram et al., 1992; Khot et al., 2003)
(D'Elia et al., 2024; Jones et al., 2025; UptoDate®, Lexidrug™, 2026)	

Select Adverse Effects of Nitroprusside

- Most adverse effects are dose related and secondary to the vasodilatory effects of nitroprusside.
- Tachycardia may occur as a normal sympathetic reflex response secondary to vasodilation, leading to hypotension. It is crucial to meticulously observe BP and HR, particularly when the HR is elevated upon the initiation of nitroprusside. Continuous monitoring of BP and HR is required.

- ♦ Bradycardia, while a rare side effect, can occur with the administration of nitroprusside. Clinical reports indicate nitroprusside infusion can stimulate a prostaglandin biosynthesis which can result in a reflex bradycardia (Hintze et al., 1984; Lukacsko, 1982).
- ♦ Hypotension, which can be significant, is listed as a US Boxed Warning.
  - The package insert requires the use of continuous BP monitoring by experienced personnel during the duration of the nitroprusside infusion.
  - With severe hypotension, end organ hypoperfusion can occur resulting in ischemia and organ death. This is the reason other vasodilating agents are used prior to nitroprusside.

(Exela Pharma Sciences, 2017; Namigen, 2016; UptoDate®, Lexidrug™, 2024)

- ♦ Increased intracranial pressure may occur during the use of nitroprusside. Nitroprusside should only be used with extreme caution in situations where increased intracranial pressure is suspected.
- ♦ Although the true incidence is unknown, coronary steal has been associated with the use of nitroprusside. Patients with CAD may develop ischemia from coronary steal while receiving nitroprusside.
- ♦ Thiocyanate toxicity and cyanide toxicity can occur with the administration of IV nitroprusside. See the Advanced Concept Focus section below on cyanide toxicity associated with nitroprusside.

(Exela Pharma Sciences, 2017; Namigen, 2016; UptoDate®, Lexidrug™, 2024)

Coronary Steal

- Nitroprusside may induce coronary steal in patients with an area of the myocardium with reduced flow secondary to a narrowed coronary artery.
- Coronary Steal Syndrome occurs when blood flow is "stolen" from one are of the heart in favor of another area leaving an area with ischemia.
- A narrowed coronary artery is typically maximally dilated to compensate for the reduced flow across the vessel.
  - Nitroprusside causes resistance vessels (arteries and arterioles) to dilate.
  - Since narrowed coronary arteries are already fully dilated, further arterial vasodilation leads to a redistribution of blood flow away from the narrowed artery resulting in ischemia.
- During nitroprusside infusion, patients with known CAD should be carefully monitored for any signs of myocardial ischemia (chest pain, arrhythmias, ST segment elevations).
- Some patients with no previous history may have undiagnosed CAD and should likewise be monitored for the development of myocardial ischemia.
- Achieving BP control while avoiding hypotension can be helpful in preventing coronary steal.

(Achim et al., 2021; Hottinger et al., 2014; Mann et al., 1978)

Advanced Concept Focus:

Cyanide Toxicity Associated with Nitroprusside

- ♦ There are many other causes of cyanide toxicity. This Advanced Concept Focus section only covers the assessment, diagnosis and treatment of toxicity secondary to nitroprusside use.
- ♦ Nitroprusside is comprised of ferrous iron complexes with one ferrous ion binding to 4 cyanide ligands and 1 nitrosyl ligand.
- ♦ Nitroprusside administration increases the risk of cyanide toxicity because it contains cyanide ligands. Thiocyanate toxicity can occur because cyanide is metabolized into thiocyanate.
- ♦ Nitroprusside IV gives rise to potentially dangerous quantities of cyanide except when used only briefly or at very low doses (< 2 mcg/kg/min). Cyanide particles can reach poisonous and even potentially lethal levels.

- In the blood nitroprusside interacts with oxyhemoglobin to produce methemoglobin while releasing nitric oxide and cyanide into the system. There are two important things that occur with cyanide: 1) cyanide can bind to methemoglobin, and 2) cyanide is neutralized and detoxified by rhodanese.
  - Cyanide and methemoglobin:
    - Methemoglobin is an attractive binding site for cyanide. When cyanide binds to methemoglobin it forms cyanohemoglobin which is less toxic than cyanide and this buffers the effect of cyanide.
    - However, this buffering effect is limited because the amount of cyanide can exceed the methemoglobin capacity when the body is exposed to approximately 500 mcg/kg of nitroprusside. According to the manufacturer's prescribing information, this amount can be reached in less than an hour at infusion rates of 10 mcg/kg/min (Namigen, 2016).
  - Cyanide neutralization and detoxification:
    - Most of the cyanide is neutralized and detoxified through interaction with the enzyme rhodanese which is found throughout the body but is most prevalent in the liver.
    - Rhodanese adds a sulfur ion, thiosulfate, to the cyanide molecule to create thiocyanate.
    - The availability of thiosulfate in the body can be a limiting factor in the detoxification of cyanide when higher or prolonged doses of nitroprusside are used. With normal stores of thiosulfate, the body can process infusions of nitroprusside at a rate of approximately 2 mcg/kg/min.
    - Thiocyanate is then cleared from the body through urinary excretion.
    - However, clearing of thiocyanate is a slow process because after filtering by the kidneys most (about 90%) of the thiocyanate is reabsorbed back into the blood.
      - This leads to a long elimination half-life.
      - This elimination half-life in healthy people is approximately 3 days and in patients with kidney failure the elimination half-life is about 9 days.

    (Schulz et al., 1979)
- Thiocyanate toxicity can occur because of how slowly thiocyanate is cleared from the body.
- Cyanide toxicity can occur due to diminished thiosulfate levels and thus the inability to convert cyanide to thiocyanate.
- Cyanide toxicity, while a rare occurrence when nitroprusside is used appropriately, can be fatal. Early recognition and treatment are essential if mortality is to be prevented.
- The risk of cyanide toxicity increases in the following situations:
  - Prolonged exposure to nitroprusside with infusions lasting greater than 24 to 48 hours.
  - Infusions at high doses (8 to 10 mcg/kg/min) for greater than 10 minutes.
  - Infusions at rates greater than the ability of the body to detoxify cyanide (rates greater than 2 mcg/kg/min).
  - Patients with renal function impairment.
  - Patients with hepatic dysfunction or failure.
  - A malnourished state.
  - Patients with Leber optic atrophy or tobacco amblyopia (see contraindications below).
  - Prolonged bypass time when nitroprusside is used during coronary artery bypass graft surgery (increased erythrocyte shearing and intracellular cyanide release).
  - Receiving targeted temperature management with temperatures in the therapeutic hypothermia range.
  - Patients with vitamin B12 deficiency have a higher risk of toxicity since one pathway for cyanide detoxification involves the formation of cyanocobalamin (Vitamin B12). Cyanide molecules have a high affinity for cyanocobalamin, allowing for detoxification with excretion through the urine.
- When higher doses of nitroprusside are used (4 to 10 mcg/kg/min) for an extended period sodium thiosulfate can be given along with nitroprusside to prevent cyanide toxicity.

The combination of nitroprusside and thiosulfate remains physically and chemically stable as a single compounded dose for up to 48 hours when kept at room temperature and protected from light (Shulz et al., 2010). However, toxicity may still occur even with this approach (Rindone & Sloane, 1992).

- ♦ Nitroprusside should be immediately discontinued with any suspicion of toxicity. As part of the US Boxed Warning, an infusion at the maximum dose of nitroprusside should never last for more than 10 minutes. If BP is not well controlled after 10 minutes of the infusion at maximum rate, the infusion should be immediately discontinued.
- ♦ S&S of thiocyanate toxicity can be vague and nonspecific in a critically ill patient. The most common sign of serious thiocyanate toxicity is a change in mental status. Any mental status change (i.e. confusion, agitation) should raise suspicion for toxicity in patients at high risk for toxicity. Nausea, abdominal pain and weakness may also be early signs.
- ♦ S&S of cyanide toxicity include:
  - ♦ Altered mental status can range from simple confusion progressing to lethargy and even coma with seizures. Note: Change in mental status is also a sign of thiocyanate toxicity.
  - ♦ Tachycardia is often seen early in cyanide toxicity. Bradycardia can occur later in toxicity and may precede CV collapse.
  - ♦ Metabolic acidosis with no other clear etiology points to cyanide toxicity.
  - ♦ Hypoxemia, respiratory distress, and respiratory arrest.
  - ♦ Methemoglobinemia, although very rare, can occur in concert with cyanide toxicity.
- ♦ Laboratory testing may be beneficial to evaluate for the presence of toxicity, especially in those at highest risk.
  - Acid-base balance and venous O_2 concentrations are routinely monitored during nitroprusside therapy. However, these indicators are imperfect in their ability to diagnose drug toxicity. Therefore, nurses should diligently observe for S&S of toxicity in patients who are at high risk.
  - Serum thiocyanate levels can be helpful to confirm suspected thiocyanate toxicity.
    - Symptoms may appear with thiocyanate levels of > 35 mcg/mL.
    - More serious signs of toxicity are not expected until levels are > 100 mcg/mL.
    - While these levels are not useful in determining cyanide toxicity, they are able to identify thiocyanate toxicity and early treatment strategies can be implemented.
    - Normal thiocyanate levels in nonsmokers are 1 to 4 mcg/L while normal levels in smokers are higher at 3 to 12 mcg/L.
  - The use of serum cyanide levels, in most situations, is not practical due to the length of time to receive results. While cyanide levels provide a definitive diagnosis of cyanide toxicity serum lactate levels are used as a surrogate marker in clinical practice.
  - Serum lactate levels increase as cyanide accumulates in the body. Cyanide interacts with cytochrome C, inhibiting aerobic metabolism and leading to lactic acidosis. Serum lactate levels serve as a surrogate marker but cannot conclusively diagnose cyanide toxicity. However, elevated lactate levels in the presence of unexplained metabolic acidosis may point to the diagnosis in high-risk patients receiving IV nitroprusside.
  - Mixed venous O_2 saturation levels or venous O_2 levels can identify venous hyperoxemia, which occurs in patients with cyanide toxicity as O_2 extraction by the cells is decreased. Bright red venous blood is a clinical sign of venous hyperoxemia. Venous hyperoxemia can also cause flushed skin that is "cherry red" in color.
  - The presence of cyanide toxicity can result in renal failure, hepatic failure, rhabdomyolysis, and pulmonary edema. Additional testing that would support diagnosis of any of these complications may be helpful when evaluating and implementing treatment strategies.

- There is only a rare possibility that methemoglobinemia can occur with the use of nitroprusside. However, it is considered reasonable to evaluate carboxyhemoglobin and methemoglobin levels to rule out other dyshemoglobinemias in patients demonstrating signs of toxicity.

♦ Treatment of cyanide toxicity should occur promptly as cyanide poisoning can rapidly become fatal.
  - Since results of cyanide levels are not quickly available anecdotal treatment should begin quickly if the clinical picture and lab work raise the suspicion of cyanide poisoning.
  - Nitroprusside infusions must be stopped upon notice of any S&S of thiocyanate or cyanide toxicity.
  - The ABCs of resuscitation should be urgently implemented when needed.
  - Anecdotal treatment for cyanide toxicity includes the use of one or more agents that will bind cyanide, induce methemoglobinemia, or add sulfur doners to the system.
  - The use of hydroxocobalamin (binding agent) is the primary drug of choice if it is available. When not available a combination of sodium nitrite (induction of methemoglobinemia) and sodium thiosulfate (sulfur doner) is used for the acute treatment of cyanide poisoning.
  - Hydroxocobalamin is a precursor to Vitamin B12 and enhances cyanide binding. When infused into the system, one molecule of hydroxocobalamin can bind with one cyanide ion. This combination forms cyanocobalamin (a synthetic form of vitamin B12), which is then excreted in the urine. Cyanide is more likely to bind with hydroxocobalamin than to cytochrome C. Cyanide binding with cytochrome C is the reaction leading to lactate production.
    - Administration of hydroxocobalamin may result in a reddish discoloration of the skin, plasma, urine and mucous membranes which may last for several days.
    - Administration of hydroxocobalamin may affect creatine, lactate, aspartate aminotransferase (AST) and alanine aminotransferase (ALT), bilirubin, and magnesium levels as well as co-oximetry measurements of total hemoglobin, carboxyhemoglobin, methemoglobin, and oxyhemoglobin.
    - Administration of hydroxocobalamin may also affect urinary glucose, protein, ketones, leukocyte and erythrocyte counts.
    - Hydroxocobalamin may be used in combination with sodium thiosulfate (see below) in acute situations. If 2 doses of hydroxocobalamin have been administered without significant patient improvement a third dose can be administered followed by a dose of sodium thiosulfate.
  - The induction of methemoglobinemia occurs with the administration of sodium nitrite. This buffering agent converts hemoglobin to methemoglobin. Methemoglobin provides a binding site that is an alternative to cytochrome C for available cyanide ions.
    - In most patients the level of methemoglobin that develops is usually at safe levels however each patient responds differently.
    - It is important to remember that excess methemoglobin decreases O_2 delivery to the tissues as it shifts the oxyhemoglobin curve to the left.
    - In patients who are anemic lower doses of sodium nitrite should be given to prevent levels of methemoglobin that will be detrimental to the patient.
    - The use of sodium nitrite can also induce vasodilation through the release of nitric oxide with a potential for hypotension. So careful monitoring of BP should be maintained. One benefit of vasodilation is the increased perfusion to key organs such as the liver which assists with cyanide metabolism.
    - Sodium nitrite is used in combination with sodium thiosulfate when hydroxocobalamin is not available.
  - Sodium thiosulfate is the sulfur doner the enzyme rhodanese adds to the cyanide molecule to detoxify cyanide. This process creates thiocyanate which is then excreted in the urine.
    - The addition of sodium thiosulfate increases the availability of sulfur doners to support rhodanese in the detoxification of cyanide.

- With an onset of action of about 30 minutes sodium nitrite is to be given first followed immediately by sodium thiosulfate.
- This drug is relatively safe, however patients with renal insufficiency may have slower removal and may develop symptoms of an overaccumulation of thiocyanate which include psychosis, arthralgias, vomiting, and myalgias. In the presence of acute renal failure hemodialysis may be necessary to remove thiocyanate accumulation in the symptomatic patients.
- There is some support for the coadministration of nitroprusside and sodium thiosulfate to allow the sodium thiosulfate to function as a prophylactic agent. The agents can be mixed, or sodium thiosulfate can be given as an intermittent bolus. Thiocyanate levels are noted to rise which if high enough may cause thiocyanate toxicity. The likelihood of this occurrence increases in those with renal dysfunction.

(D'Elia et al., 2025; Desai & Su, 2024; Exela Pharma Sciences, 2017; Holme & Sharman, 2023; Hottinger et al., 2014; Leavesley et al., 2010; Lockwood et al., 2010; Mann et al., 1978; Morris et al., 2017; Namigen, 2016)

> ***Linking Knowledge to Practice***
>
> ✓ *Nurses caring for patients with infusions exceeding 2 mcg/kg/min for 3 or more days should be alert for signs of thiocyanate or cyanide toxicity. See Advanced Concept Focus section above on cyanide toxicity associated with nitroprusside. The risk of cyanide toxicity doubles and triples in those with poor kidney function and at higher doses.*
>
> *(Exela Pharma Sciences, 2017; Namigen, 2016; UptoDate®, Lexidrug™, 2024)*

Contraindication Highlights for Nitroprusside

- ♦ Consult manufacturer recommendations for use in children, pregnant women, and nursing women.
- ♦ Avanafil must be held for 12 hours, sildenafil and vardenafil for 24 hours, and tadalafil for 48 hours prior to any nitroprusside use (Rao et al., 2025). Severe hypotension can occur. Concomitant use with PDE-5 inhibitors and riociguat (soluble guanylate cyclase stimulator) is also contraindicated.
- ♦ Not to be used in clinical situations when HTN is a necessary compensatory mechanism (e.g., coarctation of the aorta and arteriovenous shunting).
- ♦ Not to be used during surgery in patients with inadequate cerebral circulation or in patients with a low chance of survival requiring emergent surgical intervention for possible survival.
- ♦ Not to be used in acute HF or shock states when reduced SVR is present such as sepsis.
- ♦ Patients with the congenital disorder Leber's optic atrophy lack the enzyme rhodanese which is essential to convert cyanide to thiocyanate. They should not receive nitroprusside as the risk of toxicity is high and treatment for toxicity is dependent on the presence of the rhodanese enzyme (Hottinger et al., 2014).
- ♦ Patients with tobacco amblyopia (also called tobacco optic neuropathy) have been found to have elevated cyanide levels secondary to exposure to chronic tobacco smoke.
  - This is true even when serum thiocyanate levels are not particularly elevated.
  - This baseline cyanide elevation increases the risk of cyanide toxicity when nitroprusside is used, and it should be avoided in these patients.

  (Jestico et al., 1984).

Special Considerations & Monitoring with Nitroprusside

- ♦ Cyanide toxicity is a US Boxed Warning associated with nitroprusside administration. See the Advanced Concept Focus section above on cyanide toxicity associated with nitroprusside.
- ♦ Nitroprusside carries a high risk of sudden, severe hypotension that can lead to irreversible ischemia or death. Careful patient monitoring is essential.

- Methemoglobinemia can occur in patients receiving high doses of nitroprusside.
  - Although methemoglobin is a byproduct of cyanide detoxification, levels are usually not high enough to cause methemoglobinemia.
  - Patients on high doses of nitroprusside should be monitored for signs of methemoglobinemia.
  - Methylene blue is the recommended treatment.
- Anemia should be addressed prior to administration in nonurgent cases, such as in scheduled surgery requiring BP control, to mitigate the risk of methemoglobinemia.
- Impaired liver function can hinder detoxification due to the potential deficiency of the enzyme rhodanese, thereby elevating the risk of toxicity. Nitroprusside should be used with extreme caution in patients with hepatic impairment.

> ***Linking Knowledge to Practice***
>
> ✓ *Once reconstituted, protect the nitroprusside solution from light by covering it with an opaque covering or foil. The drip chamber and tubing do not need to be covered. When covered properly the solution can be used for 24 hours.*
>
> ✓ *The solution should be evaluated for its color and clarity.*
> - *The solution should be free of any sediment or particles, and the color should be colorless or a slight red/brown color (dry sodium nitroprusside powder has a reddish-brown color).*
> - *If the solution has sediment or is blue, green or bright red it should be discarded.*
>
> *(Exela Pharma Sciences, 2017; Namigen, 2016; UptoDate®, Lexidrug™, 2024)*

Key Pharmacokinetics & Pharmacodynamics Information for Nitroprusside

- The onset of action is very fast with a hypotensive effect in under 2 minutes.
- The BP lowering effect can last for 1 to 10 minutes after discontinuation.
- The circulatory elimination half-life is under 2 minutes which accounts for the short duration of the BP lowering effect.
- The elimination of thiocyanate (a byproduct of cyanide detoxification) is approximately 3 days. This elimination time can extend up to 9 days in those with renal dysfunction.

> ***Linking Knowledge to Practice***
>
> ✓ *The FDA and drug manufacturers recommend the use of nitroprusside only when continuous BP evaluation is available due to the high risk for sudden and significant hypotension that can result in irreversible ischemia and even death.*
>
> ✓ *With an onset of action of < 2 minutes hypotension can occur quickly. Small adjustments in dosage can result in big changes in blood pressure.*
>
> ✓ *Monitor BP continuously for first the 5 minutes after initiation or up titration and then every 15 to 30 minutes for the duration of the infusion.*
>
> *(Exela Pharma Sciences, 2017; Namigen, 2016; UptoDate®, Lexidrug™, 2024)*

Important Medication Interactions with Nitroprusside

- As noted in contraindications, nitroprusside should not be used with PDE-5 inhibitors or riociguat (soluble guanylate cyclase stimulator) as the risk of hypotension is great.
- Isocarboxazid an MOA inhibitor may enhance the hypotensive effects of nitroprusside. Concomitant use of nitroprusside should be avoided.

- ♦ Use of any medication that lowers BP should be used with extreme caution in combination with nitroprusside.

Appendix 11 provides additional details regarding sodium nitroprusside.

Direct Smooth Muscle Relaxants

Hydralazine and minoxidil are compared in Table 23 in the areas of 1) mechanism of action, 2) indications, 3) special dosing information, 4) select adverse effects, 5) special considerations and monitoring, 6) key pharmacokinetic and pharmacodynamic information, and 7) important medication interactions.

Table 23

Comparison of Direct Smooth Muscle Relaxants Part 1

	Hydralazine	Minoxidil
Mechanism of Action of Direct Smooth Muscle Relaxants	▪ Causes direct vasodilation of arterioles resulting in decreased SVR, little impact on veins. ▪ Thought to inhibit calcium release from the sarcoplasmic reticulum in muscle cells and inhibit myosin phosphorylation in arterial smooth muscle cells. ▪ Reduces both systolic and diastolic BP but diastolic BP is reduced to a greater degree. ▪ Reduction in SVR leads to a compensatory baroreceptor mediated release of epinephrine and norepinephrine resulting in increased venous return, HR, and subsequent CO.	▪ Opens adenosine triphosphate-controlled potassium channels in vascular smooth muscle cells. K+ efflux results in relaxation of vascular smooth muscle. ▪ Has little impact on veins. ▪ Reduces both systolic and diastolic BP. ▪ Stimulates hair growth secondary to vasodilation, increased cutaneous blood flow and stimulation of resting hair follicles. ▪ Triggers a baroreceptor (carotid and aortic) mediated activation of the peripheral SNS resulting in increased HR and CO and increased plasma renin activity leading to sodium and water retention.
Indications for Direct Smooth Muscle Relaxants	▪ HFrEF for patients who cannot take a RAAS inhibitor. ▪ Chronic HTN as alternate agent only; not a first-line agent. ▪ Perioperative HTN as an alternate agent. ▪ Hypertensive emergency as an alternate agent. ▪ Hypertensive emergency in pregnancy or postpartum [off label].	▪ HTN as an alternative agent. ▪ Reserve for patients who do not respond to maximum dose of a diuretic along with 2 other antihypertensive agents.
Special Dosing Information for Direct Smooth Muscle Relaxants	▪ No manufacturer recommendations based on renal function. ▪ If eGFR < 10 mL/min/1.73 m^2 give usual dose every 8 to 12 hours. ▪ No recommendations based on hepatic function, but the drug undergoes extensive hepatic metabolism.	▪ Manufacturer suggests patients with renal failure or on dialysis may require a decreased dose but there are no specific recommendations. ▪ No dose recommendations from manufacturer based on hepatic function. Use with caution because area under the curve (AUC) is increased and clearance is decreased with hepatic impairment.

Table 23 Comparison of Direct Smooth Muscle Relaxants Part 2		
	Hydralazine	**Minoxidil**
Select Adverse Effects of Direct Smooth Muscle Relaxants	▪ Cardiac stimulation resulting in tachycardia and palpitations. ▪ See Advanced Concept Section below on hydralazine induced lupus. ▪ Antineutrophil cytoplasmic antibody (ANCA): positive vasculitis involving the kidney. ▪ Hypotension that may last longer than the circulating half-life. ▪ Additional most common adverse effects: H/A, N&V, and diarrhea. ▪ Multiple other potential adverse effects. Consult drug reference.	▪ US Boxed Warning**:** Can exacerbate angina and cause pericardial effusion occasionally progressing to tamponade. ▪ ST segment depression / abnormal T waves on ECG (common) (may resolve after several months). ▪ Fluid retention (edema & weight gain). ▪ Hypertrichosis (common). ▪ Multiple other potential adverse effects. Consult drug reference.
Contraindication Highlights for Direct Smooth Muscle Relaxants Consult manufacturer recommendations for use in children, pregnant women, and nursing women.	▪ CAD: can cause myocardial stimulation resulting in anginal attacks and produce ECG changes consistent with myocardial ischemia. May potentially be an option if used with a beta blocker. ▪ High output HF and dissecting aortic aneurysm: due to cardiac stimulation. ▪ Mitral valve rheumatic heart disease and cor pulmonale: may cause a paradoxical increase in pulmonary artery pressures. ▪ Idiopathic SLE.	▪ Pheochromocytoma: due to potential catecholamine release. ▪ Pulmonary HTN associated with mitral stenosis and severe hepatic impairment: contraindications per Canadian labeling.
Special Considerations & Monitoring with Direct Smooth Muscle Relaxants	▪ Avoid administration before dialysis in patients at risk for hypotension during treatment. ▪ Often combined with a beta blocker to block the compensatory SNS response.	▪ Use only with close supervision. ▪ Usually given with a beta blocker to prevent tachycardia. ▪ Most often it must be given with a loop diuretic to prevent fluid accumulation.

Linking Knowledge to Practice

✓ *Although hydralazine is not used as a first-line antihypertensive agents, it is a recommended treatment option in combination with isosorbide dinitrate in HFrEF in patients self-identified as African American. For this reason, cardiac RNs and APRNs need to be aware of the potential for hydralazine induced lupus.*

✓ *Hydralazine is contraindicated in aortic dissection because it causes cardiac stimulation which can worsen the tear in the aorta. In aortic dissection the preferred initial treatment is a beta blocker to decrease the force of LV contraction to prevent further tearing of the aorta as blood is ejected.*

✓ *Although IV hydralazine is effective in lowering systolic and diastolic HTN, IV agents should only be used in situations where there is evidence of HTN induced end organ damage.*

Table 23 Comparison of Direct Smooth Muscle Relaxants Part 3		
	Hydralazine	**Minoxidil**
Key Pharmaco-kinetic & Pharmaco-dynamic Information for Direct Smooth Muscle Relaxants	▪ IV: onset of action of 5 to 80 minutes; duration of 2 to12 hours; unpredictable effect on BP and unpredictable dose response. ▪ Oral: rapidly absorbed; ↓ in BP in 20 to 30 minutes; time to peak 1 to 2 hours; duration 2 to 4 hours. ▪ 90% serum concentration is protein bound. ▪ Half-life elimination: 2 to 7 hours. ▪ Unlikely to be significantly dialyzed. ▪ Metabolized in the liver through acetylation. Drug concentration, half-life and duration may be affected by acetylator status.	▪ Onset of action for decreased BP ≈ 30 minutes. ▪ Plasma peak: 1 hour. Peak effect: 2 to 3 hours. ▪ Duration: Up to 2 to 5 days. ▪ Half-life elimination: 2 to 4 hours. ▪ Hypotensive effect can last 12 to 72 hours which may allow one-time daily dosing to provide effective 24-hour BP control; may also be given in divided doses. Required frequency of administration varies between patients.
Important Medication Interactions with Direct Smooth Muscle Relaxants (Hydralazine & Minoxidil) Avoid with bromperidol and isocarboxazid. Hold for 24 hours before chemotherapy with amifostine; hold 12 hours before until 1 hour after administration of obinutuzumab.		
Campbell et al., 2011; Grossman, & Messerli, 2007; Herman, Bruss, & Tivakaran, 2023; McComb et al., 2016; Sica, 2004b; Sica & Gehr, 2001; UptoDate®, Lexidrug™, 2025.		

Advanced Concept Focus:
Implications for Hydralazine Metabolism

- ♦ Hydralazine is metabolized in the liver through a process called acetylation.
- ♦ The enzyme involved in acetylation *is* *N*-acetyltransferase 2 (*NAT2* Gene) which is found predominantly in the liver and the gut.
- ♦ Based on genetic differences there are those who are slow acetylators and those who are rapid.
- ♦ About 50% of the general population are slow acetylators.
- ♦ There is a correlation between the rate of acetylation and the concentration of hydralazine in the body.
  - Those patients who are slow acetylators will have higher plasma drug levels and may require a lower dose of medication to achieve the desired BP response.
  - Slow acetylators may also be at risk for adverse effects of hydralazine therapy.
  - Some studies have also demonstrated an association between acetylator status and hydralazine-induced lupus.
- ♦ A total daily dose of 200 mg or greater per day should be used with caution in slow acetylators.
- ♦ In fast acetylators lower doses of hydralazine will likely be ineffective. Genotype testing is available to determine if a patient is a fast or slow acetylator.
- ♦ There are other medications that are metabolized in the liver through the process of acetylation.
  - Procainamide, an antiarrhythmic, is another cardiac medication that is metabolized through the process of acetylation.
  - Other medications that undergo acetylation include isoniazid, phenelzine, dapsone, and some sulphonamides (known as sulfa drugs).

(Collins et al., 2020; McMorran et al., 2018)

Hydralazine Key Points

- Hydralazine stimulates the SNS and for this reason it is not a first-line agent in the treatment of HTN. Hydralazine can be used in HTN management as an alternative agent in select patients.
- While hydralazine is effective in lowering BP it is not as efficacious as other medications such as CCBs, thiazide diuretics, and medications that block the RAAS such as ACEIs, ARBs, and ARNIs.
- The reduction in SVR by hydralazine leads to a compensatory baroreceptor mediated release of epinephrine and norepinephrine. This results in increased venous return, tachycardia, and increased CO. This is the reason hydralazine cannot be given to patients at risk for myocardial ischemia or other conditions where cardiac stimulation would be detrimental (Campell et al., 2011).
- Hydralazine is typically given in conjunction with a beta blocker and diuretic to improve patient tolerance.
- Although hydralazine has been in use since the 1950s as an antihypertensive, its use expanded to HFrEF after the publication of the African American Heart Failure Trial in 2004. As a result of this trial and subsequent guideline recommendations, the use of hydralazine increased.
- Hydralazine along with a fixed dose long-acting nitrate (e.g. isosorbide dinitrate) is recommended for self-identified African Americans who have HFrEF (NYHA class III-IV) and are already on optimal medical therapy. This recommendation is to improve symptoms and reduce mortality and morbidity (Heidenreich et al., 2022).
  - The African American Heart Failure trial demonstrated a 43% reduction in mortality from any cause with the use of hydralazine and isosorbide dinitrate compared to placebo (Taylor et al., 2004).
  - A more recent study of demonstrated benefit of hydralazine and isosorbide dinitrate in African Americans with HFrEF but the mortality benefit was not as great as that seen in the African American Heart Failure trial (Ziaeian, Fonarow, & Heidenreich, 2017).
- There are potentials dangers to treating severe uncomplicated HTN with IV agents including hydralazine. IV agents should not be used in the treatment of severe HTN without symptoms related to HTN or evidence of end organ damage.
  - When there is not new or worsening target organ damage, guidelines recommend restarting or intensifying oral medications and arranging follow up (Jones et al., 2025).
  - In a retrospective study of 94 patients at a university teaching hospital, only 2% of the patients who received IV hydralazine for HTN had clinical evidence of an urgent hypertensive condition. Seventeen patients experienced an adverse event, the most common being hypotension (Campbell et al., 2011).
  - It is important to remember that BP responses to hydralazine can be variable and harm can occur if IV hydralazine is prescribed and given to patients with HTN who are not symptomatic or demonstrating evidence of end organ damage.
- Hydralazine may result in clinical deterioration in patients with cor pulmonale.
  - While hydralazine lowers SVR, it can cause a paradoxical increase in pulmonary artery pressure because it may not effectively lower PVR. An elevated pulmonary artery pressure is less likely to occur in patients who are also receiving beta blocker therapy.
  - Patients with cor pulmonale already have elevated PVR and may have clinical deterioration with the use of hydralazine.
  - Additionally, the increase in CO seen with hydralazine may not be beneficial in the setting of cor pulmonale.

(McCombs et al., 2016; Sica & Gehr, 2001)

- Patients with CKD often require several medications to achieve BP control. Hydralazine has been shown to increase renal blood flow without changes in GFR indicating that this medicine may be used in patients with kidney dysfunction. However, when used in a patient with a CrCl less than 20 mL/min the half-life may be substantially prolonged (McCombs et al., 2016).

Advanced Concept Focus:

Hydralazine Induced Lupus

- ♦ Hydralazine is one of several drugs that can trigger an autoimmune response.
- ♦ Hydralazine and other medications induce autoantibodies in many patients, but not all patients have symptoms of autoantibody associated disease.
- ♦ Some patients affected by drug induced autoantibodies can develop clinical symptoms that resemble idiopathic SLE.
- ♦ When symptoms like SLE are caused by a medication the condition is called drug-induced lupus.
- ♦ The probability of a patient expressing drug induced autoantibodies that result in symptomatic lupus increase as the dose and duration of the drug increase.
- ♦ Drug-induced lupus has some similarities to idiopathic SLE but there are also clinical and immunological differences. There are also differences in clinical patterns of drug-induced lupus among different medications.
- ♦ It is estimated there are between 15,000 and 30,000 cases of drug-induced lupus each year in the United States.
- ♦ For most medications drug-induced lupus occurs equally among males and females and is more common in older adults and in the White population.
- ♦ Procainamide and hydralazine are the 2 medications with the highest risk for drug induced lupus.
  - With procainamide the risk is approximately 15 to 20%.
  - With hydralazine this adverse effect occurs in approximately 5 to 13% of patients.
- ♦ The mechanism or mechanisms involved in the development of drug induced lupus are not fully understood.
  - Differences in drug metabolism may play a role.
  - Immunogenetic characteristics of individual patients may also play a role.
  - See Advanced Concept Focus section above on implications for hydralazine metabolism.
  - Multiple other mechanisms within the immune system have also been proposed as contributing to the development of drug induced lupus.
- ♦ Several risk factors identified for the development of hydralazine induced lupus include:
  - High doses of hydralazine (more than 200 mg per day); hydralazine therapy greater than 3 months; or a cumulative dose of more than 100 g.
  - Prolonged exposure time: In a small cohort study 83% of the patients were exposed to hydralazine for more than 12 months (Timlin et al., 2019).
  - Female sex: Although in a small cohort study of 7 patients, 57% were male. (Timlin et al., 2019).
  - White race.
  - Slow hepatic acetylation.
  - Immunogenetic factors / specific phenotypes.
  - Family history of autoimmune disease.
- ♦ Patients on low doses of hydralazine however can still develop hydralazine-induced lupus.
- ♦ The result of drug induced lupus includes autoimmunity with target organs suffering immune mediated effects. However, compared to idiopathic SLE there are usually not major end organ threatening complications.
- ♦ S&S of drug-induced lupus usually develops after months or years of drug exposure. However, there can also be an abrupt onset of symptoms.

- The most common S&S of drug induced lupus include:
  - Fever.
  - Myalgias.
  - Arthralgias / arthritis (most common in hands and wrists).
  - Rash.
  - Serositis (inflammation of serous tissues lining the lungs, heart and abdomen).
- Severe cases of hydralazine induced lupus can result in glomerulonephritis (lupus nephritis), vasculitis, and pulmonary failure from pulmonary renal syndrome.
  - Hydralazine induced lupus nephritis is not common.
  - However, in small cohort study of 7 patients with hydralazine induced lupus, 4 of the 7 patients had biopsy proven lupus nephritis (Timlin et al., 2019).
  - Hydralazine-induced lupus nephritis occurs most commonly in conjunction with systemic vasculitis; however isolated lupus nephritis can also occur in the setting of hydralazine-induced lupus.
- Cutaneous effects are less common with drug-induced lupus compared to idiopathic SLE.
  - A subset of patients with drug-induced lupus will however have S&S of a drug-induced subacute cutaneous lupus erythematosus (SCLE).
  - The skin is involved in about $^1/_3$ of patients with hydralazine induced lupus.
- Hydralazine induced lupus may rarely present in an atypical manner such as with pleural or pericardial effusions (Iyer et al., 2017; Jerome et al., 2024)
- Clinical S&S of drug induced lupus occur in approximately 5 to 13% of patients taking hydralazine.
  - Low doses of hydralazine do not eliminate the risk for drug-induced lupus.
  - If the patient is a slow acetylator, there is the potential for development of drug-induced lupus even at a dose of only 100 mg per day.
- If drug induced lupus is suspected a CBC with differential, a complete metabolic panel, and a urinalysis should be ordered.
  - There are also several antibody panels that need ordered.
  - Consult a medical reference on drug-induced lupus for complete information on a diagnostic workup to differentiate drug-induced lupus from idiopathic SLE and other potential differentials.
- The most common immunological lab findings include:
  - Positive antinuclear antibody
  - Positive anti-histone antibody
- In a small cohort study the presence of other antibodies (anti-myeloperoxidase antibody and anti-proteinase antibody) were associated with more severe disease, such as involvement of the kidneys, lungs, or both organs (Timlin et al., 2019).
- Abnormal antibodies should resolve after stopping the hydralazine. Resolution can occur within 3 to 12 months, but abnormal antibodies can persist for over 12 months.
- Common hematological abnormalities include anemia, leukopenia, and a positive Combs.
- The common immunological and hematological findings, however, are nonspecific because they are also associated with idiopathic lupus.
- If the diagnosis is confirmed the treatment is to stop the medication.
- The prognosis for drug-induced lupus is favorable.
- S&S should resolve after stopping the medication.
  - Initial improvement in S&S can occur early (day to weeks) after stopping the medication.
  - Complete resolution of S&S can take weeks to months.

- Patients may also temporarily receive treatment for the manifestations of drug-induced lupus with the same therapies used in idiopathic SLE and in SCLE.
  - Arthritis and arthralgia may be treated with NSAIDs.
  - Hydroxychloroquine may be used temporarily if musculoskeletal, cutaneous, or constitutional symptoms do not resolve within 4 to 8 weeks of drug discontinuation.
  - Systemic glucocorticoids or topical corticosteroids may be needed to treat specific clinical manifestations.
  - Mycophenolate mofetil has also been used in the treatment of hydralazine induced lupus

♦ For patients who develop lupus nephritis additional treatment options include plasmapheresis, hemodialysis, and cyclophosphamide (chemotherapeutic agent).

(Khan et al., 2020; Merola, 2024; Timlin et al., 2019; Yokogawa & Vivino, 2009)

Minoxidil Key Points

- Minoxidil is only used in the treatment of resistant or refractory HTN that does not respond to maximal treatment using 4 agents. Renal dysfunction is one reason for resistant HTN.
- Minoxidil is a more potent vasodilator than hydralazine. However, because the mechanism of action is predominantly arterial with no venous vasodilation, postural hypotension is rare (Sica, 2004; Sica & Gehr, 2001)
- Minoxidil triggers a baroreceptor mediated activation of the peripheral SNS which results in an increase in HR and CO.
- Minoxidil also increases plasma renin activity leading to sodium and water retention. One specific mechanism by which minoxidil leads to sodium and water retention is activation of the potassium channel in the thick ascending limb of the loop of Henle which results in increased sodium and chloride reabsorption.
- ST segment depression and T wave inversion are common with minoxidil therapy. These changes may spontaneously resolve after several months continued minoxidil therapy.
  - ST / T wave changes may also reflect minoxidil induced myocardial ischemia (minoxidil increases HR and CO which increase MVO_2) or worsening of LV hypertrophy (fluid retention can contribute to the development of LV hypertrophy).
  - The coadministration of an ACEI or an ARB should be used as adjunctive therapy to mitigate the worsening the LV hypertrophy associated with minoxidil therapy.
- A potential complication of minoxidil is pericardial effusion with an incidence of about 3%.
  - Some effusions may spontaneously resolve.
  - It is important to know that this complication may occur more commonly in patients with renal dysfunction, especially those with uremic syndrome.
  - Other risk factors for pericardial effusion in the setting on minoxidil include connective tissue disease, HF, or any substantial amount of fluid retention. In some cases, the development of pericardial effusion is a manifestation of generalized volume overload.
  - However, it is important to remember that pericardial effusion may also occur with minoxidil in patients with no risk factors. If a patient develops pericardial effusion in the absence of volume overload, then minoxidil must be permanently discontinued.
- Hypertrichosis is an adverse effect of minoxidil and limits its use to male patients. See Advanced Concept Focus section below on hypertrichosis versus hirsutism.
- Other adverse effects such as tachycardia, fluid retention, and potential pericardial effusion limit its consideration to only those patients with refractory HTN that is symptomatic or involves end organ damage and is not responsive to a combination of medications including at minimum a CCB, an ACEI or an ARB, and a diuretic.

(McComb et al., 2016; Sica & Gehr, 2001)

Prescribing Pearls for Minoxidil Part 1

Use in Refractory HTN

- Minoxidil is only used in cases of severe refractory HTN.
- A HTN specialist should be making the decision to prescribe minoxidil
- Minoxidil is effective regardless of the level of renal function and is often the last option in patients with CKD who are non-responsive to other antihypertensive agents.
  - In most patients with HTN and normal renal function, minoxidil does not alter renal function.
  - Renal function should be carefully monitored when minoxidil is used to treat malignant HTN in a patient with CKD.
    - In this setting there may be a decline in GFR due to the sudden change in BP with minoxidil therapy.
    - Also, in this setting the GFR may also recover once a normal BP is established and maintained.
- In some studies, in patients with renal dysfunction, there was a stabilization or even reversal of declining renal function when BP was effectively controlled.
- An accelerated dosing schedule of minoxidil is effective in rapidly lowering diastolic BP when a patient is symptomatic with a diastolic BP > 120 mmHg. This treatment is not a replacement for IV therapy in patients with symptomatic HTN. However, it can be used under close medical supervision in conjunction with IV therapy to facilitate the transition to oral therapy.

Prescribing Pearls for Minoxidil Part 2

Adverse Effects

The adverse effects of tachycardia and fluid retention are dose dependent.

Management strategies include:

- Combining minoxidil with either a beta blocker (most common) or a centrally acting $alpha_2$ agonist like clonidine, or a CCB with HR control (verapamil or diltiazem) can help to counteract the reflex increase in HR and CO.
- A beta blocker or other HR lowering medication should be started prior to the initiation of minoxidil.
- Dividing the minoxidil dose may also help with managing the tachycardia.
- Using minoxidil with a diuretic (typically a loop diuretic) can help counteract minoxidil's sodium retaining quality and thus enhance BP lowering. Occasionally, a combination of a loop diuretic with a thiazide diuretic or aldosterone antagonist will be necessary to control volume.
- Dose adjustments of the beta blocker and diuretic are often needed to achieve the desired HR and volume status.
- Fluid retention may be substantial enough to warrant stopping the medication. Patients should be instructed to weigh daily to track fluid retention.

(Sica, 2004; Sica & Gehr, 2001)

Advanced Concept Focus:

Hypertrichosis versus Hirsutism

- Hypertrichosis is the condition of diffusely increased hair growth that involves the total body.
- Hypertrichosis is a rare condition that is usually medication induced. In addition to minoxidil, other medications associated with hypertrichosis include phenytoin, cyclosporine, penicillamine, and diazoxide.

- In about 80% of patients taking minoxidil, thickening and enhanced pigmentation of fine body hair begins within 3 to 6 weeks of starting the medication.
  - One possible explanation for the increased hair growth is related to increased blood flow to affected areas. There is also some evidence that increased hair growth is related to the opening of potassium channels which is the mechanism of action of minoxidil.
  - Hypertrichosis limits the ability to use this medication in women and children.
  - Hair growth typically starts over the temples and eyebrows, extending next to between the eyebrows and the hairline or sideburn region. The final areas of hair growth are on the scalp, trunk, and extremities. Hair growth can also occur in the ear canal to the extent that it affects hearing.
  - Hair growth will stop when the medication is discontinued, and hypertrichosis starts to disappear within a few weeks, it may take up to 6 months for the patient's appearance to return to normal.
- Hypertrichosis can also occur in some disease processes including but not limited to malnutrition, anorexia nervosa, and hypothyroidism.
- Hirsutism is different from hypertrichosis. In most cases of hirsutism there is excessive androgen mediated terminal hair growth. Terminal hair is that which is pigmented, long, and course.
  - Androgen is not needed for the growth of hair on the scalp, eyebrows, and eyelashes. However, androgen is involved in hair growth on the face, ears, axilla, pubis, arms, legs, and trunk.
  - Androgen excess in women involves hair growth on upper lip, chin, midsternum, upper abdomen, back, and buttocks.
  - Hirsutism results from the interaction of serum androgens, local growth factors and the sensitivity of hair follicles to the androgens and growth factors.
  - The androgens testosterone, dehydroepiandrosterone, and androstenedione can be excreted in excess.
  - Hirsutism may affect between 5% to 10% of females in the reproductive age range.
  - Polycystic ovarian disease is the most common reason for hirsutism.

(Barbieri & Ehrmann, 2023; McComb et al., 2016; Sica & Gehr, 2001)

Appendix 11 provides additional details regarding direct smooth muscle relaxants.

Selective Alpha$_1$ Blockers

Mechanism of Action of Selective Alpha$_1$ Blockers

- Alpha$_1$ receptors are part of the SNS and respond to the neurotransmitters epinephrine and norepinephrine. These receptors are found within vascular smooth muscle and are essential in modulating the tone of small arterioles, thereby influencing SVR and BP. Activation of $\alpha 1$ receptors increases intracellular calcium levels, which induces smooth muscle contraction and results in peripheral vasoconstriction.
- Alpha$_1$ receptor blockers function by inhibiting these receptors, thus preventing peripheral vasoconstriction. Blocking $\alpha 1$ receptors leads to vasodilation of veins and arterioles, which lowers SVR and BP (Nachawati et al., 2025). Medications with the suffix of "osin" are classified as selective alpha$_1$ blockers. They may also be referred to as alpha$_1$ antagonists. They are called selective because they block only $\alpha 1$ receptors and do not influence $\alpha 2$ receptors.

Indications for Selective Alpha$_1$ Blockers

- Selective alpha$_1$ blockers are used in the treatment of HTN. They may also be used in the treatment of benign prostatic hypertrophy (BPH), reducing the sympathetic tone-induced component of urethral stricture that drives BPH symptoms.
- Doxazosin, prazosin, and terazosin are the 3 agents approved for the indication of resistant HTN and are the only agents in this class that will be discussed in this section.

- ♦ Doxazosin and terazosin are also indicated for the treatment of BPH which makes them appealing for the treatment of resistant HTN in the presence of BPH.
- ♦ Table 24 outlines details about the indications of these 3 medications.

Special Dosing Information for Selective Alpha$_1$ Blockers

- ♦ Alpha$_1$ blockers are typically taken at bedtime to avoid the orthostatic hypotension that may occur with the administration of these medications. Any dose adjustments should also occur at bedtime.
- ♦ There are no manufacturer recommendations for dose adjustment with doxazosin, prazosin, or terazosin in patients with altered kidney function.
  - Drug pharmacokinetics are unchanged with an eGRF of < 60 mL/min/1.73 m^2, however, the BP lowering effect may be enhanced.
  - If renal impairment exists, the initial dose should be lower, and the medication should be titrated cautiously.
  - Selective alpha$_1$ blockers are highly bound to protein and are not readily dialyzable. Therefore, no dose adjustments are recommended for patients on dialysis.
- ♦ There are no manufacturer recommendations for dose adjustment with doxazosin, prazosin, or terazosin in patients with mild to moderate liver impairment.
  - Selective alpha$_1$ blockers are highly metabolized in the liver and hepatic dysfunction will increase the exposure to these medications. Cautious use is required in patients with active liver disease.
  - Doxazosin is not recommended to be used in severe liver impairment (Pfizer, 2021).
- ♦ While not absolutely contraindicated in the elderly, selective alpha$_1$ blockers should be started at low doses with close monitoring due to the risk of orthostatic hypotension and dizziness and associated increased fall risk. The American Geriatrics Society Beers Criteria recommends avoiding these drugs in older adults for this reason (American Geriatrics Society Beers, 2023).
- ♦ Doxazosin is available in two preparations, IR and ER.
  - In the United States the IR preparation is approved for the treatment of HTN.
  - Doxazosin ER preparation is not approved for the treatment of HTN in the United States. However, there is emerging evidence outside of the United States suggesting that ER doxazosin is an acceptable option for the treatment of HTN.
  - Doxazosin ER preparation is approved for use in BPH in the United States.

(Abbott Laboratories, 2009; Li et al., 2022, Pfizer, 2021)

Table 24

Indications for Selective Alpha$_1$ Blockers

	Doxazosin	Prazosin	Terazosin
Indications for Individual Agents	▪ BPH: Mono or combination therapy in patients with moderate to severe symptoms. ▪ Ureteral stone expulsion [off label]. For stones ≥ 5 to ≤ 10 mm.	▪ Post-traumatic stress disorder related nightmares and sleep disruption [off label]. ▪ Raynaud phenomenon [off label].	▪ BPH: Mono or combination therapy in patients with moderate to severe symptoms. ▪ Ureteral Stone Expulsion [off label]. For stones ≥ 5 to ≤ 10 mm.
Indications for All Agents	▪ HTN as an additional agent; not first-line therapy. ▪ Resistant HTN as add on therapy in patients who do not respond to combination therapy with preferred agents.		

(Abbott Laboratories, 2009; Basquez & Pippin, 2023; Pfizer, 2021; Pfizer, 2009; UptoDate®,Lexidrug™ 2025)

Select Adverse Effects of Selective Apha$_1$ Receptor Antagonists

Hypotension / Orthostatic Hypotension

- Selective α1 blockers are reported to have a greater effect on BP and subsequently HR in the standing position compared to the supine position. This may contribute to the development of orthostatic hypotension.
- First dose orthostatic hypotension may develop within minutes to hours to days after initiation, depending on the medication's onset of action.
  - This effect can also occur if therapy is interrupted for several days and restarted.
  - See the box below on first dose hypotension.
- Syncope can occur secondary to severe orthostasis. In some cases, the syncopal episode may be preceded by significant tachycardia when the HR is 120 to 160 BPM.

> ***Linking Knowledge to Practice***
>
> ✓ *Diuretics, antihypertensives, or the combination of these agents will enhance the BP lowering effect of a selective alpha$_1$ blocker.*
> - *Manufacturers suggest that the dose of prazosin be decreased prior to initiation of another antihypertensive or diuretic.*
> - *Once the new agent has been established, the desired dose of prazosin should be reestablished with careful up titration and BP monitoring.*
>
> *(Pfizer, 2021)*

Intraoperative Floppy Iris Syndrome

- Intraoperative floppy iris syndrome (IFIS) is a complication of cataract surgery linked to selective alpha$_1$ blockers. The highest risk is associated with the use of tamsulosin (Wang et al., 2022).
- Stopping these medications before surgery offers no benefit, but surgical techniques can be adjusted to prevent this complication in patients currently or previously on a selective alpha$_1$ blocker.
- Generally, use of a selective alpha$_1$ blocker for 3 months or longer is associated with an increased risk of IFIS.

(Abbott Laboratories, 2009; Cantrell et al., 2008; Christou et al., 2020; Pfizer, 2009; Pfizer, 2021; UptoDate®, Lexidrug™ 2025)

CNS Depression

- The use of a selective alpha$_1$ blocker can result in impaired physical or mental abilities.
- Patients should be cautioned about participating in tasks that require mental acuity such as driving a car or operating machinery until the impact of the drug is fully understood.

Priapism

- Priapism (painful penile erection) sustained for hours and unrelieved by sexual intercourse or masturbation can occur.
- Although this adverse effect is extremely uncommon with these medications, it is a serious complication requiring immediate medical intervention.
- Male patients should be advised of this potential risk to ensure timely management if symptoms arise.

(Abbott Laboratories, 2009; Pfizer, 2009; Pfizer, 2021; UptoDate®,Lexidrug™ 2025)

Contraindication Highlights for Selective Alpha$_1$ Blockers

- Consult manufacturer recommendations for use in children, pregnant women, and nursing women.
- Do not use in patients with quinazoline sensitivity or with other quinazoline ("osins").
- In a Scientific Statement published in 2016 by the AHA, selective alpha$_1$ blockers (doxazosin, prazosin, terazosin) were highlighted as medications that may worsen underlying myocardial dysfunction and should be avoided in patients with HF (Page et al., 2016).

"First Dose" Orthostatic Hypotension

- Orthostatic hypotension is a potential concern with any antihypertensive agent but the risk of first dose orthostasis is of particular concern with selective alpha$_1$ blockers and centrally acting alpha$_2$ agonists. This adverse effect contributes to the decision to not use these medications as first, second or even third-line agents for the treatment of HTN.
- Patients can experience orthostatic hypotension as quickly as with the first dose (within 60 minutes) or within the first few days of initiation.
- Orthostasis has also been reported with rapid drug up-titration, or with the addition of a new antihypertensive medication to a current regiment that includes a selective alpha$_1$ blocker or a centrally acting alpha$_2$ agonist.
- If the selective alpha$_1$ blocker or centrally acting alpha$_2$ receptor agonist antihypertensive medication is temporarily stopped for several days "first dose" orthostatic hypotension can occur with reinitiation of the medication. Reintroduction of the medication should begin with the lowest dose.
- It is recommended that initiation of these medications occurs at bedtime starting with the lowest dose to avoid the orthostatic hypotension that occurs when up and about during waking hours.
- Slow up-titration will also help reduce the incidence of orthostatic hypotension.
- Patients should be advised to move slowly from a lying to standing position to avoid the development of orthostatic hypotension. This is especially important upon wakening.
- The risk for orthostatic hypotension can be increased in the elderly, especially the frail elderly, and alternatives to selective alpha$_1$ blockers or centrally acting alpha$_2$ agonists should be considered.

(Li et al., 2022; Nachawati et al., 2025; Wang et al., 2022; Welsh & Mitchell, 2023)

Linking Knowledge to Practice

- ✓ *Primary aldosteronism is present in approximately 15% of the patients with resistant HTN.*
- ✓ *The accurate calculation of the aldosterone-to-renin ratio is essential for diagnosing primary aldosteronism.*
- ✓ *When screening a patient for primary aldosteronism it is important to avoid antihypertensives that alter aldosterone and renin levels as many antihypertensive agents do.*
- ✓ *Selective alpha$_1$ blockers can be used temporarily for BP control to allow for a more accurate measurement of plasma aldosterone and renin levels in patients with resistant HTN being evaluated for primary aldosteronism.*

(Li et al., 2022; Welsh & Mitchell, 2023)

Special Considerations & Monitoring with Selective Alpha$_1$ Blockers

- There is no recommended specific monitoring of laboratory values.
- Selective alpha$_1$ blockers require careful BP and HR monitoring during initiation and dose changes.
- Increased BP monitoring should occur when adding other drugs affecting BP.
- Monitor for mental status changes:

- Selective $alpha_1$ blockers may cause significant drowsiness, dizziness, and low blood pressure, which can impair the ability to drive or operate heavy machinery.
- Patients should be advised to wait to drive until the effects of the medication are known.

Key Pharmacokinetic & Pharmacodynamic Information for Selective $Alpha_1$ Blockers

See Table 25 for key pharmacokinetic and pharmacodynamic information for selective $Alpha_1$ blockers.

Table 25

Key Pharmacokinetic & Pharmacodynamic Information for Selective $Alpha_1$ Blockers

Doxazosin	Prazosin	Terazosin
▪ Plasma Peak: √ IR: 2 to 3 hours. √ ER: 8 to 9 hours. ▪ Duration: > 24 hours. ▪ Half-life Elimination: √ IR: 22 hours. √ ER: 15 to 19 hours. ▪ 98% protein bound. ▪ Extensive hepatic metabolism. ▪ Excreted in feces.	▪ Onset of Action: 2 hours. ▪ Plasma Peak: 2 to 4 hours. ▪ Duration: 10 to 24 hours. ▪ Half-life Elimination: 2 to 3 hours. ▪ 97% protein bound. ▪ Extensive hepatic metabolism. ▪ Excreted in feces.	▪ Onset of Action: 15 minutes. ▪ Plasma Peak: 2 to 3 hours. ▪ Duration: 24 hours. ▪ Half-life Elimination: 12 hours. Increased to 14 hours in adults ≥ 70 years. ▪ 90-94% protein bound. ▪ Hepatic metabolism. ▪ Excreted in feces (60%). ▪ Excreted in the urine (40%).
(Abbott Laboratories, 2009; Pfizer, 2009; Pfizer, 2021; UptoDate®,Lexidrug™ 2025)		

Important Medication Interactions with Selective $Alpha_1$ Blockers

See Table 26 for important medications interactions with selective $alpha_1$ blockers.

Table 26

Important Medication Interactions with Selective $Alpha_1$ Blockers

Doxazosin	Prazosin	Terazosin
▪ Strong substrate of CYP3A4. Strong CYP3A inhibitors may increase serum concentration of doxazosin. ▪ PDE-5 inhibitors can result in additive BP lowering effects and symptomatic hypotension. ▪ MOA inhibitors may increase antihypertensive effect.	▪ MOA inhibitors may increase antihypertensive effect. ▪ PDE-5 inhibitors can result in additive BP lowering effects and symptomatic hypotension.	▪ MOA inhibitors may increase antihypertensive effect. ▪ PDE-5 inhibitors can result in additive BP lowering effects and symptomatic hypotension. ▪ Use with verapamil can increase the body's exposure to terazosin and worsen the hypotensive effect.
(Abbott Laboratories, 2009; Pfizer, 2009; Pfizer, 2021; UptoDate®,Lexidrug™ 2025)		

Appendix 11 provides additional details regarding selective $alpha_1$ blockers.

Centrally Acting $Alpha_2$ Agonists

Centrally acting $alpha_2$ agonists are medications primarily used for treating resistant HTN in adults. These medications were approved decades ago, and newer antihypertensive agents have replaced their routine use.

- Although no longer first-line therapy for chronic HTN, this class can be employed as add on therapy for the treatment of resistant HTN. They have been deemed helpful in treating resistant HTN produced by anxiety.
- In addition to HTN, centrally acting alpha$_2$ receptor agonists may be used for the treatment of severe cancer pain, ICU sedation, and alleviating opioid withdrawal symptoms. The sedating effect of some formulations have led to their use in anesthesia to reduce anesthesia requirements by potentiating anesthetic agents. They are also used as a sedative in the ICU when patients are transitioned off IV dexmedetomidine.
- Additionally, some of these medications are used solely for the treatment of disorders in children including attention deficit hyperactivity disorder (ADHD), Tourette syndrome, and post-traumatic stress disorder. The only use covered in this writing is HTN treatment in adults.

(Kamibayashi et al., 1997; UptoDate®,Lexidrug™ 2025)

Mechanism of Action of Centrally Acting Alpha$_2$ Agonists

- When stimulated, α_2 adrenergic receptors in the CNS inhibit the release of neurotransmitters, primarily norepinephrine.
- Centrally acting alpha$_2$ agonists enhance the ability of α_2 adrenergic receptors, primarily in the brain stem and spinal cord, to slow SNS activity.
- Reduced norepinephrine release lowers BP, HR, and peripheral vascular resistance. The reduction on systolic BP and diastolic BP has been found to be equal.
- Despite the vasodilator effect reflex tachycardia is rarely an issue. Minor reductions in CO and renal blood flow may occur but most often these remain normal without any effect on perfusion.
- Centrally, alpha$_2$ agonists can produce sedation, relaxation, pain relief, and cognitive improvement.
- There are three receptor subtypes, α2-A, α2-B and α2-C, present in the brain, kidneys, heart, and vasculature.
  - Each uniquely influences BP and sympathetic transmission.
  - The impact on the individual α2 adrenergic receptor subtypes varies based on the formulation of each medication. Therefore, not all centrally acting alpha$_2$ agonists have the same indications due to varying pharmacodynamics.
- This section will address those centrally acting alpha$_2$ agonists that are primarily used in the treatment of HTN. These agents are clonidine, methyldopa, and guanfacine IR.

(Giovannitti et al., 2015; Kamibayashi et al., 1997; Schwartz et al., 2022; Sica, 2007).

Indications for Centrally Acting Alpha$_2$ Agonists

See Table 27 for a comparison of indications for the 3 centrally acting alpha$_2$ agonists.

Special Dosing Information for Centrally Acting Alpha$_2$ Receptor Agonists

- See Prescribing Pearls for clonidine and methyldopa for additional information.
- Centrally acting alpha$_2$ receptor agonists are most often initiated at bedtime.
  - Bedtime dosing helps mitigate the risk of orthostatic hypotension.
  - Initiating and adjusting doses at night results in peak drowsiness that typically coincides with sleep.
  - Nighttime dosing of these agents has been associated with reducing the typical early morning BP surge associated with catecholamine and neurohormonal activation upon awakening.
    - The early morning BP surge is part of the normal circadian rhythm.
    - Guanfacine is especially effective due to a longer duration of action.

  (Bilo et al., 2018; Sica, 2015)

- While not absolutely contraindicated in the elderly, centrally acting $alpha_2$ receptor agonists should be started at low doses with close monitoring due to risks of orthostatic hypotension, dizziness, and drowsiness that increase fall risk. The American Geriatrics Society Beers Criteria recommends avoiding these drugs in older adults for this reason (American Geriatrics Society Beers, 2023).
- There are no recommendations for dose adjustment for clonidine, methyldopa or guanfacine with chronic hepatic impairment. However, careful monitoring is recommended when used in patients with chronic stable liver disease. Methyldopa is contraindicated in acute hepatic dysfunction such as acute hepatitis or acute cirrhosis.
- In the presence of altered renal function the starting dose should be lower, and the medication should be carefully titrated to response because worsening kidney function may enhance drug effects. Methyldopa is recommended to be given at different dosage intervals based on creatinine clearance.
    - If CrCl > 50 mL/min methyldopa is administered every 8 hours.
    - If CrCl 10 to 50 mL/min methyldopa is administered every 8 to 12 hours.
    - If CrCl < 10 mL/min methyldopa should be taken no more frequently than every 12 to 24 hours.
- Dosage adjustments are not necessary for patients receiving dialysis. Methyldopa is dialyzable and should be administered following dialysis. Clonidine and guanfacine are not significantly removed by dialysis and may be given before, during, or after the treatment based on the patient's BP.
- Tolerance may occur with methyldopa about 2 to 3 months after initiation of therapy. Tolerance is addressed by increasing the dose or adding a thiazide diuretic if the patient is not currently taking one.
- Guanfacine tablets are manufactured in two different preparations, IR and ER tablets.
    - In the United States guanfacine ER is not approved for the treatment of HTN.
    - The only indication for IR guanfacine in the United States is HTN.
    - IR and ER tablet dosages are not interchangeable. They possess different pharmacokinetic profiles.
- Centrally acting $alpha_2$ receptor agonists should not be abruptly stopped due to the risk of withdrawal syndrome and the potential to develop significant rebound HTN. See Advanced Concept Focus section below on centrally acting $alpha_2$ agonists and withdrawal syndrome.

Table 27

Indications for Centrally Acting $Alpha_2$ Agonists

Medication	Indication
Clonidine	▪ HTN (resistant) as an additional agent; not first-line therapy. √ Oral (IR and ER): hypertensive urgency or chronic HTN. √ Transdermal: chronic HTN. ▪ Severe cancer pain management. √ For intractable pain not responsive to opioids. √ Epidural use only and under the care of a pain management specialist. ▪ Off label use: √ ICU sedation (transition from dexmedetomidine to clonidine). √ Treatment of opioid withdrawal. √ Vasomotor symptoms (flushing) associated with menopause.
Methyldopa & Guanfacine IR	▪ HTN as an additional agent; not first-line therapy. Often reserved for "last line" therapy due to side effect profile.
(Actavis Pharma, 2023; Athena Bioscience, 2021; Boehringer Ingelheim International, 2009, 2024; Chartwell RX, 2024, 2025; TruPharma, 2024; UptoDate®,Lexidrug™ 2025)	

Clonidine Key Points

- Clonidine hydrochloride (clonidine) is a centrally acting $alpha_2$ agonist that works in the brain stem and spinal cord.
- This medication is unique because it is a dominant $alpha_2$ *agonist* yet also exerts an $alpha_2$ *antagonist* effect, working differently in the anterior hypothalamus than the posterior hypothalamus.
  - The anterior hypothalamus serves as the primary control center for the parasympathetic nervous system and when activated inhibits the sympathetic outflow of excitatory CV neurons. Clonidine works as an $alpha_2$ *agonist* by further inhibiting the inhibition of the sympathetic outflow of excitatory CV neurons, primarily norepinephrine.
  - The posterior hypothalamus is the primary control center for the SNS and when activated it increases the release of excitatory CV neurons, primarily norepinephrine. Clonidine works as an $alpha_2$ *antagonist* in the posterior hypothalamus inhibiting the release of excitatory CV neurons.
- With the dual impact on the release of excitatory CV neurons BP is reduced with a decrease in SVR, along with decreased renal vascular resistance and a lower HR.
  - CO may decrease initially; however, this decrease is not usually significant and will normalize soon after drug initiation.
  - While there is usually a lowering of HR noted with clonidine initiation there does not appear to be any impact on the normal HR response with activity.

(Isaac, 1980; Yasaei & Saadabadi, 2023)

- In addition to resistant HTN, clonidine can be used as a short-term solution for severe asymptomatic hypertensive urgency. While not usually a first-line agent, this oral medication can be beneficial in this nonemergency situation due to its short onset of action of 30 to 60 minutes.
  - Severe HTN is defined as systolic BP $\geq$180 or diastolic BP $\geq$120 mmHg.
  - Oral clonidine, among other agents, has been found to be safely used as a short-term solution for severe asymptomatic HTN in the ambulatory setting. It allows for treatment without hospitalization for most patients.
  - The overall short-term BP reduction goal is usually $\leq$160 / $\leq$100 mmHg, remembering that the MAP should not be lowered more than 5 to 30% in the first few hours.
  - IR oral clonidine begins to take effect in 30 to 60 minutes with a maximum reduction of BP in 2 to 4 hours.
  - All patients treated in this manner will need frequent dosing and close outpatient follow up as well as a long-term treatment plan.
  - With an onset of action of 30 to 60 minutes oral clonidine is not an appropriate choice in hypertensive emergency when symptoms of end organ failure are present and hospitalization is required.

(Karachalios, 1986; Mirdamadi et al., 2022; Varon & Elliott, 2025)

- Clonidine has been used off label in the ICU as an alternative for sedation due to the CNS effects associated with clonidine. Patients can be transitioned from IV sedation with dexmedetomidine to oral sedation with clonidine.
  - This practice has not demonstrated an improvement in outcomes including ventilation time, ICU LOS, or ICU morality.
  - The use of clonidine does appear to reduce narcotic use but is associated with an increased incidence of clinically significant hypotension.
  - While the lower cost of clonidine over dexmedetomidine is appealing, the risk of significant hypotension appears to out weight the cost benefit.

(Srivastava, 2014; Wang et al., 2017; Yasaei & Saadabadi, 2023)

Prescribing Pearls for Clonidine

- Clonidine is available as a weekly transdermal patch, oral tablet, or extended-release tablet. There is an injectable suspension available for epidural use in treating cancer pain which is beyond the scope of this publication.
- Oral clonidine is clonidine hydrochloride while the transdermal patch is referred to as clonidine base.
- Dosages are not interchangeable between the transdermal patch, IR, or ER tablets.
- The transdermal patch is not indicated for acute situations.
- For transitions between the patch or oral formulas see Prescribing Pearls for the clonidine transdermal system patch.
- The transdermal patch has some advantages over oral dosing; however, the cost of the patch may prohibit its use.
    - The patch deliverers a continuous steady dose once therapeutic levels have been achieved. This steady state is without the peaks and troughs experienced with oral dosing and mimics that of a continuous IV infusion.
    - The patch may help eliminate missed doses that can occur with poor adherence to oral regimens.
    - The transdermal patch is associated with less dry mouth and less excessive drowsiness than oral tablets.
- Clonidine dosing should continue through the perioperative period in patients requiring surgical procedures to prevent rebound HTN.
    - If oral clonidine cannot be resumed immediately in the postoperative period, a transition to a transdermal patch 3 or more days prior to surgery should be considered to prevent postoperative withdrawal syndrome.
    - Patients taking the extended-release formulation should take their last dose 28 hours prior to surgery and it should be restarted on postoperative day 1.
    - In patients taking IR clonidine the drug should be continued up to 4 hours prior to surgery then resumed as soon as possible after surgery.
    - Anesthesia requirements may be reduced in patients taking clonidine.
- Clonidine must be tapered gradually when the drug is discontinued to prevent withdrawal symptoms associated with abrupt discontinuation. Significant rebound HTN can occur if the medication is not tapered appropriately.
- See Advanced Concept Focus section below on centrally acting $alpha_2$ agonists and withdrawal syndrome.

(Actavis Pharma, 2023: Athena Bioscience, 2021; Boehringer Ingelheim International, 2009, 2023; TruPharma, 2024; UptoDate®,Lexidrug™ 2025; Yasaei & Saadabadi, 2023)

Linking Knowledge to Practice

- ✓ *Patients should be instructed that it takes about 2 days after starting the first clonidine patch for full BP effect to take place. BPs taken as part of home monitoring within the first 48 hours after starting a clonidine patch for the first time will not reflect the full therapeutic effect of the clonidine patch.*
- ✓ *Just as with oral clonidine, patients need to know that they should not abruptly discontinue the clonidine patch. If there are concerns about continuing an ordered patch, patients should notify a provider for instructions on how to safely discontinue the patch as well as to receive instructions for alternative medication(s) for BP control.*

Prescribing Pearls Specific to the Clonidine Transdermal System Patch

- The amount of medication delivered is directly proportional to the size of the patch. The larger the patch the more drug administered. The patch will deliver 0.1, 0.2, or 0.3 mg of clonidine per day based on the size of the patch.
- The term clonidine patch refers to the patch containing the medication clonidine. This differs from the cover patch that comes with the clonidine patch. Use of the cover patch is described below.
- After the clonidine patch is applied and adheres to the skin surface the medication will be administered to the capillaries of the skin based on a concentration gradient.
  - Clonidine will flow from the patch, which is highly concentrated, through a rate controlling membrane to the skin.
  - The skin will always have a lower concentration of clonidine. The patch is dosed to always have more drug than the rate that is being delivered if the patch is changed at appropriate intervals.
- Continuous drug delivery occurs if the patch is at least 40% saturated with the drug. The system is designed to not drop below this level for up to an average of 9 days after application.
- The full pharmacodynamic effect of the drug will be known 3 days after the first patch is applied.
- Repeat application of the same dose in 7-day intervals will maintain the level of drug in the body at a steady state.
- The full effect of the drug will continue for approximately 8 hours after the patch is removed. It will then begin to taper if a new patch is not applied.
- The cover patch is supplied with each clonidine medicated patch. This cover patch can be used for two purposes. Firstly, it can be used to cover the clonidine patch and promote adherence if there is not adequate adherence to the skin. It can also be used to administer a partial dose of the clonidine patch. For example, to give ½ the normal dose of a prescribed clonidine patch the following steps would be used:
  - The cover patch is cut into 2 halves. If the cover patch is not available, the same principles can be applied using an adhesive bandage cut to the same size. Set aside or discard ½ of the cover patch.
  - The adhesive backing should be removed from the ½ cover patch being used and applied directly to the skin in a location appropriate for clonidine patch application.
  - Once the cover patch is in place the entire clonidine patch should be place on top of the cover patch with ½ of the medicated patch directly applied to the skin and the other ½ of the medicated patch on top of the cover patch. This will allow only ½ of the normal dose to be delivered.
- The clonidine medicated patch should <u>never</u> be cut as this will alter the drug distribution system.
- When transitioning from oral clonidine to a clonidine patch, apply the patch on day one and have the patient take the full prescribed dose of oral clonidine.
  - On day 2 the oral dose of clonidine should be 50% of the prescribed oral dose.
  - On day 3 the patient should receive 25% of the prescribed oral dose.
  - On day 4 the oral dose should be discontinued.
- When transitioning from transdermal patch to oral clonidine the new oral dose should not be initiated any sooner than 8 hours after the patch was removed. Drug effect from the patch can continue for up to 24 to 48 hours or longer after removal. BP monitoring is required during the transition.
- The patch should not be removed for surgical procedures. Anesthesia must be aware of the patch for appropriate BP monitoring.
- Most clonidine patches have an aluminum component which can result in skin burns during an MRI therefore it is recommended by the manufacturer that the patch is removed prior to this procedure.

(Actavis Pharma, Inc, 2023; Boehringer Ingelheim International 2023; Sica & Grubbs, 2005)

Clonidine Transdermal Patch Administration and Patient Education

- The patch should be replaced every seven days and applied to a new, clean, dry, hairless area on the chest wall or upper outer arms.
  - For optimal drug absorption, avoid wrinkled, injured (areas with open wounds, rashes, or unhealed scratches), or freshly shaven skin.
  - Early clinical trials demonstrated that placement on the chest or upper arms results in superior drug absorption compared to application on the legs.
- The patch is designed to be waterproof, allowing the patient to bathe, shower or swim.
- If the patch becomes loose and is no longer adhering tightly to the skin, there is a white round adhesive cover patch supplied with each medicated patch that can applied over the patch to assure the patch has full skin contact. The adhesive cover is supplied for this reason to help assure the patient can use the patch for a full 7 days.
- If the patch and adhesive cover are unable to maintain complete skin contact, the patch should be removed and replaced with a new one. This will reset the 7-day treatment period.
- The patch can cause local skin irritation.
  - Rotating sites weekly can help limit skin irritation.
  - If the irritation is significant, the patch can be removed and a new patch placed in a new location. This will reset the 7-day treatment period.
  - The application of a corticosteroid spray prior to applying the patch has been suggested to mitigate the skin irritation. The skin must completely dry from the corticosteroid spray before applying the patch.
- Upon removal, the patch should be folded so that the adhesive sides stick together and then disposed of in a secure location not accessible to children. The patch retains residual medication, which may be harmful if ingested or applied by infants or children.

(Actavis Pharma, 2023; Sica, 2007; Sica & Grubbs, 2005)

Linking Knowledge to Practice

✓ *Correct use of the clonidine patch is essential for its effectiveness. Patients should receive clear instructions to ensure they apply the patch properly, allowing the medication to work safely and as intended.*

Linking Knowledge to Practice

✓ *Clonidine patches should be removed prior to cardioversion or defibrillation due to the risk of altered electrical conductivity.*

Advanced Concept Focus:
Centrally Acting Alpha$_2$ Agonists and Withdrawal Syndrome

- The sudden cessation of chronic therapy with a centrally acting alpha$_2$ agonist can result in what is referred to as withdrawal syndrome.
- Withdrawal syndrome is most frequently discussed in relation to clonidine, most likely due to its shorter onset of action and duration but is recognized as a possibility with all centrally acting alpha$_2$ receptor agonists. Most information in the literature is specific to clonidine withdrawal.
- Manufacturers warn of the importance of tapering these medications to prevent withdrawal syndrome.

- ♦ Withdrawal symptoms include H/A, agitation, insomnia, and palpitations when chronic therapy is stopped without a gradual taper of these medications.
- ♦ In the worst-case scenario sudden cessation of the drug may cause severe rebound HTN, potentially leading to an acute hypertensive crisis with risks of stroke, encephalopathy, cardiac ischemia, HF, or pulmonary edema.
- ♦ Rebound HTN results from the abrupt termination of blockade of adrenal catecholamine secretion, leading to an increase in circulating catecholamine levels.
  - This sympathetic surge typically manifests within 8 to 12 hours following sudden discontinuation of clonidine, though its onset may be delayed up to 3 days depending on the specific drug formulation administered.
  - Guanfacine sympathetic surge can present as late as 2 to 4 days due to a half-life that is longer than clonidine.
- ♦ The recommended rate for tapering varies. A reduction over several days may still lead to rebound HTN depending on the dose and the length of use. Generally, tapering over weeks rather than days helps to lower the likelihood of rebound HTN.
- ♦ In patients experiencing unfavorable non-urgent clonidine side effects a taper over 6 to 10 days is considered a faster taper and would include a reduction of the dose by $^{1}/_{2}$ every 2nd to 3rd day. Tapering over several weeks would provide a safer taper if able.
- ♦ Both the duration of medication usage and the dosage administered are critical factors when establishing an appropriate tapering schedule. Either a higher dose or a longer period of administration typically requires a more gradual reduction over a longer timeframe.
- ♦ Withdrawal syndrome has also been noted with discontinuation of the clonidine transdermal patch.
  - Withdrawal syndrome with the patch is reported less frequently than with oral dosing and is thought to be due to the slow decline in the drug level after patch removal.
  - Drug levels begin to decline about 8 hours after patch removal. This is followed by a gradual decrease in the drug levels over several days.
  - This gradual decrease in drug level is further slowed due to residual drug that remains in the skin where the patch was last placed. This residual drug provides an auto tapering effect which further slows the drug removal from the system (Sica & Grubbs, 2005).
  - If HTN occurs during transdermal patch down titration, oral clonidine can be used to treat the rebound HTN. Once the BP is stable, slow titration of the oral dose can begin. See Prescribing Pearls for the clonidine transdermal system patch which discusses how to decrease dosing with the patch.
- ♦ Monitoring BP at home is essential during a centrally acting $alpha_2$ agonist taper. Patients should be advised to report any elevation in BP or other signs of withdrawal as this may necessitate reverting to the previous dose and implementing a slower tapering schedule.
- ♦ If the patient is on a beta blocker in addition to clonidine the beta blocker should be withdrawn several days before beginning the clonidine taper (UptoDate®,Lexidrug™, 2025).
  - This allows for the reactivation of the beta response in a patient that has been experiencing beta blockade.
  - Nonselective beta blockers block both ß1 and ß2 receptors. ß2 activation is responsible for peripheral vascular relaxation and when these receptors are blocked peripheral vasoconstriction can occur resulting in an increase in peripheral vascular resistance.
  - Cardioselective beta blockers mainly target ß1 receptors with little effect on ß2. However, all beta blockers should be discontinued before weaning clonidine.
  - Discontinuing the beta blocker reactivates ß2 receptors, allowing peripheral vascular relaxation including arterial vasodilation, which can help counteract rebound HTN and reduce its effects.

➢ If a centrally acting $alpha_2$ agonist must be stopped faster than desired because of severe side effects, another antihypertensive can be started during the taper to keep BP controlled. However, beta blockers should be avoided in this situation to allow for stimulation of ß2 receptors.

(Actavis Pharma, 2023; Athena Bioscience, 2021; Boehringer Ingelheim International, 2009, 2023; Chartwell RX, 2024, 2025; Elliott, 2025; Geyskes et al., 1979; Hart et al., 1981; Hunyor et al., 1973; Sica, 2015; Sica & Grubbs, 2005; Tru-Pharma, 2024; UptoDate®,Lexidrug™ 2025; Vanholder et al., 1977)

Linking Knowledge to Practice

✓ *Patients on long-term clonidine treatment who develop resistant HTN should be assessed for medication adherence.*

✓ *Patients on long-term clonidine therapy who miss doses can also experience rebound HTN. These patients will have variable BPs due to inconsistent dosing of clonidine.*

(Elliott, 2025)

Select Adverse Effects of Centrally Acting $Alpha_2$ Agonists

Hypotension

- As with all antihypertensive medications, hypotension is a potential adverse effect. The risk for hypotension is greater with the use of centrally acting $alpha_2$ agonists.
- Orthostatic hypotension is of particular concern due to the ability of the centrally acting $alpha_2$ agonist to impact both supine and standing blood pressure.
- The onset of hypotension varies based on onset of action and peak effect. With clonidine, hypotension can occur as early as 30 minutes after administration with the most noted effects within 1 to 4 hours after administration. A hypotensive response to a clonidine patch usually does not occur until approximately 2 days after application of the first patch.
- Factors that increase the risk of developing hypotension include dehydration, use with other antihypertensive medications, history of hypotension, bradycardia, or CV disease.

Bradycardia

- Low HRs from sinus bradycardia as well as more significant arrhythmias including sinus node arrest, junctional bradycardia, high degree AV block can occur. If there is an unknown sinus arrhythmia or AV block this can worsen with the addition of a centrally acting $alpha_2$ receptor agonist.
- Clonidine should not be used in patients with known arrhythmias.
- HR decreases of up to 5 BPM can be expected with the routine use of a centrally acting $alpha_2$ receptor agonists but there is no appreciable change in cardiac output.
- Arrhythmias typically occur at higher doses, while lower doses usually have less impact on HR.
- Possible additive effects, including bradycardia and AV block may occur when used in combination with agents that influence sinus node function or AV nodal conduction, such as digitalis, CCBs, and beta blockers.

General Reported Adverse Effects

Clinical trials have identified the general side effects listed below as the most frequent reasons for patient withdrawal of therapy. These adverse effects tend to intensify with increasing drug dosages. Some symptoms may diminish over time when lower dosages are administered.

- Dry mouth (less frequent with transdermal patch).

- Somnolence (excessive tiredness, daytime sleepiness).
- Dizziness.
- Fatigue and weakness.
- Constipation.
- Edema is a documented adverse effect associated with multiple antihypertensive agents, particularly methyldopa. This is more likely to occur with the clonidine patch which is associated with higher sodium and water retention than oral clonidine. Management often involves the concurrent administration of a diuretic.

> ***Linking Knowledge to Practice***
>
> ✓ *Contact lens users should be aware that treatment with oral clonidine tablets may cause dryness of eyes. The use of additional wetting solutions may be needed.*

Methyldopa Specific Adverse Effects

- Rare occurrences of hematologic abnormalities are reported with the use of methyldopa requiring periodic laboratory monitoring of the CBC.
  - These rare occurrences include granulocytopenia and thrombocytopenia. In each of these abnormalities blood counts return to normal with drug cessation.
  - The use of methyldopa may also result in a methyldopa-induced direct Coombs-positive hemolytic anemia that can occur between 6 and 12 months of drug use. See Advanced Concept Focus section below on methyldopa induced Coombs-positive hemolytic anemia.
- Hepatotoxicity and fatal hepatic necrosis have been documented and considered a hypersensitivity reaction to methyldopa use. Although hepatotoxicity is uncommon, prompt intervention is essential, as discontinuation of the medication may reverse its effects.
  - Any occurrence of unexplained fever or jaundice should immediately trigger laboratory assessment for acute liver injury, and the drug should be withdrawn without delay.
  - Cholestasis can occur within the first 2 to 3 months of therapy resulting in jaundice, with or without fever.
- Additionally, HF may develop, potentially related to sympathetic system suppression. The onset of edema warrants a thorough evaluation for HF.

(Actavis Pharma, Inc, 2023; Athena Bioscience, 2024; Boehringer Ingelheim International 2009, 2023; Chartwell RX, 2024, 2025; Gupta & Khalili, 2023; Muluk, 2025; Sica, 2015; TruPharma, 2024; UptoDate®,Lexidrug™ 2025; Yasaei & Saadabadi, 2025)

Advanced Concept Focus:

Methyldopa Induced Coombs-Positive Hemolytic Anemia

- Approximately 10 to 20% of patients taking methyldopa will develop a positive direct Coombs test.
- Not all patients who develop a positive direct Coombs test on methyldopa therapy will develop hemolytic anemia, but a positive Coombs test should prompt an evaluation for hemolytic anemia.
- The manufacturer notes that having a positive direct Coombs test before or during methyldopa therapy, without evidence of hemolytic anemia, does not preclude the use of methyldopa.
- This hypersensitivity occurs when the drug triggers the immune system to produce IgG antibodies that attach to the red blood cells. A positive direct Coombs test indicates these antibodies are present.
- The development of autoimmune hemolytic anemia because of methyldopa therapy is very rare and reported to only be between 1 and 2% of those with a positive direct Coombs test result.

- ♦ Prior to initiation of methyldopa, a CBC should be completed to assess for anemia and establish a baseline.
- ♦ Manufacturers recommend periodic evaluation of CBCs performed during the first 12 months of therapy. Important measures include hematocrit, hemoglobin, and red blood cell count. Direct Coombs is recommended prior to initiation, and again at 6 months and 12 months.
- ♦ If a patient develops a positive direct Coombs test during methyldopa therapy and hemolytic anemia is confirmed, methyldopa should be discontinued and not restarted.
- ♦ Direct Coombs positive hemolytic anemia generally resolves within weeks to months after discontinuation of the drug. If early resolution does not occur and corticosteroids are required for management, alternative causes of this disorder should be considered.
- ♦ In patients receiving methyldopa who require blood transfusion, it is advisable to conduct both direct and indirect Coombs tests. A positive direct Coombs test does not impede blood cross-matching; however, a positive indirect Coombs test may present cross-matching challenges. In such instances, it is recommended to consult a hematologist or transfusion specialist for further guidance.

(Carstairs et al., 1966; Chartwell RX, 2025; Gupta & Khalili, 2023; UptoDate®,Lexidrug™ 2025)

Contraindication Highlights for Centrally Acting Alpha$_2$ Agonists

Table 28 lists contraindications to centrally acting alpha$_2$ agonists.

Table 28

Contraindication Highlights for Centrally Acting Alpha$_2$ Agonists

Clonidine	Methyldopa	Guanfacine IR
▪ No absolute contraindications. ▪ If allergic reaction from transdermal patch occurs the substitution of oral clonidine will most often result in the development of a skin rash. Substitution is not advised. ▪ Use with caution in severe CAD, conduction disturbances, recent MI, cerebrovascular disease or CKD due to possibility of hypotension and bradycardia.	▪ Contraindications include: √ Concurrent MAO inhibitor use. √ Active hepatic disease. √ Previous direct Coombs positive hemolytic anemia. √ Pheochromocytoma. ▪ Use with caution in CKD which results in accumulation of methyldopa and enhances hypotensive effect. Lower doses are encouraged.	▪ No absolute contraindications. ▪ Caution advised with kidney impairment and liver impairment. ▪ Use with caution in severe CAD, conduction disturbances, recent MI, cerebrovascular disease or CKD secondary to possibility of hypotension and bradycardia.

Note: Consult manufacturer recommendations for use in children, pregnant women, and nursing women.
(Actavis Pharma, 2023; Athena Bioscience, 2021; Boehringer Ingelheim International, 2009, 2023; Chartwell RX, 2024, 2025; TruPharma, 2024; UptoDate®,Lexidrug™ 2025)

Linking Knowledge to Practice

- ✓ *Dry mouth is a frequently reported side effect of centrally acting alpha$_2$ agonists. This is likely caused by an α2-mediated decrease in saliva production. This leads to hyposalivation, which over time raises the risk for dental caries, periodontal disease, and oral candidiasis.*
- ✓ *Encourage patients to try foods or drinks that help increase salivation such as sugar-free gums and candies.*
- ✓ *Clonidine has the highest report of dry mouth. Dry mouth is reported less often with the clonidine transdermal patch. Therefore, transition from oral to the patch may be helpful in reducing this adverse effect.*

(Sica 2015)

Methyldopa Key Points

- Methyldopa, introduced over 60 years ago, is now considered a last-line treatment option for resistant HTN in adults.
- Methyldopa remains a viable treatment option for pregnancy-induced HTN. While there may be other more effective agents with a lower side effect profile, the use of methyldopa during pregnancy has not demonstrated any apparent adverse effects on the fetus, and the associated improvement in maternal BP is linked to better fetal outcomes (Arshad et al., 2024; August, 2025; Gupta & Al Khalili, 2019; Molvi et al., 2012; Spitalewitz et al., 1983).
- Methyldopa, a centrally acting $alpha_2$ agonist, has a mechanism of action that differs from the other two centrally acting $alpha_2$ agonists.
  - α-methyldopa is a prodrug that requires biotransformation in the body to an active form before it can exert a therapeutic effect.
  - When introduced to the body, α-methyldopa converts to α-methyl norepinephrine. α-methyl norepinephrine is considered a "false" neurotransmitter that attaches to the α2 adrenergic receptors in the brainstem replacing the action of norepinephrine.
  - α-methyl norepinephrine mimics the actions of norepinephrine but with substantially less impact then the "true" much more potent neurotransmitter norepinephrine.
  - This "false" transmitter, released via the sympathetic pathways, decreases the sympathetic outflow to the heart, kidneys and peripheral vasculature.
  - With the release of α-methyl norepinephrine there is less SNS impact resulting in a reduction in SVR without significant changes in cardiac output.
  - Additionally, there appears to be a selective reduction in renal vascular resistance improving glomerular flow.
  - There is also a reduction in renin release with methyldopa that is not present with other antihypertensive medications. This fact is felt to play an important role in the drugs ability to lower blood pressure.
- Methyldopa may cause urine samples to exhibit fluorescence at wavelengths commonly used for urine catecholamine detection, potentially leading to falsely elevated urinary catecholamine results. This interference can complicate the diagnostic process for pheochromocytoma; therefore, alternative diagnostic methods should be considered.
- Patients taking methyldopa may need reduced anesthesia during surgery. It is recommended to continue the medication before surgery and assure the anesthesia team is aware of the medication.
- Methyldopa is typically dosed 2 to 4 times a day to achieve the desired BP.
- If administered with other antihypertensives the total initial daily dose of methyldopa should not exceed 500 mg (in divided doses) until response to the drug is known. There may be a need to adjust the other antihypertensives to allow for the safe administration of methyldopa.
- There is no adjustment needed when methyldopa is used with a thiazide diuretic. Methyldopa and thiazide diuretics function synergistically to reduce HTN. While methyldopa decreases sympathetic output in the brain to lower BP through vasodilation, thiazide diuretics act on the kidneys to increase the excretion of sodium and water reducing BP by decreasing blood volume and fluid retention. Since methyldopa lowers plasma renin activity it counteracts the rise in plasma renin activity that occurs with diuretics resulting in better BP control.

(Bellomo, 2022; Chartwell RX, 2025; Kaplan, 1979; UptoDate®,Lexidrug™ 2025)

Special Considerations & Monitoring for Centrally Acting $Alpha_2$ Agonists

- ♦ Centrally acting $alpha_2$ agonists require careful BP and HR monitoring during initiation and dose changes. Increased BP monitoring should occur when adding other drugs affecting BP.
- ♦ Monitor for mental status changes.

- ♦ Methyldopa requires the following lab monitoring:
  - A CBC prior to initiation and at 6 and 12 weeks.
  - A direct Coombs test prior to admission and at 6 and 12 months.
  - Liver enzymes at 6 and 12 weeks after drug initiation or with any unexplained fever or jaundice.
- ♦ No specific monitoring of laboratory tests are required for clonidine or guanfacine IR.

Key Pharmacokinetic and Pharmacodynamic Information for Centrally Acting Alpha$_2$ Agonists

Table 29 lists key pharmacokinetic and pharmacodynamic information for centrally acting alpha$_2$ agonists.

Table 29

Key Pharmacokinetic & Pharmacodynamic Information for Centrally Acting Alpha$_2$ Agonists

Clonidine	Methyldopa	Guanfacine IR
▪ Onset of Action: √ IR: 0.5 to 1 hour. √ Patch: 2 to 3 days. ▪ Plasma Peak: √ IR: 1 to 3 hours. ▪ Half-life Elimination: √ IR: 12 to 16 hours. ▪ Patch: 20 hours after patch removed. ▪ Half-life increases with altered kidney function. Can extend to 41 hours with severe impairment. ▪ About 50% of absorbed dose is metabolism in the liver. ▪ Poorly bound to protein. ▪ Excreted by the kidneys.	▪ Onset of Action: 3 to 6 hours. ▪ Plasma Peak: 2 to 4 hours. ▪ Duration: √ Single Dose: 12 to 24 hours. √ Multiple-dose: 24 to 48 hours. ▪ Half-life Elimination: 1.5 to 2 hours. ▪ Metabolized by the liver. ▪ Poorly bound to protein. ▪ Excreted by the kidneys. ▪ Half-life increases with altered kidney function.	▪ Plasma Peak: 1 to 4 hours (2.6 hours on average). ▪ Half-life Elimination: 17 hours. ▪ 50% of clearance is hepatic via CYP3A4. ▪ 70% bound to protein. ▪ 50% renally cleared. ▪ Half-life increases with altered kidney function.
(Actavis Pharma, 2023; Athena Bioscience, 2021; Boehringer Ingelheim International, 2009, 2023; Chartwell RX, 2024, 2025; TruPharma, 2024; UptoDate®,Lexidrug™ 2025)		

Important Medication Interactions with Centrally Acting Alpha$_2$ Agonists

- ♦ Table 30 below lists key medication interactions with centrally acting alpha$_2$ agonists.
- ♦ The following CNS depressants should be avoided in combination with clonidine or guanfacine.
  - Alcohol.
  - Azelastine (nasal).
  - Benzodiazepines.
  - Carbinoxamine.
  - Kratom.
  - Nabilone.
  - Olopatadine (nasal).
  - Opioid agonists.
  - Paraldehyde.

Appendix 11 provides additional details regarding individual centrally acting alpha$_2$ agonists.

Table 30 Centrally Acting Alpha$_2$ Agonists		
Important Medication Interactions		
Clonidine	**Methyldopa**	**Guanfacine IR**
▪ Concomitant use with other antihypertensive agents can enhance antihypertensive effect. Careful monitoring is recommended. ▪ Possible additive effects, including bradycardia and AV block may occur when used in combination with digitalis, CCBs, and ß-blockers. Careful monitoring is recommended. ▪ MAO inhibitors may increase antihypertensive effect. ▪ The use of tricyclic antidepressants may reduce effectiveness requiring higher doses to achieve BP goals. ▪ Can enhance the sedative effects of other CNS depressants. Concomitant use with any CNS depressants should be monitored or alternative therapies considered. ▪ See list above of CNS depressants that should be avoided in combination with clonidine.	▪ Concomitant use with other antihypertensive agents can enhance antihypertensive effect. Careful monitoring is recommended. ▪ Possible additive effects, including bradycardia and AV block may occur when used in combination with digitalis, CCBs, and ß-blockers. Careful monitoring is recommended. ▪ MOA inhibitors may increase antihypertensive effect. ▪ Not recommended to be given with ferrous sulfate or ferrous gluconate as this decreases the availability of methyldopa in the body.	▪ Substrate of CYP3A4 (Major) ▪ Concomitant use with other antihypertensive agents can enhance antihypertensive effect. Careful monitoring is recommended. ▪ Possible additive effects, including bradycardia and AV block may occur when used in combination with agents that influence sinus node function or AV nodal conduction, such as digitalis, CCBs, and ß-blockers. Carefully monitor when used concomitantly. ▪ The use of tricyclic antidepressants may reduce effectiveness requiring higher doses to achieve BP goals. ▪ Concomitant use with grapefruit juice/products can result in increased serum concentrations of guanfacine. ▪ See list above of CNS depressants that should be avoided in combination with guanfacine IR.
(Actavis Pharma, 2023; Athena Bioscience, 2021; Boehringer Ingelheim International, 2009, 2023; Chartwell RX, 2024, 2025; TruPharma, 2024; UptoDate®,Lexidrug™ 2025)		

FINAL THOUGHTS

Congratulations on completing this learning journey. Your commitment to learning and applying new knowledge makes a difference in the lives of the patients you serve.

We hope you have gained knowledge and feel equipped to implement what you have learned in your clinical practice. We also hope you have been inspired to engage in lifelong learning and to pursue excellence in all you do for patients and families.

We want to personally say thank you for the important and challenging work you do. We have learned the value of nursing excellence not only through our own clinical practices, but also through observing the power of nurses to transform the atmosphere during the multiple times we have been on the receiving end of healthcare walking with friends and family on their health journeys. With absolute assurance we can say that excellence in nursing practice matters.

Continue to deliver care with wisdom, care, and intentionality. It indeed makes all the difference.

ACE Inhibitors (Appendix 1)			
Drug Name	**Drug Specific Pharmacokinetics**	**Dosing Information (Note: Dosing for select FDA labeled cardiovascular indications and key "off label" cardiovascular indications are covered below. Consult a drug reference manual for dosing recommendations for other FDA labeled and "off label" non-cardiac indications and for recommended dosing in patients receiving renal replacement therapy or for women who are pregnant or nursing).**	**Administration Information**
Benazepril	• Peak Effect of single dose on BP is 2 to 4 hrs. • Duration 24 hrs. • $T_{1/2}$ 10 to 11 hrs.	• HTN: Initial dose 10 mg once daily. Consider lower initial dose in older adults. Titrate up to 40 mg once daily in 1 or 2 divided doses. • Altered Kidney Function: If CrCl < 30 mL/min: Initial dose 5 mg once daily, maximum dose 40 mg once daily. • Liver Impairment: Should be avoided in cirrhosis and in those with ascites. Can precipitate hepatorenal syndrome.	• Administer without regard to food.
Captopril	• Onset of Action within 15 mins. • Peak Effect 1 to 1.5 hrs. • Duration dose related. May take several weeks for full BP lowering effect. • $T_{1/2}$ 4 to 6 hrs (up to 21 hrs with severe renal impairment).	• HFrEF and ACS: Initial dose 6.25 mg 3 times daily. Titrate to a target dose 50 mg 3 times daily. • HTN: Initial dose 6.25 to 25 mg 2 or 3 times daily. Titrate to maximum dose of 50 mg 3 times daily. Consider transitioning to longer acting agent to improve patient adherence. • Altered Kidney Function: ♦ If CrCl 10 to < 50 mL/min: Administer the dose every 12 to 24 hrs. Maximum dose 50 mg every 12 hrs. ♦ If CrCl < 10 mL/min: Administer the dose every 24 hrs. Maximum dose 50 mg every 24 hrs. • Liver Impairment: Should be avoided in cirrhosis and in those with ascites. Can precipitate hepatorenal syndrome.	• Take at least 1 hr before meals or 2 hrs after meals.
Enalapril	• Onset of Action ≈1 hr. • Peak Effect 4 to 6 hrs. • Duration 12 to 24 hrs. • $T_{1/2}$ 2 hrs in healthy adult; ≈ 3.5 to 6 hrs in patients with HF.	• HFrEF: Initial dose 2.5 mg 2 times daily. Titrate to target dose 10 to 20 mg 2 times daily. • HTN: Initial dose 5 to 10 mg once daily. Maximum dose is 40 mg, either once daily or 20 mg 2 times daily. • Altered Kidney Function: ♦ If CrCl 10 to 30 mL/min: Initial dose 2.5 mg once daily or 1.25 mg 2 times daily. Maximum dose 20 mg daily. ♦ If CrCl < 10 mL/min: Consider alternate therapy. If used initial dose of 1.25 mg once daily or 2.5 mg every other day. Maximum dose 10 mg daily. • Liver Impairment: Should be avoided in cirrhosis and in those with ascites. Can precipitate hepatorenal syndrome.	• Administer without regard to food.

Enalaprilat IV	• Onset of Action ≤15 mins. • Peak Effect 1 to 4 hrs. • Duration ≈ 6 hrs. • $T_{1/2}$ ≈ 35 hrs.	• HTN: Initial dose 1.25 mg IV every 6 hrs. If patient is on a diuretic start with a lower dose of 0.625 mg IV. If the lower dose is used reassess BP in 1 hr. If the 0.625 mg dose was not effective repeat the dose of 0.625 mg IV, then begin dosing 1.25 mg IV every 6 hrs starting 6 hrs after the second dose of 0.625 mg. Maximum dose is 5 mg every 6 hrs. • Altered Kidney Function: If CrCl ≤ 30 mL/min: Initial dose of 0.625 mg IV. If after 6 hours the 0.625 mg dose was not effective repeat the dose of 0.625 mg IV, then begin dosing 1.25 mg IV starting at the next 6 hr interval if needed. • Liver Impairment: No adjustments recommended.	• Give each dose over 5 mins.
Fosinopril	• Onset of Action 1 hr. • Peak Effect ≈ 3 hrs. • Duration 24 hrs. • $T_{1/2}$ 12 hrs in adults. In adults with HF 14 hrs.	• HFrEF: Initial dose 5 to 10 mg once daily. Titrate to target dose of 40 mg once daily. • HTN: Initial dose 10 mg once daily. Titrate to a usual dose of 10 to 40 mg once daily. Maximum dose 80 mg once daily. • Altered Kidney Function: ♦ Mild impairment: No dosage adjustment. ♦ Moderate to severe impairment: Initial dose reduction to 5 mg once daily in patient with HF. • Liver Impairment: Should be avoided in cirrhosis and in those with ascites. Can precipitate hepatorenal syndrome.	• Administer without regard to food. • Take antacids 2 hrs apart from drug.
Lisinopril	• Onset of Action ≈ 1 hr. • Peak Effect ≈ 7 hrs. • Duration 24 hrs. • $T_{1/2}$ 12 hrs.	• HFrEF: Initial dose 2.5 to 5 mg once daily. Titrate to target dose of 20 to 40 mg once daily. • ACS: Initial dose 2.5 to 5 mg once daily within 24 hrs of presentation. Titrate to 10 mg once daily or higher. Maximum dose of 40 mg once daily. • HTN: Initial dose 5 to10 mg once daily. Titrate to a maximum dose of 40 mg once daily. • Altered Kidney Function: ♦ If CrCl 10 to < 30 mL/min: Initial dose 2.5 mg once daily (HFrEF) and 5 mg once daily (HTN). Titrate as tolerate while not exceeding maximum dose of 40 mg once daily. ♦ If CrCl < 10 mL/min: Consider alternative therapy. • Liver Impairment: Should be avoided in cirrhosis and in those with ascites. Can precipitate hepatorenal syndrome.	• Administer without regard to food.
Moexipril	• Onset of Action 2 hrs. • Peak Effect 3 to 6 hrs. • Duration 24 hrs. • $T_{1/2}$ 1.3 hrs.	• HTN: Initial dose 3.75 to 7.5 mg once daily. Titrate to 30 mg daily in 1 or 2 divided doses. • Altered Kidney Function: If CrCl ≤ 40 mL/min: Initial dose of 3.75 mg once daily with a maximum dose of 15 mg daily. • Liver Impairment: No dosage adjustments recommended. Hepatic impairment noted to increase exposure to Moexipril and should be used with caution in those with ascites due to cirrhosis.	• Take on an empty stomach 1 hr before a meal.
Perindopril	• Peak Effect 1 to 2 hrs. • $T_{1/2}$ Parent Drug 1.5 to 3 hrs. • Effective $T_{1/2}$ 3 to 10 hrs.	• HFrEF: Initial dose of 2 mg once daily. Titrate to target dose of 8 to 16 mg once daily. • HTN: Initial dose of 4 mg once daily. Titrate to maximum dose of 16 mg once daily. • Stable CAD: Initial dose of 4 mg once daily. Titrate to target does of 8 mg once daily. • Altered Kidney Function: ♦ If CrCl ≥ 30 to ≤ 80 mL/min: Initial dose of 2 mg once a day with maximum dose of 8 mg once daily.	• Take 1 hr before meal.

	• Plasma levels higher in renal/hepatic impairment and in patients age >70.	♦ If CrCl < 30 mL/min: Use not recommended. Dose of 2 mg every 48 hrs may be considered with careful monitoring. • Liver Impairment: Should be avoided in cirrhosis and in those with ascites. Can precipitate hepatorenal syndrome.	
Quinapril	• Onset of Action 1 hr. • Peak Effect 2 to 4 hrs. • Duration 24 hrs. • $T_{1/2}$ 0.8-3 hrs (longer if renal impairment).	• HFrEF: Initial dose 5 mg 2 times daily. Titrate to target dose of 20 mg 2 times daily. • HTN: Initial dose 10 to 20 mg once daily. Titrate to maximum dose of 80 mg daily in 1or 2 divided doses. • HFrEF with renal impairment: ♦ CrCl > 30 mL/min: Initial dose 5 mg once daily. ♦ CrCl 10 to 30 mL/min: Initial dose 2.5 mg once daily. ♦ CrCl < 10 mL/min: Manufacturer reports insufficient data to make recommendations. • HTN with renal impairment: ♦ CrCl > 60 mL/min: Maximum initial dose 10 mg once daily. ♦ CrCl 30 to 60 mL/min: Maximum initial dose 5 mg once daily. ♦ CrCl 10 to 30 mL/min: Maximum initial dose 2.5 mg once daily. ♦ CrCl < 10 mL/min: Manufacturer reports insufficient data to make recommendations. • Liver Impairment: No adjustments provided by manufacturer. Use contraindicated in ascites.	• Administer without regard to food.
Ramipril	• Onset of Action 1-2 hrs. • Peak Effect 1 hr. • Duration 24 hrs. • $T_{1/2}$ 13-17 hrs.	• HFrEF: Initial dose 1.25 to 2.5 mg once daily. Titrate to target dose of 10 mg once daily. • HTN: Initial dose of 2.5 mg once daily. Titrate to maximum dose of 20 mg daily in 1 or 2 divided doses. • Altered Kidney Function: ♦ If eGRF 15 to 30 mL/min/1.73 m^2: Initial dose 1.25 mg once daily with maximum dose of 5 mg daily in 1 or 2 divided doses. ♦ If eGRF < 15 mL/min/1.73 m^2: Alternative agents should be considered. • Liver Impairment: Should be avoided in cirrhosis and in those with ascites. Can precipitate hepatorenal syndrome.	• Can mix contents of capsule with water, apple juice or applesauce.
Trandolapril	• Peak Effect ≈ 1 hr. • $T_{1/2}$ ≈ 6 hrs.	• HTN: Initial dose 1 mg once daily. Titrate to maximum dose of 4 mg once daily. • Post MI with HF or LV Dysfunction: Initial dose 1 mg once daily. Titrate to maximum dose of 4 mg once daily. • HFrEF (off label): Initial dose 1 mg once daily. Titrate to maximum dose of 4 mg once daily. • Altered Kidney Function: If CrCl < 30 mL/min: Initial dose 0.5 mg once daily and titrate to optimal response. • Liver Impairment: Should be avoided in cirrhosis and in those with ascites. Can precipitate hepatorenal syndrome.	• Administer without regard to food.

Angiotensin Receptor Blockers (Appendix 2)			
Drug Name	**Drug Specific Pharmacokinetics**	**Dosing Information (Note: Dosing for select FDA labeled cardiovascular indications and key "off label" cardiovascular indications are covered below. Consult a drug reference manual for dosing recommendations for other FDA labeled and "off label" non-cardiac indications and for recommended dosing in patients receiving renal replacement therapy or for women who are pregnant or nursing).**	**Administration Information**
Azilsartan	• Peak Serum 1.5 to 3 hrs. • $T_{1/2} \approx 11$ hrs.	• HTN: Initial dose 40 mg once daily. Titrate to maximum dose of 80 mg once daily. • Altered Kidney Function: No dose adjustment recommended. • Liver Impairment: Should be used with caution in those with ascites due to cirrhosis.	• Administer without regard to food.
Candesartan	• Onset of Action 2 to 3 hrs. • Peak Effect 6 to 8 hrs; maximum antihypertensive effect 4 to 6 weeks. • Duration > 24 hrs. • $T_{1/2}$ 5-9 hrs (dose dependent).	• HFrEF: Alternative agent in patients who cannot tolerate ARNI or ACE I due to cough or angioedema. Initial dose 4 to 8 mg once daily. Titrate to target dose 32 mg once daily. • HTN: Initial dose 8 mg once daily. Titrate to maximum dose of 32 mg once daily. • ACS NSTEMI / STEMI (off label): Alternative agent in patients who cannot tolerate ACE I due to cough or angioedema. Initial dose 8 mg once daily. Titrate to target dose 32 mg once daily. • Altered Kidney Function: If CrCl < 30 mL/min: Initial dose of 4 mg once daily with maximum dose of 16 mg once daily. • Liver Impairment: ♦ Mild Impairment: No dose adjustment. ♦ Severe Impairment: Should be used with caution in those with ascites due to cirrhosis.	• Administer without regard to food.
Irbesartan	• Peak Effect 1 to 2 hrs. • Duration > 24 hrs. • $T_{1/2}$ 11 to 15 hrs.	• HTN: Initial dose 150 mg once daily. Titrate to maximum dose of 300 mg once daily. • ACS NSTEMI / STEMI (off label): Alternative agent in patients who cannot tolerate ACE I due to cough or angioedema. Initial dose 150 mg once daily. Titrate to maximum dose of 300 mg once daily. • Altered Kidney Function: No dose adjustment recommended. • Liver Impairment: Should be used with caution in those with ascites due to cirrhosis.	• Administer without regard to food.
Losartan	• Onset of Action ≈ 6 hrs. • Peak Serum 3.5 hrs. • $T_{1/2}$ 2.1 hrs ± 0.7 hrs.	• HTN: Initial dose 25 to 50 mg once daily. Titrate to maximum dose of 100 mg daily in 1 or 2 divided doses. • ACS NSTEMI / STEMI (off label): Alternative agent in patients who cannot tolerate ARNI or ACE I due to cough or angioedema. Initial dose 25 to 50 mg once daily. Titrate to maximum dose of 100 mg once daily. • HFrEF (off label): Alternative agent in patients who cannot tolerate ACE I due to cough or angioedema. Initial dose 25 to 50 mg once daily. Titrate to maximum dose of 150 mg once daily. • Altered Kidney Function: No dose adjustment necessary. • Liver Impairment: Should be used with caution in those with ascites due to cirrhosis.	• Administer at the same time daily with or without food. • Recommend consistent administration related to meals • Food slows absorption.
Olmesartan	• Peak Effect 1 to 2 hrs. • $T_{1/2}$ 13 hrs.	• HTN: Initial dose 20 mg once daily. Titrate to maximum dose of 40 mg once daily. • ACS NSTEMI / STEMI (off label): Alternative agent in patients who cannot tolerate ACE I due to cough or angioedema. Initial dose 20 mg once daily. Titrate to maximum dose of 40 mg once daily. • Altered Kidney Function: If CrCL < 20 mL/min: Initial dose 10 to 20 mg once daily. Maximum dose 20 mg once daily.	• Administer without regard to food.

		• Liver Impairment: No dosage adjustments recommended. Hepatic impairment noted to increase exposure to Olmesartan by approximately 60% in moderate impairment. Should be used with caution in those with ascites due to cirrhosis.	
Telmisartan	• Onset of Action 1 to 2 hrs. • Peak Serum 0.5 to 1 hr. • Duration 24 hrs. • $T_{1/2}$ 24 hrs. • Plasma concentrations 2 to 3 times higher in women than men.	• HTN: Initial dose 20 to 40 mg once daily. Titrate to maximum dose of 80 mg once daily. • CV Risk Reduction: Initial dose 80 mg once daily. Doses < 80 mg once daily may not reduce CV risk. • Altered Kidney Function: No dosage adjustments recommended. Increased monitoring of BP, kidney function and potassium recommended as kidney function worsens. • Liver Impairment: Initiate therapy with low doses and increase monitoring.	• Administer without regard to food.
Valsartan	• Onset of Action ≈ 2 hrs. • Peak Serum 2 to 4 hrs. • Duration 24 hrs. • $T_{1/2}$ ≈ 6 hrs (35% longer in elderly patients).	• HFrEF: Alternative agent in patients who cannot tolerate ACE I due to cough or angioedema. Initial dose 20 to 40 mg 2 times daily. Titrate to target dose of 160 mg 2 times daily. • HTN: Initial dose 80 to 160 mg once daily. Titrate to maximum dose of 320 mg once daily. • ACS: Alternative agent in patients who cannot tolerate ACE I due to cough or angioedema. Initial dose 20 mg 2 times daily. Titrate to target of 160 mg 2 times daily. • Monitor kidney function and potassium with renal impairment especially with Cr Cl < 30 mL/min/1.73m^2. No medication adjustments are recommended. • Liver Impairment: Should be used with caution in those with ascites due to cirrhosis.	• Administer without regard to food. • Recommend consistent administration related to meals. • High fat, high calorie meals decrease drug absorption. This is greatest when the <u>oral solution</u> is used.

Angiotensin Receptor Blocker / Neprilysin Inhibitor (ARNI) (Appendix 3)			
Drug Name	**Drug Specific Pharmacokinetics**	**Dosing Information (Note: Dosing for select FDA labeled cardiovascular indications and key "off label" cardiovascular indications are covered below. Consult a drug reference manual for dosing recommendations for other FDA labeled and "off label" non-cardiac indications and for recommended dosing in patients receiving renal replacement therapy or for women who are pregnant or nursing).**	**Administration Information**
Sacubitril / Valsartan	• Sacubitril is converted to active metabolite LBQ657. • Peak Effect Sacubitril 0.5 hr, LBQ657 2 hrs; valsartan 1.5 hrs. • $T_{1/2}$ Sacubitril 1.4 hrs; LBQ657 11.5 hrs; valsartan 9.9 hrs.	• HFrEF: If previously taking a moderate to high dose of ACEI or ARB initial dose is usually sacubitril 49 mg/valsartan 51 mg 2 times daily. If previously taking a low dose of ACEI or ARB or if not previously on an ACEI or ARB, the initial dose is sacubitril 24 mg/valsartan 26 mg 2 times daily. The target maintenance dose is sacubitril 97 mg/valsartan 103 mg 2 times daily. • HFpEF: Initial dose is either sacubitril 24 mg/valsartan 26 mg 2 times daily or sacubitril 49 mg/valsartan 51 mg 2 times daily depending on the patient's baseline BP. The target maintenance dose is sacubitril 97 mg/valsartan 103 mg 2 times daily. • Altered Kidney Function: ♦ eGFR < 30 ml/min/1.73 m^2: Initial dose sacubitril 24 mg/valsartan 26 mg 2 times daily. ♦ eGFR is < 20 ml/min/1.73 m^2: Limited safety and efficacy data available. • Liver Impairment: ♦ Moderate Impairment: Initial dose sacubitril 24 mg/valsartan 26 mg 2 times daily. ♦ Should be used with caution in those with ascites due to cirrhosis. ♦ Severe Impairment: Avoid use.	• Administer without regard to food. • Allow 36 hrs after stopping ACEI and before starting this combo drug.
Renin Inhibitor (Appendix 4)			
Aliskiren	• Peak Serum 1 to 3 hrs; maximum antihypertensive effect within 2 weeks. • $T_{1/2}$: Average 24 hrs; range 16 to 32 hrs. • Max antihypertensive effect within 2 weeks.	• HTN: Initial dose 150 mg once daily. May increase to maximum dose of 300 mg once daily. • No renal dosing adjustments per manufacturer recommendations. However, use with caution if CrCl is < 30 mL/min due to risk of hyperkalemia and worsening renal impairment.	• Administer at the same time daily with or without food. • Consistent administration related to meals is recommended. • High fat meals reduce absorption. • Grapefruit juice may decrease serum drug concentration.

Mineralocorticoid Receptor Antagonists (Appendix 5)			
Drug Name	**Drug Specific Pharmacokinetics**	**Dosing Information (Note: Dosing for select FDA labeled cardiovascular indications and key "off label" cardiovascular indications are covered below. Consult a drug reference manual for dosing recommendations for other FDA labeled and "off label" non-cardiac indications and for recommended dosing in patients receiving renal replacement therapy or for women who are pregnant or nursing).**	**Administration Information**
Eplerenone (Also a Potassium Sparing Diuretic)	• Peak Serum 1.5 to 2 hrs. • May take up to 4 weeks for full antihypertensive effect. • $T_{1/2}$ 3 to 6 hrs.	• Prior to initiation: Assure serum potassium < 5 mEq/L AND either serum creatinine ≤ 2.5 mg/dL (males) or ≤ 2 mg/dL (females) OR eGFR < 30 mL/min/1.73 m^2. • Post MI with reduced LVEF: Initial dose 25 mg once daily. Maximum target dose of 50 mg once daily. • HTN: 50 mg once daily. Maximum dose of 50 mg 2 times daily. Not recommended for initial management of HTN but may be considered for additional therapy for resistant HTN. • HFrEF and HFpEF (both off label): Initial dose 25 mg once daily. Titrate to target dose of 50 mg once daily. • When used post MI with reduced LVEF or when used off label in HFrEF or HFpEF: ♦ eGFR 31 to 49 mL/min/1.73 m^2: Initial dose of 25 mg every other day. Maximum dose 25 mg once daily. ♦ eGFR < 30 mL/min/1.73 m^2: Use is not recommended. • When used for HTN: Use is contraindicated if CrCl is < 50 mL/min or if serum creatinine is > 2.0 mg/dL in men or > 1.8 mg/dL in women.	• Administer without regard to food.
Finerenone (Also a Potassium Sparing Diuretic)	• Peak Effect 0.5 to 1.25 hrs. • $T_{1/2}$ 2 to 3 hrs.	• Prior to initiation verify potassium is ≤ 5 mEq/L. Dosing for both indications based on potassium and eGFR. Do not initiate if potassium > 5.0 mEq/L or eGFR < 25 mL/min/1.73 m^2. • HFrEF and HFmrEF: ♦ Initial Dose: ▪ If eGFR ≥ 60 mL/min/1.73 m^2 20 mg once daily. Target dose 40 mg once daily. ▪ If eGFR ≥ 25 to < 60 mL/min/1.73 m^2 10 mg once daily. Target dose 20 mg once daily. ♦ Titration and Maintenance: ▪ Assess potassium 4 weeks after initiation and 4 weeks after dosage changes. ▪ If potassium is < 5.0 mEq/L increase dose from 10 mg to 20 mg once daily. If on the 20 mg dose continue this dose if the eGFR < 60 mL/min/1.73 m^2. If the eGFR ≥ 60 mL/min/1.73 m^2 increase the dose to 40 mg once daily. If prescribed the 40 mg dose maintain this dose. ▪ If potassium is ≥ 5.0 to < 5.5 mEq/L continue the current dose (10, 20 or 40 mg) and reassess potassium. ▪ If potassium is ≥ 5.5 to < 6.0 stop 10 mg dose. Decrease 20 mg dose to 10 mg once daily. Decrease 40 mg dose to 20 mg once daily. Consider restarting or up titrating when potassium < 5.5 mEq/L. ▪ If potassium is ≥ 6.0 mEq/L stop therapy. Restart at 10 mg once daily when potassium is < 5.5 mEq/L. ▪ If eGFR decreases by > 30% maintain current dose. • CKD associated with DMT2: ♦ Initial Dose:	• Administer without regard to food. • Grapefruit juice increases drug concentration. Avoid use.

		▪ If eGFR $\geq$ 60 mL/min/1.73 m^2 20 mg once daily. Target dose 20 mg once daily. ▪ If eGFR $\geq$ 25 to < 60 mL/min/1.73 m^2 10 mg once daily. Target dose 20 mg once daily. ♦ Titration and Maintenance: ▪ Assess potassium 4 weeks after initiation and 4 weeks after dosage changes. ▪ If potassium is $\leq$ 4.8 mEq/L increase from 10 mg to 20 mg once daily. Maintain 20 mg dose. ▪ If potassium is > 4.8 to 5.5 mEq/L: Maintain current dose of either 10 mg or 20 mg once daily. ▪ If potassium is > 5.5 mEq/L discontinue therapy. Restart at 10 mg once daily when potassium is < 5.0 mEq/L. ▪ If eGFR decreases by > 30% maintain a 10 mg once daily dose.	
Spironolactone (Also a Potassium Sparing Diuretic)	• Peak Serum 2.6 to 4.3 hrs. • Duration 2-3 days. • $T_{1/2}$ 1.4 hrs; up to 16.5 hrs for multiple metabolites.	Prior to initiation: Assure serum potassium < 5 mEq/L AND either serum creatinine $\leq$ 2.5 mg/dL (males) or $\leq$ 2 mg/dL (females) OR eGFR < 30 mL/min/1.73 m^2. • HFrEF: Initial dose 12.5 to 25 mg once daily. Maximum target dose 50 mg once daily in 1 to 2 divided doses. • HFpEF (off label): Initial dose 12.5 mg once daily. Titrate to target dose of 50 mg once daily. • Resistant HTN: Initial dose 25 mg once daily and titrated to maximum dose of 100 mg once daily. Some experts recommend a lower starting dose of 12.5 mg once daily and do not exceed 50 mg once daily. Not recommended for initial management of HTN but may be considered for additional therapy for resistant HTN. • Altered Kidney Function: ♦ In HFrEF and HFpEF: ▪ eGFR 30 to 50 mL/min/1.73 m^2: Initial dose is 12.5 mg once daily, target maximum dose of 25 mg once daily. ▪ Not recommended if eGFR < 30 mL/min/1.73 m^2. ♦ In HTN: No renal dose recommendations given.	• Administer without regard to food. • Consistent administration related to meals is recommended. • Food increases bioavailability of unmetabolized spironolactone by 90 to 95%.

Beta Blockers (Appendix 6)

Drug Name	Drug Specific Pharmacokinetics	Dosing Information (Note: Dosing for select FDA labeled cardiovascular indications and key "off label" cardiovascular indications are covered below. Consult a drug reference manual for dosing recommendations for other FDA labeled and "off label" non-cardiac indications and for recommended dosing in patients receiving renal replacement therapy or for women who are pregnant or nursing).	Administration Information
Acebutolol β1 selective ISA	• Onset of Action 1 to 2 hrs. • Peak Effect 2 to 4 hrs. • Duration 12 to 24 hrs. • $T_{1/2}$ of parent drug 3 to 4 hrs; metabolite 8 to 13 hrs.	• HTN or PVCs: 200 to 400 mg daily in 1 or 2 divided doses. Titrate to 200 to 800 mg daily (usual dose range) in 2 divided doses. Max dose 1200 mg daily in 2 divided doses. Note: Do not use in overt heart failure.	• Administer without regard to food although peak serum levels may be slightly decreased if taken with food.
Atenolol β1 selective	• Onset of Action ≤ 1hr. • Peak Effect 2 to 4 hrs. • Duration 12 to 24 hrs. • $T_{1/2}$ 6 to 7 hrs with normal renal function, prolonged with renal impairment.	• Angina (chronic stable): Initial dose 50 mg once daily, usual dose range 50 to 100 mg once daily. • A Fib/Flutter for rate control (off label): Initial dose 25 mg once daily. Maximum dose 100 mg once daily. • HTN: Used for treating HTN only in patients with specific comorbid conditions such as ischemic heart disease or arrhythmias. Initial dose 25 mg 1 or 2 times daily. Maximum dose is 100 mg daily in 1 or 2 divided doses. • Post Myocardial Infarction (early treatment/secondary prevention): Initiation of beta blocker recommended within the first 24 hrs of presentation with MI. Initial dose 25 to 50 mg 2 times daily. Maximum daily dose 100 mg/day in 1 or 2 divided doses. • SVT for rate control (off label): Initial dose 25 to 50 mg 2 times daily. Maximum daily dose 100 mg once daily. • Ventricular arrhythmia or PVCs (off label): Initial dose 25 mg once daily. Maximum dose 200 mg daily in 1 or 2 divided doses. Usual dose range 25 mg to 100 mg per day in 1 or 2 divided doses. • Altered Kidney Function: ♦ If CrCl 10 to 30 mL/min: Maximum dose 50 mg once daily. ♦ If CrCl < 10 mL/min: Maximum dose is 25 mg once daily.	• Administer without regard to food although serum concentrations may be reduced when taken with food.
Betaxolol β1 selective	• Onset of Action 1 to 1.5 hrs. • Peak Effect 1.5 to 6 hrs. • $T_{1/2}$ 14 to 22 hrs. Prolonged in hepatic or renal failure.	• HTN: Used for treating HTN only in patients with specific comorbid conditions such as ischemic heart disease or arrhythmias. Initial dose 5 to 10 mg once daily. Maximum dose 20 mg once daily. • Altered Kidney Function: If severe renal impairment the initial dose is 5 mg once daily and then titrate to a maximum of 20 mg once daily based on BP effect.	• Administer without regard to food.

Bisoprolol β1 selective	• Onset of Action 1 to 2 hrs. • Peak Effect 2 to 4 hrs. • $T_{1/2}$ 9-12 hrs. Prolonged in hepatic or renal failure.	• Angina (chronic stable) (off label): Initial dose 5 to 10 mg once daily. Titrate as needed with maximum dose of 20 mg once daily. • A Fib/Flutter for rate control (off label): Initial dose 2.5 to 5 mg once daily. Maximum dose 20 mg once daily. • HFrEF (off label but guideline recommended): Initial dose 1.25 mg once daily. Titrate to target dose of 10 mg once daily. • HTN: Used for treating HTN only in patients with specific comorbid conditions such as ischemic heart disease or arrhythmias. Initial dose 2.5 to 5 mg once daily. Usual range 2.5 to 10 mg once daily. Maximum dose 20 mg once daily. • Ventricular Arrhythmias (off label): Initial dose 2.5 to 5 mg once daily. Usual range 2.5 to 10 mg once daily. Maximum dose 20 mg once daily. • Altered Kidney Function: If CrCl < 20 mL/min: Start with a low dose (1.25 to 2.5 mg once daily) with a maximum dose of 10 mg once daily.	• Administer without regard to food.
Carvedilol Nonselective (vasodilating) Immediate Release (IR) Extended Release (ER)	• Onset of Action Beta-blockade within 1 hr; alpha-blockade 30 mins. • Peak antihypertensive effect ≈ 1 to 2 hrs. • Peak serum level of ER 5 hrs. • $T_{1/2}$ 7 to 10 hrs.	• Angina (chronic stable) (off label): Initial dose 12.5 mg 2 times daily. Usual dosage range 25 to 50 mg 2 time daily (IR). • A Fib/Flutter for rate control (off label): Initial dose 3.125 mg 2 times daily. Maximum dose 25 mg 2 times daily (IR). • HFrEF: ♦ IR: Initial dose 3.125 mg 2 times daily. Target dose 25 mg once daily (if ≤ 85 kg) or 50 mg 2 times daily (if > 85 kg). ♦ ER: Initial dose 10 mg once daily. Target dose 80 mg once daily. • HTN: Used for treating HTN only in patients with specific comorbid conditions such as ischemic heart disease or arrhythmias. ♦ IR: Initial dose 6.25 mg 2 times daily. Maximum dose 50 mg/day in 2 divided doses. ♦ ER: Initial dose 20 mg once daily. Maximum dose 80 mg once daily. • Nonsustained VT or PVCs (off label): Initial dose 3.125 mg 2 times daily. Maximum dose 25 mg 2 times daily (IR). • Post Myocardial Infarction (early treatment / secondary prevention) (off label): Initiation of beta blocker recommended within the first 24 hrs of presentation with MI. Initial dose 3.125 to 6.25 mg 2 times daily. Titrate to 25 mg 2 times daily (IR).	• Administer with food to avoid hypotension.
Esmolol β1 selective	• Onset of Action 2 to 10 mins (quickest when loading dose used). • Duration of hemodynamic effects 10 to 30 mins. Prolonged	• IV dosing only. • Acute Aortic Syndromes/Acute Aortic Dissection (off label): Control pain and manage HR (60 to 80 bmp) prior to addressing SBP (target SBP≤ 120 mm Hg without hypoperfusion). ♦ Initial bolus: 500 mcg/kg over 1 min ♦ Continuous Infusion: 25 to 50 mcg/kg/min. Titrate every 5 mins to achieve clinical goals (target HR and BP). To enhance BP control, consider repeat loading bolus. Maximum infusion 300 mcg/kg/min. • A Fib/Flutter (acute rate control): ♦ Loading Dose (optional): 500 mcg/kg over 1 min followed by continuous infusion.	• Use large bore IV cannula when possible. Infusion into small veins can cause thrombophlebitis. • Vesicant: ensure proper needle or catheter

	with extended duration of use. • $T_{1/2}$ 9 mins.	♦ Continuous Infusion: 50 mcg/kg/min. Increase in increments of 50 mcg/kg/min at ≥ 4-min intervals to a maximum of 300 mcg/kg/min. To achieve a faster response, repeat bolus prior to increasing the continuous infusion rate. • HTN Emergency (off label): ♦ Initial bolus: 250 to 500 mcg/kg over 1 min. ♦ Continuous Infusion: 25 to 50 mcg/kg/min. Titrate every 5 mins to achieve clinical goals (target BP while maintaining HR). To enhance BP control, consider repeat loading bolus prior to each up titration. Maximum infusion 300 mcg/kg/min. • Intra and post op tachycardia and/or HTN: ♦ Immediate Control: Initial bolus: 1,000 mcg/kg over 30 seconds, followed by a 150 mcg/kg/min infusion, if needed. Adjust infusion rate up to 300 mcg/kg/min as needed. ♦ Gradual Control: Initial bolus: 500 mcg/kg over 1 min, followed by a 50 mcg/kg/min continuous infusion for 4 mins. Infusion may be continued at 50 mcg/kg/min or titrated upward in 50 mcg/kg/min increments at ≥ 4-min intervals to a maximum of 200 mcg/kg/ min for tachycardia and 250 to 300 mcg/kg/min for HTN. May administer an optional loading dose of 500 mcg/kg over 1 min prior to each increase in infusion rate to achieve faster results. • Sinus Tachycardia – Inappropriate/non-compensatory: ♦ Loading Dose (optional): 500 mcg/kg over 1 min followed by continuous infusion. ♦ Continuous Infusion: 50 mcg/kg/min. Increase in increments of 50 mcg/kg/min at ≥ 4-min intervals to a maximum of 300 mcg/kg/min. To achieve a faster response, repeat bolus prior to each increase in the continuous infusion rate. • SVT: Consider for hemodynamically stable patients with lack of response to vagal maneuvers and/or adenosine administration. Avoid use in pre-excitation or when SVT suspected to be associated with an accessory pathway. ♦ Loading Dose: 500 mcg/kg over 1 min followed by continuous infusion. ♦ Continuous Infusion: 50 mcg/kg/mins. Increase in increments of 50 mcg/kg/min at ≥ 4-min intervals to a maximum of 300 mcg/kg/min. To achieve a faster response, repeat bolus prior to increasing the continuous infusion rate. • When transferring esmolol to oral beta blocker or calcium channel blocker, reduce infusion by 50% 30 min after first dose of alternative drug. If control is adequate 1 hr after the second dose of alternative drug, infusion can be discontinued.	placement prior and during infusion to avoid extravasation.
Labetalol Nonselective (vasodilating)	• Onset of Action Oral 20 min to 2 hrs; IV within 5 mins. • Peak Effect Oral 2 to 4 hrs; IV 5 to 15 mins.	• Acute Aortic Syndrome / Acute Aortic Dissection (off label): Control pain and manage HR (target HR 60-80 bmp) prior to addressing SBP (target SBP < 120 mm Hg without hypoperfusion). ♦ Intermittent IV: Initial dose 20 mg over 2 mins. Repeat IV bolus every 10 mins with a dose of 20 to 80 mg until target HR reached. May move to continuous infusion. ♦ Continuous Infusion: Start with initial IV bolus of 20 mg over 2 mins. Continuous IV infusion to follow at 0.5 to 2 mg/min. May titrate up to 10 mg/min to achieve target HR and BP control. • Acute Ischemic Stroke – BP Management with Reperfusion Strategy (off label): Prior to initiating reperfusion strategy BP should be maintained at ≤ 185/110 mm Hg.	• Administer without regard to food. • Administer in a consistent manner with regard to meals.

	• Duration (BP response) Oral 8 to12 hrs; IV 16 to 18 hrs. • $T_{1/2}$ Oral 6 to 8 hrs; IV ≈ 5.5 hrs.	♦ Prior to Reperfusion Therapy: IV bolus 10 to 20 mg over 1 to 2 mins. ♦ During and After Reperfusion Therapy: IV bolus 10 to 20 mg over 1 to 2 mins. Then initiation of continuous infusion of 2 to 8 mg/min. Not recommended to exceed a cumulative dose of 300 mg. • HTN Chronic / Resistant: Not recommended for initial management of HTN. Can be considered as adjunct therapy when HTN is resistant on combination therapy with recommended agents. Initial oral dose of 100 mg 2 times daily. Titrate to desired response. Titration increments not to exceed 200 mg 2 times daily. Usual dosage range 200 to 800 mg/day in 2 divided doses. • HTN Emergency / Urgency: ♦ IV Push (Intermittent Dosing): Initial dose of 10 to 20 mg IV push over 1 to 2 mins; may give additional boluses of 20 to 80 mg (double dose with each bolus) every 10 mins until target SBP goal is reached. Cumulative dose should not exceed 300 mg. Can follow with continuous infusion. ♦ IV Continuous Infusion: Initial loading dose of 10 to 20 mg over 2 mins (if not using intermittent dosing to begin with). Continuous infusion to follow loading dose at a rate of 0.5 to 2 mg/min. Titration up to maximum continuous dose of 10 mg/min. • Intracerebral Hemorrhage – Acute BP Management (off label): ♦ Intermittent IV: Initial dose bolus 5 to 20 mg over 2 mins. Repeat bolus every 10 to 15 mins with a dose of 20 mg and increased incrementally to 80 mg until SBP < 160 mm Hg or MAP < 100 mm Hg. ♦ IV Continuous Infusion: Begin with 0.5 to 2 mg/mins. Titrate based on response. • Subarachnoid Hemorrhage – Acute BP Management (off label): ♦ Intermittent IV: Initial dose bolus of 10 to 20 mg over 2 mins. Repeat bolus every 10 to 15 mins with a dose of 20 to 80 mg until SBP < 160 mm Hg or MAP < 100 mm Hg. ♦ IV Continuous Infusion: Begin with 0.5 to 2 mg/mins. Titrate based on response.	
Landiolol β1 selective	• $T_{1/2}$ 4.5 mins.	• IV dosing only. • SVT: Short-term use for the reduction of ventricular rate in SVT including atrial fibrillation and flutter. Short term use is defined as 24 hrs or less as there is limited data on infusions > 24 hrs. ♦ Normal Cardiac Function: Initial dose (no bolus) 9 mcg/kg/min. Titrate every 10 mins in increments of 9 mcg/kg/min to achieve desired HR goal. Maximum dose: 36 mcg/kg/min. ♦ Impaired Cardiac Function (not defined): Initial dose (no bolus) 1 mcg/kg/min. Titrate every 15 mins in increments of 1 mcg/kg/min to achieve desired HR goal. Maximum dose: 36 mcg/kg/min. ♦ Transition from IV to oral beta blocker (after HR control achieved): Ten minutes after oral beta blocker administered reduce IV infusion rate by 50% over the next hour monitoring for continued HR rate control. Further titration and discontinuation can then occur with continued HR control over the next hour. • With Liver Impairment: ♦ Mild hepatic impairment, more conservative titrations recommended. ♦ With moderate to severe hepatic impairment avoid use.	• May be administered via central or peripheral line. • FDA approved for use in the critical care setting.

Metoprolol Tartrate Immediate Release (IR) **β1 selective** **Metoprolol Succinate** Extended Release (ER) β1 selective	• Onset of Action Oral IR within 1 hr; IV ≈ 20 mins when infused over 10 mins. • Peak Effect Oral IR 1 to 2 hrs. • Duration of IR is dose dependent from 3.3 to 6.4 hrs; ER ≈ 24 hrs. • $T_{1/2}$ 3 to 4 hrs, delayed in hepatic impairment or in poor CYP2D6 metabolizers.	• Angina (chronic stable): ♦ IR: Initial dose 50 mg 2 times daily. Usual dose range 50 to 200 mg 2 times daily. Maximum dose 400 mg per day in 2 divided doses. ♦ ER: Initial dose 100 mg once daily. Maximum dose 400 mg once a day. • A Fib/Flutter for Rate Control (off label): ♦ Acute Ventricular Rate Control: Initial IV bolus 2.5 to 5 mg over 5 mins. May repeat dose every 5 mins as needed. Maximum cumulative dose 15 mg. ♦ Maintenance Rate Control (Oral): ▪ IR: Initial dose 25 mg 2 times daily. Titrate, as needed, up to 200 mg per day in 2 to 4 divided doses. ▪ ER: Initial dose 25 to 50 mg once daily. Titrate, as needed, up to 200 mg per day in 1 to 2 doses. • A Fib/Flutter Prevention Post Cardiac Surgery (off label): Preferably initiate 48 hrs prior to surgery. ♦ IR: Initial dose 25 to 50 mg orally 2 times daily. Maximum dose 200 mg per day in divided doses. ♦ ER: Initial dose 50 mg orally once daily. Maximum dose 200 mg per day in 1 or 2 divided doses. • HFrEF: ER Only (for long term mortality benefit): Initiate 12.5 to 25 mg once daily. Titrate to target dose of 200 mg once daily. IR dosing not recommended for mortality benefit. • HTN: Used for treating HTN only in patients with specific comorbid conditions such as ischemic heart disease or arrhythmias. ♦ IR: Initial dose 50 mg 2 times daily. Titrate to maximum dose of 400 mg daily in 2 divided doses. ♦ ER: Initial dose 25 to 100 mg once daily. Titrate to maximum dose of 400 mg once daily. Usual dose 50 to 100 mg once daily. • Post Myocardial Infarction (early treatment / secondary prevention): Initiation of beta blocker recommended within the first 24 hrs of presentation with MI. ♦ IV: For persistent HTN and/or ongoing ischemia in STEMI. Initial dose 5 mg IV push undiluted over 1 min Repeat dose every 5 mins to maximum cumulative dose of 15 mg. Initiate oral therapy 15 to 30 mins after last IV dose. ♦ Oral IR: Initial dose 25 to 50 mg every 6 to 12 hrs in acute setting. Consider lower starting dose based on patient stability. Transition to ER for outpatient therapy with a target dose of 200 mg once daily. ♦ Oral ER: Initial dose 25 to 50 mg once daily. Titrate to target dose of 200 mg once daily. • SVT (off label): Consider for hemodynamically stable patients with lack of response to vagal maneuvers and/or adenosine administration. Avoid use in pre-excitation or when SVT suspected to be associated with an accessory pathway. ♦ Acute Treatment: Initial IV bolus 2.5 to 5 mg over 5 mins. May repeat dose every 5 mins as needed. Maximum cumulative dose 15 mg. ♦ Maintenance Therapy (Oral):	• IR and ER: administer with or immediately after meals.

		▪ IR: Initial dose 25 mg 2 times daily. Maximum dose 400 mg daily in 2 to 4 divided doses. ▪ ER: Initial dose 25 to 50 mg once daily. Maximum dose 400 mg per day in 1 or 2 divided doses.	
Nadolol Nonselective	• Peak Effect 3 to 4 hrs. • Duration 17 to 24 hrs. • $T_{1/2}$ 20 to 24 hrs.	• Angina (chronic stable): Initial dose 40 mg once daily. Titrate in 40 to 80 mg increments to maximum dose of 240 mg once daily. Usual dose 40 to 80 mg once daily. • A Fib/Flutter for Rate Control (off label): Dosage range 10 to 240 mg once daily. Start at lower dose and titrate to affect. • HTN: Used for treating HTN only in patients with specific comorbid conditions present such as ischemic heart disease or arrhythmias. Initial dose 40 mg once daily. Titrate in 40 to 80 mg increments to maximum dose of 320 mg once daily. Usual dose 40 to 120 mg once daily. • SVT (off label): Consider for hemodynamically stable patients with lack of response to vagal maneuvers and/or adenosine administration. Avoid use in pre-excitation or when SVT suspected to be associated with an accessory pathway. Initial oral dose 40 mg once daily. Titrate to response with maximum dose 320 mg once daily. • VT Prevention / PVCs (off label): Initial dose 40 mg once daily. Titrate to response with maximum dose 320 mg once daily. • Altered Kidney Function: ♦ If CrCl > 50 mL/min: Administer every 24 hrs. ♦ If CrCl 31 to 50 mL/min: Administer every 24 to 36 hrs. ♦ If CrCl 10 to 30 mL/min: Administer every 24 to 48 hrs. ♦ If CrCl < 10 mL/min: Administer every 40 to 60 hrs.	• Administer without regard to food.
Nebivolol β1 selective (vasodilating)	• Peak Serum 1.5 to 4 hrs. • $T_{1/2}$ 12 to 19 hrs.	• HTN: Used for treating HTN only in patients with specific comorbid conditions such as ischemic heart disease or arrhythmias. Initial dose 5 mg once daily. Maximum dose of 40 mg once daily. • Altered Kidney Function: If CrCl < 30 mL/min decrease initial dose to 2.5 mg once daily. If initial response is inadequate increase dose cautiously.	• Administer without regard to food.
Pindolol Nonselective ISA	• Peak Effect ≈1 hr. • $T_{1/2}$ 3 to 4 hrs; elderly 7 up to 15 hrs; cirrhosis 2.5 to 30 hrs.	• HTN: Not recommended as 1st line therapy for HTN. Initial dose 5 mg 2 times daily. Titrate by 10 mg increments to a maximum dose of 30 mg 2 times daily.	• Administer without regard to food.
Propranolol Nonselective IV Oral Immediate Release (IR)	• Onset of Action Oral 1 to 2 hrs; IV ≤ 5 mins. • Peak Effect IR 1 to 4 hrs; ER 12 to 14 hrs. • Peak hypertensive effect a few days to several weeks.	• Angina (chronic stable): Initial dose 80 mg/day in 1 to 4 divided doses based on drug formulation used (ER or IR). Dosage range 80 to 320 mg/day in 1 to 4 divided doses based on drug formulation used. • A Fib/Flutter (rate control): ♦ IV Bolus (acute rate control): 1 mg over 1 min, repeat every 2 mins up to a maximum of 3 doses. ♦ Oral (maintenance rate control): ▪ IR: Initial dose 10 mg 3 to 4 daily with maximum dose 40 mg 3 to 4 daily. ▪ ER: Initial dose 60 mg once daily with maximum dose of 160 mg once daily.	• Administer extended-release capsules without regard to food. However, maintain a consistent pattern if taking with or without food.

Extended Release (ER)	• Duration IR 6 to12 hrs; ER 24 to 27 hrs. • $T_{1/2}$ IR 3 to 6 hrs; ER 8 to10 hrs.	• HTN: Used for treating HTN only in patients with specific comorbid conditions such as ischemic heart disease or arrhythmias. Initial dose 80 mg/day in 1 to 4 divided doses with maximum dose 80 to 160 mg/day in 1 to 4 divided doses based on chosen formulation (ER or IR). • Post Myocardial Infarction (secondary prevention): Initiation of beta blocker recommended within the first 24 hrs of presentation with myocardial infarction. Initial dose (IR) 60 to 120 mg/day in 2 to 3 divided doses. Titrate to maximum dose to of 240 mg/day in 2 to 3 divided doses. • SVT (off label): ♦ IV Bolus (acute treatment): 1 mg over 1 min, repeat every 2mins up to a maximum of 3 doses. ♦ Oral Therapy (maintenance therapy): IR initial dose 30 to 60 mg/day in 1 or 3 divided doses. Maximum dose 160 mg/day. • Ventricular Tachycardia (acute, incessant): IV 1 to 3 mg every 5 mins up to a total dose of 5 mg (to be used in combination with an IV antiarrhythmic. • Ventricular Tachycardia Prevention or Nonsustained VT or PVCs: ♦ IR: 10 to 40 mg every six hrs. Some recommend beginning with 10 mg every eight to twelve hrs and titrating based on response. Maximum dose 320 mg/day in divided doses every six hrs. ♦ ER: Initial dose 80 mg once daily. Maximum dose 320 mg once daily.	• IR tablets should be taken on empty stomach.
Sotalol Nonselective (Class III antiarrhythmic agent)	See Cardiovascular Pharmacology Volume 2 for Information regarding Sotalol.		
Timolol Nonselective	• Onset of Action 15 to 45 mins. • Peak Effect 0.5 to 2.5 hrs. • Duration ≈ 4 hrs. • $T_{1/2}$ 2 to 2.7 hrs.	• For HTN: Used for treating HTN only in patients with specific comorbid conditions such as ischemic heart disease or arrhythmias. Initial dose 10 mg 2 times daily. Titrate to maximum dose of 60 mg/day in 2 divided doses. Usual range 20 to 40 mg/day in 2 divided doses. • Post Myocardial Infarction (early treatment / secondary prevention): Initiation of beta blocker recommended within the first 24 hrs of presentation with myocardial infarction. Initial dose 5 mg 2 times daily with a target does of 10 mg 2 times daily.	• Administer with food at the same time each day.

Calcium Channel Blockers (Appendix 7)			
Drug Name	**Drug Specific Pharmacokinetics**	**Dosing Information (Note: Dosing for select FDA labeled cardiovascular indications and key "off label" cardiovascular indications are covered below. Consult a drug reference manual for dosing recommendations for other FDA labeled and "off label" non-cardiac indications and for recommended dosing in patients receiving renal replacement therapy or for women who are pregnant or nursing).**	**Administration Information**
Heart Rate Lowering (Non-dihydropyridines)			
Diltiazem IV Oral Immediate Release (IR) Extended Release (ER 12) 12-hr dose Extended Release (ER 24) 24-hr dose	• Onset of Action IR 30 to 60 mins; IV bolus 3 mins. • Peak Effect IR 2 to 4 hrs; ER tablet 11 to 18 hrs; ER capsule 10 to 14 hrs. • Duration IV bolus 1 to 3 hrs; continuous infusion 0.5 to 10 hrs after discontinuation. • $T_{1/2}$ IR tablets 3 to 4.5 hrs; ER tablet 6 to 9 hrs; ER capsules 4 to 9.5 hrs; IV single dose ≈ 3.4 hrs; continuous infusion 4 to 5 hrs.	• Angina (chronic stable) and Vasospastic Angina: Beta blockers are preferred for initial therapy for chronic stable angina. Calcium channel blockers can be added if ongoing angina persists on beta blocker therapy alone. Calcium channel blockers are the preferred treatment for vasospastic angina and can be used with or without nitrates. ♦ IR: Initial dose 30 mg 4 times daily. Titrate to maximum dose of 240 to 360 mg/day in 3 to 4 divided doses. ♦ Twice Daily Formulas (ER 12): Initial dose 60 mg 2 times daily. Titrate to maximum dose of 240 to 360 mg 2 times daily. ♦ Once Daily Formulas (ER 24): Initial dose 120 to 180 mg once daily. Titrate to maximum dose of 240 to 360 mg once daily. • A Fib/Flutter (acute rate control): IV only (chronic oral rate control is off label). ♦ Bolus Dosing: Initial dosing 0.25 mg/kg (actual body weight) over 2 mins. Average bolus approximately 20 mg. Lower doses can be used when concern for hypotension is present. May repeat bolus with a dose of 0.35 mg/kg (average 25 mg) over 2 mins if initial response insufficient. ♦ Continuous Infusion: Begin after 1 to 2 bolus doses with noted ventricular response. Initial dose of 5 to 10 mg/hr. May increase by 5 mg/hr up to a maximum dose of 15 mg/hr. The potential for drug accumulation occurs if infusion rate exceeds 15 mg/hr or if infusion runs for > 24 hrs. • HTN: Non-dihydropyridine calcium channel blockers are best used in the treatment of HTN in patients with relative comorbid conditions that have indications for calcium channel blockers. They should be in combination with other medications indicated as primary treatment for HTN. ♦ Twice Daily Formulas (ER 12): Initial dose 60 to 120 mg 2 times daily. Titrate to maximum dose of 240 to 360 mg 2 times daily. ♦ Once Daily Formulas (ER 24): Initial dose 120 to 180 mg once daily. Titrate to maximum dose of 240 to 360 mg once daily. • Nonsustained VT / PVCs (off label): Beta blocker is preferred initial treatment. Diltiazem can be added to beta blocker therapy or used if beta blocker cannot be used. Initial dose 120 to 180 mg once daily or divided doses (based on drug formulation used). Titrate to usual dose of 240 to 360 mg/day. Maximum dose 480 mg/day.	• IR tablets administer before meals and at bedtime. • Long-acting forms should be administered at the same time each day either morning or evening. • Grapefruit juice may increase the serum concentration of diltiazem.

		• SVT: Consider for hemodynamically stable patients with lack of response to vagal maneuvers and/or adenosine administration. Avoid use in pre-excitation associated with an accessory pathway (can lead to ventricular arrhythmias). IV bolus of 0.25 mg/kg (actual body weight) over 2 mins. If response is inadequate over 15 mins repeat bolus with a dose of 0.35 mg/kg over 2 mins. If response remains insufficient after second bolus, consider alternative therapy.	
Verapamil IV Oral Immediate Release (IR) Extended Release (ER)	• Peak Effect Oral IR 1 to 2 hrs; ER 4 to 9 hrs (based on brand); IV bolus 3 to 5 mins. • Duration Oral IR 6 to 8 hrs; IV 0.5 to 6 hrs. • $T_{1/2}$ IV 2 to 5 hrs; Oral IR single dose 2.8 to 7.4 hrs or multiple doses 4.5 to 12 hrs; ER ≈12 hrs; with hepatic impairment 14 to 16 hrs.	• Angina (chronic stable) and Vasospastic Angina: Beta blockers are preferred for initial therapy for chronic stable angina. Calcium channel blockers can be added if ongoing angina persists on beta blocker therapy alone. Calcium channel blockers are the preferred treatment for vasospastic angina and can be used with or without nitrates. ♦ IR: Initial dose 80 to 120 mg 3 times a day. Maximum dose 480 mg/day divided into 3 equal doses. ♦ ER: Initial dose 180 mg once daily. Maximum dose 480 mg/day administered as 1 or 2 doses. • A Fib/Flutter: Rate control in hemodynamically stable patients. DO NOT use in preexcitation associated with accessory pathways – can lead to ventricular arrhythmias. ♦ Acute Ventricular Rate Control IV Bolus: Initial bolus of 5 to 10 mg over ≥ 2 mins. Repeat bolus once after 15 to 20 mins if response is inadequate. If no response with 1 or 2 bolus doses begin continuous infusion. ♦ Acute Ventricular Rate Control IV Infusion: Initial infusion after 1 to 2 bolus doses at rate of 5 mg/hr. Titrate to HR goal up to a maximum dose of 20 mg/hr. ♦ Chronic Ventricular Rate Control IR: Initial dose of 40 mg 3 to 4 times daily. Maximum dose 480 mg/day divided into 3 to 4 doses. ♦ Chronic Ventricular Rate Control ER: Initial dose 120 to 180 mg once daily. Maximum dose of 480 mg/day given in 1 to 2 divided doses. • HTN: Non-dihydropyridine calcium channel blockers are best used in the treatment of HTN in patients with relative comorbid conditions that have indications for calcium channel blockers. They should be in combination with other medications indicated as primary treatment for HTN. ♦ IR: Initial dose 40 to 80 mg t3 times a day. Maximum dose 480 mg/day divided into 3 equal doses. Usual dosage: 120 to 360 mg/day in 3 divided doses. ♦ ER: Initial dose 120 to 180 mg once daily. Maximum dose 480 mg/day administered as 1 or 2 divided doses. Usual dosage: 120 to 360 mg/day in 1 or 2 divided doses. ♦ ER (Delayed Onset / PM Formula): Initial dose 100 to 200 mg once daily at bedtime. Maximum dose 400 mg once daily at bedtime. Usual dose 100 to 300 mg once daily at bedtime. • Idiopathic LV Tachycardia (off label): ♦ Acute IV Bolus: Initial dose 5 to 10 mg over 2 mins. May give an additional 10 mg bolus if no response 15 to 30 mins after initial bolus. ♦ Oral Treatment for Prevention: ▪ IR: 120 mg 3 times a day. ▪ ER: 240 to 480 mg/day in 1 to 2 divided doses.	• Grapefruit juice may increase the serum concentration of verapamil. • Verapamil may increase blood ethanol levels.

		• Nonsustained VT / PVCs (off label): ♦ IR: Initial dose 40 to 80 mg 3 times a day. Maximum dose 360 mg/day divided into 3 to 4 divided doses. ♦ ER: Initial dose 120 to 180 mg once daily. Maximum dose 360 mg/day administered as 1 or 2 divided doses. • SVT Chronic Maintenance (Acute IV treatment is off label): ♦ IR: Initial dose 40 mg 3 to 4 times daily. Maximum dose 480 mg/day divided into 3 to 4 doses. ♦ ER: Initial dose 120 mg once daily. Maximum dose 480 mg/day divided into 1 to 2 doses.	
Dihydropyridines			
Amlodipine	• Onset of antihypertensive effect 24 to 48 hrs. • Peak Effect 6-12 hrs. • Duration at least 24 hrs; can extend to 72 hrs after 6 to 7 weeks of treatment. • $T_{1/2}$ 30 to 50 hrs; prolonged with liver failure.	• Angina (chronic stable) and Vasospastic Angina: Beta blockers are preferred for initial therapy for chronic stable angina. Calcium channel blockers can be added if ongoing angina persists on beta blocker therapy alone. Calcium channel blockers are the preferred treatment for vasospastic angina and can be used with or without nitrates. Initial dose 5 to 10 mg once daily. • HTN: For treatment of HTN for those needing combination therapy and already on other appropriate antihypertensive agents (ACEIs, ARB, thiazide diuretic) used for the treatment of HTN. Initial dose 2.5 to 5 mg once daily. Titrate to maximum dose of 10 mg once daily.	• Administer without regard to food.
Clevidipine	• Onset of Action 2 to 4 mins. • Duration 5 to 15 mins. • $T_{1/2}$ 15 mins.	• Acute Ischemic Stroke - BP Management with Reperfusion Strategy (off label): Prior to initiating reperfusion strategy BP should be maintained at ≤ 185/110 mm Hg. Continuous IV Infusion: Initial dose 1 to 2 mg/hr. Titrate with doubling of dose as needed every 90 seconds. Slow titration rate to every 5 to 10 mins as SBP approaches goal. Every 1 to 2 mg/hr increase should reduce SBP by 2 to 4 mm Hg. Maximum dose 21 mg/hr. Maximum dose limited by maximum volume of one L/day due to restrictions on lipid load. • Hypertensive Emergency: Continuous IV Infusion: Initial dose 1 to 2 mg/hr. Titrate with the doubling of dose as needed every 90 seconds. Slow titration rate to every 5 to 10 mins as SBP goal approaches. Every 1 to 2 mg/hr increase should reduce SBP by 2 to 4 mm Hg. Usual maintenance dose 4 to 6 mg/hr with maximum dose averaging 21 mg/hr over 24 hrs. Maximum dose limited by maximum volume of one L/day due to restrictions on lipid load.	• Do not dilute. • Invert vial gently several times to ensure uniformity of emulsion prior to initiation.
Felodipine	• Onset of antihypertensive action 2 to 5 hrs. • Peak Effect 2.5 to 5 hrs.	• Angina (chronic stable) (off label): Beta blocker therapy is preferred initial therapy. Felodipine can be used as additive therapy or if beta blockers are contraindicated. Initial dose 5 mg once daily. Maximum dose 10 mg once daily. • HTN: For treatment of HTN for those needing combination therapy and already on other appropriate antihypertensive agents (ACEIs, ARB, thiazide diuretic) used for the treatment of HTN. Initial dose 5 mg once daily. Maximum dose 10 gm once daily.	• Administer without food or with a small meal low in fat and carbohydrate. • Grapefruit juice and /or high fat, high

	• Duration of antihypertensive effect 24 hrs. • $T_{1/2}$ 11 to 16 hrs.		carbohydrate meals may increase peak plasma concentrations two-fold. This may result in enhanced vasodilator effects resulting in hypotension or ischemia.
Isradipine	• Onset of Action 2 to 3 hrs. • Peak Effect 1 to 1.5 hrs. • Duration >12 hrs. • $T_{1/2}$ 8 hrs.	• HTN: For treatment of HTN in those needing combination therapy and already on other appropriate antihypertensive agents (ACEIs, ARB, thiazide diuretic) used for the treatment of HTN. Initial dose 2.5 mg 2 time daily. Titrate to maximum dose of 5 mg 2 times daily.	• Administer without regard to food.
Nicardipine	• Onset of Action IV mins; oral 0.5 to 2 hrs. • Peak Effect Oral 1 to 2 hrs. • Duration IV ≤ 8 hrs, 50% decrease in effect seen ≈ 30 mins after discontinuation; oral ≤ 8 hrs. • $T_{1/2}$ Oral 8.6 hrs; prolonged with severe hepatic impairment.	• Acute Aortic Syndrome / Acute Aortic Dissection (off label): Control pain and manage HR (target HR 60-80 bmp) prior to addressing SBP (target SBP < 120 mm Hg without hypoperfusion). Initial continuous IV infusion dose 5 mg/hr. Titrate as needed every 5 to 15 mins in increments of 2.5 mcg/kg/min. Maximum dose 15 mg/hr. • Acute Ischemic Stroke – BP Management with Reperfusion Strategy (off label): Prior to initiating reperfusion strategy BP should be maintained at ≤ 185/110 mm Hg. Initial continuous IV dose 5 mg/hr. Titrate as needed every 5 to 15 mins in increments of 2.5 mcg/kg/min. Maximum dose 15 mg/hr. • Angina (chronic stable): Beta blockers are preferred for initial therapy for chronic stable angina. Calcium channel blockers can be added if ongoing angina persists on beta blocker therapy alone. Initial oral dose 20 mg 3 times daily. Usual oral dose 20 to 40 mg 3 times daily. • HTN: Initial oral dose 20 mg 3 times daily. Usual dose 20 to 40 mg 3 times daily. • Hypertensive Emergency: IV dosing only. Initial dose 5 mg/hr. Titrate as needed every 5 to 15 mins in increments of 2.5 mcg/kg/min. Maximum dose 15 mg/hr. • Intracerebral Hemorrhage – Acute BP Management (off label): For mild to moderate hemorrhage with initial SBP ≥ 150 mm Hg. Initial continuous IV dose 5 mg/hr. Titrate as needed every 5 to 15 mins in increments of 2.5 mg/hr. Maximum dose 15 mg/hr. • Subarachnoid Hemorrhage – Acute BP Management (off label): Initial continuous IV dose 5 mg/hr. Titrate as needed every 5 to 15 mins in increments of 2.5 mg/hr. Maximum dose 15 mg/hr.	• Invasive BP monitoring recommended with IV infusion. • Do not administer with other IV medications at the same site. • Central line or large peripheral line preferred. To minimize venous irritation, rotate sites every 12 hrs. • Administer without regard to food (oral). • Avoid grapefruit or grapefruit juice. Serum concentrations of the drug will be increased when consumed with grapefruit or

			grapefruit juice. This may result in enhanced vasodilator effect resulting in severe hypotension or ischemia.
Nifedipine	• $T_{1/2}$ 2 to 5 hrs; prolonged with liver disease and in elderly to 7 hrs.	• Use of IR nifedipine sublingually is NOT RECOMMEDED for ANY indication due to safety concerns. Nifedipine capsules SHOULD NOT be punctured, and contents of capsule SHOULD NOT be administered sublingually due to risk of severe hypotension and subsequent ischemia. • Angina (chronic stable): Beta blockers are preferred for initial therapy for chronic stable angina. A long-acting dihydropyridine calcium channel blocker can be added if ongoing angina persists on beta blocker therapy alone. ER nifedipine may also be used as alternative therapy if beta blockers are contraindicated ♦ IR nifedipine (oral or SL) is NOT recommended due to increase adverse effects. ♦ ER: Initial dose 30 to 60 mg once daily. Titrate to maximum dose of 120 mg once daily. • Vasospastic Angina: Calcium channel blockers are the preferred treatment for vasospastic angina and can be used with or without nitrates. ♦ IR nifedipine (oral or SL) is NOT recommended due to increase adverse effects. ♦ ER: Initial dose 30 to 60 mg once daily. Titrate to maximum dose of 120 mg once daily. • HTN: For treatment of HTN for those needing combination therapy and already on other appropriate antihypertensive agents (ACEIs, ARB, thiazide diuretic) used for the treatment of HTN. ♦ IR nifedipine (oral or SL) is NOT recommended due to increase adverse effects. ♦ ER: Initial dose 30 to 60 mg once daily. Titrate to maximum dose of 90 mg once daily. Doses up to 120 mg daily are reported. Consider additional therapies if BP not controlled on dose of 90 mg once daily.	• Administer without regard to food. • Avoid grapefruit or grapefruit juice. Serum concentrations of the drug will be increased when consumed with grapefruit or grapefruit juice. This may result in enhanced vasodilator effect resulting in severe hypotension or ischemia.
Nimodipine	• Peak Effect 0.25 to 1.05 hrs. • $T_{1/2}$ 1 to 2 hrs; prolonged with renal impairment.	• DO NOT administer via the IV route. Life threatening events have occurred with parenteral administration. • Subarachnoid Hemorrhage: Initial dose 60 mg every 4 hrs for 21 consecutive days. No titration. Start therapy within 96 hrs of onset of SAH.	• Capsules or oral solution: administer at least 1 hr before meals or 2 hrs after meals. • Tablets: administer without regard to food. But administer consistently with or without food. • Avoid concurrent use with grapefruit juice. This may

			result in enhanced vasodilator effect resulting in severe hypotension or ischemia.
Nisoldipine	• Peak Effect 4 to14 hrs. • Duration > 24 hrs. • $T_{1/2}$ 9 to 18 hrs.	• HTN: For treatment of HTN for those needing combination therapy and already on other appropriate antihypertensive agents (ACEIs, ARB, thiazide diuretic) used for the treatment of HTN. ♦ Oral (Geomatrix Delivery System): Initial dose 17 mg once daily. Titrate to maximum dose of 34 mg once daily. ♦ ER: Initial dose 20 mg once daily. Titrate to maximum dose of 40 mg once daily.	• Administer on an empty stomach. • Take at least 1 hr before meals or 2 hrs after meals. • Administer the same time each day to maintain serum levels. • Avoid grapefruit or grapefruit juice. Serum concentrations of the drug will be increased when consumed with grapefruit or grapefruit juice. This may result in enhanced vasodilator effect resulting in severe hypotension or ischemia.

SGLT2 Inhibitors (Appendix 8)			
Drug Name	**Drug Specific Pharmacokinetics**	**Dosing Information (Note: Dosing for select FDA labeled cardiovascular indications and key "off label" cardiovascular indications are covered below. Consult a drug reference manual for dosing recommendations for other FDA labeled and "off label" non-cardiac indications and for recommended dosing in patients receiving renal replacement therapy or for women who are pregnant or nursing).**	**Administration Information**
Bexagliflozin	• Peak Effect 2-4 hrs (5 hrs if taken with high fat, high calorie meal) • T ½ ≈12 hrs.	• DMT2: Initial dose 20 mg once daily. No titration recommended. • Altered Kidney Function: ◆ eGFR ≥ 30 mL/min/1.73 m^2: No adjustment recommended. ◆ eGFR < 30 mL/min/1.73 m^2: Use not recommended due to lack of efficacy in the treatment of DMT2.	• Administer in the morning without regard to food.
Canagliflozin	• Peak Effect 1-2 hrs. • Duration of Action 24 hrs. • Steady State: 3 days. • T½ 100mg 10.6 hrs. • T½ 300mg 13.1 hrs.	• DMT2: Initial dose 100 mg once daily prior to 1st meal. Titrate to maximum dose of 300 mg once daily. • DMT2 & ASCVD: Initial dose 100 to 300 mg once daily. • DMT2 and Diabetic Kidney Disease (urinary albumin excretion > 300 mg/day): Initial dose 100 mg once daily. No titration recommended. • Altered Kidney Function: ◆ eGFR 30 to < 60 mL/min/1.73 m^2: 100 mg once daily. ◆ eGFR < 30 mL/min/1.73 m^2 with urinary albumin excretion > 300 mg/day: Do not initiate therapy. May continue if on established therapy at a dose of 100 mg once daily prior to decline of eGFR to < 30 mL/min/1.73 m^2. ◆ eGFR < 25 to 30 mL/min/1.73 m^2 with urinary albumin excretion < 300 mg/day: Use not recommended. May continue if on established therapy at a dose of 100 mg once daily prior to decline of eGFR < 30 mL/min/1.73 m^2.	• Administer in the morning without regard to food. • Administering prior to first meal of day may delay intestinal absorption of glucose and subsequently reducing postprandial hyperglycemia.
Dapagliflozin	• Peak Effect 2 hrs. • Duration Urinary glucose excretion returns to baseline ≈ 3 days after discontinuation of 10 mg dose. • T ½ ≈12.9 hrs.	• DMT2: Initial dose 5 mg once daily. Titrate to a maximum dose of 10 mg once daily. • Diabetic Kidney Disease: Initial dose10 mg once daily. No further titration recommended. • Any HF with or without DMT2: Initial dose 10 mg once daily. No further titration recommended. • Altered Kidney Function: ◆ eGFR 25 to < 45 mL/min/1.73 m^2 with: ▪ CKD or DMT2 with CKD: No dose adjustment needed. ▪ DMT2 to Treat Hyperglycemia: Manufacturer does not recommend use since SGLT2Is have less glycemic effect as eGFR declines. ▪ DMT2 with Any HF: No dose adjustment recommended. ◆ eGFR < 25 mL/min/1.73 m^2 with: ▪ CKD and/or HF: Initiation is not recommended; however, patients may continue 10 mg once daily if already on established therapy prior to eGFR decline to < 25 mL/min/1.73 m^2.	• Administer in the morning without regard to food.

		▪ DMT2 to Treat Hyperglycemia: Manufacturer does not recommend use since SGLT2Is have less glycemic effect as eGFR declines.	
Empagliflozin	• Peak Effect 1.5 hrs. • Duration Urinary glucose excretion returns to baseline ≈ 3 days after discontinuation (10 mg and 25 mg doses). • T ½ 12.4 hrs.	• DMT2: Initial dose 10 mg once daily. Titrate up to maximum dose of 25 mg once daily. • DMT2 & ASCVD: Initial dose 10 mg once daily. May titrate to 25 mg once daily. • DMT2 and Diabetic Kidney Disease (eGFR < 45 mL/min/1.73 m^2 and/or albumin to creatinine rations > 200 mg/g): Initial dose 100 mg once daily. No titration recommended. • ANY HF with or without DMT2: Initial dose 10 mg once daily. No titration recommended for the treatment of any HF. May titrate to 25 mg once daily to achieve glycemic goals. • CKD with persistent proteinuria (with or without DMT2): Initial dose 10 mg once daily. No titration recommended for patients with CKD alone. May titrate to 25 mg once daily to achieve glycemic goals. • Altered Kidney Function: ♦ eGFR ≥ 30 mL/min/1.73 m^2: No dosage adjustment necessary. ♦ eGFR < 30 mL/min/1.73 m^2: ▪ DMT2: Not recommended to continue for glycemic control (less glycemic effect as eGFR declines). ▪ CKD: No dosage adjustment for eGFR ≥ 20 mL/min/1.73 m^2. Therapy not initiated with eGFR < 20 mL/min/1.73 m^2. ▪ Any HF: Benefit continues as long as eGFR ≥ 20 mL/min/1.73 m^2. Insufficient evidence for continuing if eGFR < 20 mL/min/1.73 m^2.	• Administer in the morning without regard to food.
Ertugliflozin	• Peak Effect 1 hr (fasting) or 2 hrs (if administered with high-fat, high calorie meal). • T ½ 16.6 hrs.	• DMT2: Initial dose of 5 mg once daily. Titrate to a maximum dose of 15 mg once daily. • Altered Kidney Function: ♦ eGFR ≥ 45 mL/min/1.73 m^2: No dosage adjustment necessary. ♦ eGFR < 45 mL/min/1.73 m^2: Use is not recommended (lack of efficiency in DMT2).	• Administer in the morning without regard to food.
Sotagliflozin Inhibits SGLT1in addition to SGLT2	• Peak Effect 2.5 to 4 hrs. • Duration 5-10 hrs. • T ½ 21 to 35 hrs.	• Any HF (to improve outcomes in HF): Initial dose 200 mg once daily. Titrate to a maximum dose of 400 mg once daily. • CKD (with or without albuminuria) with DMT2 with CV risk factors (for CV Risk Reduction not for treatment of DMT2): Initial dose 200 mg once daily. Titrate to 400 mg once daily. • Altered Kidney Function: ♦ eGFR ≥ 25 mL/min/1.73 m^2: No adjustment necessary. ♦ eGFR < 25 mL/min/1.73 m^2: No dosing adjustments provided by manufacturer; in clinical trials medication was stopped for eGFR ≤ 15 mL/min/1.73 m^2.	• Administer not more than 1 hr before the 1st meal of the day.

Diuretics Appendix 9

Drug Name	Drug Specific Pharmacokinetics	Dosing Information (<u>Note</u>: Dosing for select FDA labeled cardiovascular indications and key "off label" cardiovascular indications are covered below. Consult a drug reference manual for dosing recommendations for other FDA labeled and "off label" non-cardiac indications and for recommended dosing in patients receiving renal replacement therapy or for women who are pregnant or nursing).	Administration Information
Loop Diuretics			
Bumetanide	• Onset of Action Oral 0.5 to 1 hr; IV 2 to 3 mins. • Peak Effect Oral 1 to 2 hrs; IV 15 to 30 mins. • Duration Oral 4 to 6 hrs; IV 2 to 3 hrs. • $T_{1/2}$ 1 to 1.5 hrs.	• Edema / Volume Overload: Oral or IV bolus initial dose (naïve to loop diuretic) 0.5 to 1 mg once then titrate to effect. May repeat oral dose every 4 to 5 hrs. May repeat IV dose every 2 to 3 hrs. IV bolus administered at a rate of 0.5 to 1 mg over 1 to 2 mins. Total maximum recommended daily dose is 10 mg/day. • Refractory Edema / Acute Decompensation: ♦ IV Bolus / Intermittent Dosing: Initial bolus 1 to 2.5 times the total daily oral maintenance dose. Titrate to effect with maximum dosing 3 to 10 mg daily. Total maximum recommended daily dose is 10 mg/day. ♦ IV Continuous Infusion: Start immediately after IV bolus dose. Initial infusion rate 0.5 mg/hr. Titrate to effect up to 2 mg/hr. • Altered Kidney Function: ♦ eGFR $\geq$ 30 mL/min/1.73 m^2: No adjustment necessary. ♦ eGFR < 30 mL/min/1.73 m^2: ▪ IV Bolus / Oral Dosing: Higher doses may be required to be effective. Single oral IV doses > 8 to 10 mgs are unlikely to produce an increased diuretic effect. ▪ IV Continuous Infusion: Initial infusion rate of 1 mg/hr. If response is inadequate repeat bolus dose and increase infusion to 2 mg/hr.	• Administer without regard to food.
Furosemide	• Onset of Action: Oral 30 to 60 mins; IV 5 mins. • Peak Effect Oral 1 to 2 hrs; IV 0.5 hrs; SQ 4 hrs. • Duration Oral 6 to 8 hrs; IV ≈ 2 hrs. • $T_{1/2}$ IV or Oral 0.5 to 2 hrs with normal renal function. In ESRD 9 hrs.	• Edema / Volume Overload: ♦ Oral: Initial oral dose (naïve to loop diuretic) 20 to 40 mg then titrate as needed to affect. If response is inadequate repeat the same dose or increase dose in increments of 20 to 40 mg/dose at intervals of 6 to 8 hrs; may titrate up to 600 mg/day with severe edematous states. ♦ SQ: Preprogrammed on-body infuser. Initial dose 30 mg infused over 1 hr. Subsequent delivery is 12.5 mg/hr for 4 hrs. Total dose 80 mg over 5 hrs. Not adjustable. Not for continuous use. • Refractory Edema or Acute Decompensation: ♦ IV Bolus/Intermittent Dosing: Initial bolus 1 to 2.5 times the total daily oral maintenance dose. Titrate as needed to an effective dose. If initial bolus not effective, double the initial dose. Titration of IV bolus can occur at $\geq$ 2-hr intervals as needed in hospitalized patients. Maximum single dose 80 to 200 mg. Maximum recommended daily dose 600 mg/day.	• Administer without regard to food. • IV bolus should occur at a rate of 20 to 40 mg per min. Consider short term infusion for higher bolus doses ($\geq$ 160 mg) at a rate of 4 mg/min to avoid ototoxicity.

		♦ IV Continuous Infusion: Start immediately after IV bolus dose. Initial infusion rate is 5 mg/hr. If response is inadequate repeat IV bolus and double the infusion rate. Titrate as need to maximum infusion rate of 40 mg/hr with bolus dose prior to each up titration. • Altered Kidney Function: ♦ eGFR ≥ 30 mL/min/1.73 m^2: No adjustment recommended. ♦ eGFR < 30 mL/min/1.73 m^2: ▪ IV Bolus / Oral Dosing: Higher doses may be required to be effective. Single doses > 160 to 200 mg are unlikely to produce an increased diuretic effect. ▪ IV Continuous Infusion: Initial infusion rate of 20 mg/hr. If response is inadequate repeat bolus dose and increase infusion to 40 mg/hr.	
Torsemide	• Onset of Action Within 1 hr. • Peak Effect Diuresis 1 to 2 hr. Antihypertensive effect 4 to 6 wks. • Duration ≈ 6 to 8 hrs. • $T_{1/2}$ ≈ 3.5 hrs.	Only available as an oral preparation in the U.S. • Edema / Volume Overload: Initial dose (naïve to loop diuretic) 10 to 20 mg once daily. May increase gradually by doubling dose until the desired diuretic response is obtained. Maximum effective single dose 50 to 100 mg. Maximum daily dose is 200 mg/day in 2 divided doses. May use loop equivalent doses when changing from one loop to another. Torsemide 10 to 20 mg = bumetanide 1 mg = furosemide 40 mg. • HTN: When adding a diuretic for the treatment of HTN in patients with HF or chronic kidney disease a loop diuretic is preferred over other diuretics. Initial dose 5 mg once daily. May increase to 10 mg once daily if inadequate anti-hypertensive response after 4 to 6 weeks. • Altered Kidney Function: ♦ eGFR ≥ 30 mL/min/1.73 m^2: No adjustment recommended. ♦ eGFR < 30 mL/min/1.73 m^2: Higher doses may be required to be effective. Single doses > 50 to 100 mg are unlikely to produce an increased diuretic effect.	• May administer without regard to food. However, food will delay onset and peak action by ≈ 30 to 45 mins.
Ethacrynic Acid	• Onset of Action Oral ≈ 30 mins; IV 5 mins. • Peak Effect Oral 2 hrs; IV 30 mins. • Duration Oral 12 hrs; IV 2 to 4 hrs. • $T_{1/2}$ 2 to 4 hrs.	• Edema / Volume Overload: Reserved for patient with hypersensitivity to sulfonamide-based loop diuretics. ♦ Oral Dosing: Initial oral dose (naïve to loop diuretic) 25 to 50 mg once daily. Titrate to diuretic effect. Usual dose 50 to 200 mg/day in 1 to 2 divided doses. Maximum dose of 400 mg/day in 2 divided doses. ♦ IV Dosing: Initial IV dose (naïve to loop diuretic) 50 mg (0.5 to 1 mg/kg/dose). Maximum single IV dose 100 mg. Repeat doses not routinely recommended, but if needed can be administered after 12 hrs with up to 200 mg/day in 2 divided doses (12-hr intervals). • No dosage adjustment for kidney impairment.	• Administer after a meal. • IV bolus should occur over 5 to 20 mins to avoid ototoxicity.
Thiazide and Thiazide Like Diuretics			
Chlorthalidone	• Onset of Action ≈ 2.6 hrs. • Peak Effect 2 to 6 hrs.	• Edema or Volume Overload: Optimize therapy with loop diuretic before adding thiazide diuretic for use in diuretic resistant patients. Initial dose 12.5 to 25 mg once daily. Increase dose as needed to a maximum dose of 100 mg once daily. May also administer on alternating days or certain days of the week based on patient response.	• Take in AM with food. • Administer with scheduled loop

	• Duration Single dose 24 to 48 hrs; Long-term dosing 48 to 72 hrs. • $T_{1/2}$ Single dose 40 hrs; Long-term dosing 45 to 60 hrs.	• HTN: Usual dosage range 12.5 to 25 mg once daily. Doses > 25 mg not recommended based on minimal added antihypertensive benefit with increased risk for adverse effects. • Altered Kidney Function: ♦ If CrCL ≥ 10 mL/min: No adjustment recommended. However, with CrCL < 30 mL/min diuretic effect is diminished. ♦ If CrCL < 10 mL/min: Use not recommended due to lack of efficacy.	diuretic or shortly before.
Chlorothiazide	• Onset of Action (diuresis) Oral 2 hrs; IV 15 mins. • Peak Effect Oral ≈ 4 hrs; IV 30 mins. • Duration (diuresis) Oral ≈ 6 to 12 hrs; IV 2 hrs. • $T_{1/2}$ 45 to 120 mins.	• Edema or Volume Overload: Optimize therapy with loop diuretic before adding thiazide diuretic for use in diuretic resistant patients. Usual dose IV or Oral 250 to 1000 mg 1 or 2 times daily. May also administer on alternating days or certain days of the week based on patient response. • HTN: Initial oral dose 500 to 1000 mg daily in 1 or 2 divided doses. Maximum daily oral dose 2000 mg in 1 or 2 divided doses. • Altered Kidney Function: ♦ If CrCL < 30 mL/min: Ineffective diuretic effect unless used with a loop diuretic. ♦ If CrCL < 10 mL/min: Avoid use.	• Administer with scheduled loop diuretic or shortly before. • Do not give IM or SQ.
Hydrochloroth iazide	• Onset of Action (diuresis) Oral ≈ 2 hrs. • Peak Effect Oral ≈ 4 hrs. • Duration Oral 6 to 12 hrs. • $T_{1/2}$ ≈ 6 to15 hrs. Prolonged with altered kidney function.	• Edema or Volume Overload: Optimize therapy with loop diuretic before adding thiazide diuretic for use in diuretic resistant patients. Initial oral dose 25 to 50 mg 1 or 2 times daily. Maximum dose 200 mg/day. May also administer on alternating days or certain days of the week based on patient response. • HTN: Initial oral dose 12.5 to 25 mg once daily. Maximum dose 50 mg once daily. Doses > 25 mg not recommended based on minimal added antihypertensive benefit with increased risk for adverse effects. • Altered Kidney Function: ♦ If CrCl ≥ 10 mL/min: No adjustment recommended. However, with CrCL < 30 mL/min diuretic effect is diminished. ♦ If CrCl < 10 mL/min: Use not recommended due to lack of efficacy.	• Administer with scheduled loop diuretic or shortly before.
Indapamide	• Peak Effect 2 hrs. • $T_{1/2}$ Biphasic: 14 and 25 hrs.	• Edema or Volume Overload: Optimize therapy with loop diuretic before adding thiazide diuretic for use in diuretic resistant patients. Initial oral dose 2.5 mg once daily. Maximum dose 5 mg once daily. May also administer on alternating days or certain days of the week based on patient response. • HTN: Initial dose 1.25 mg to 2.5 mg once daily. Doses > 2.5 mg not recommended based on minimal added antihypertensive benefit with increased risk for adverse effects. • Altered Kidney Function: ♦ If eGFR ≥ 30 mL/min/1.73 m^2: No adjustment recommended. ♦ If eGFR < 30 mL/min/1.73 m^2: No adjustment recommended. However, diuretic effect is diminished as kidney function declines.	• May administer without regard to food. • Administer with food or milk to help decrease GI adverse effects.

Metolazone	• Onset of Action ≈ 60 mins. • Duration > 24 hrs. • $T_{1/2}$ 8 to 14 hrs. Accumulation can occur with severe renal impairment.	• Edema or Volume Overload: Optimize therapy with loop diuretic before adding thiazide diuretic for use in diuretic resistant patients. Initial dose 2.5 to 5 mg once daily. Maximum dose 20 mg daily in 1 or 2 divided doses. May also administer on alternating days or certain days of the week based on patient response. • No dosage adjustment for kidney impairment.	• May administer without regard to food.
Potassium Sparing Diuretics			
Amiloride	• Onset of Action within 2 hrs. • Peak Effect 6 to 10 hrs. • Peak Serum 3 to 4 hrs. • Duration ≈ 24 hrs. • $T_{1/2}$ 6 to 9 hrs. With CrCl <50 mL/min 21-144 hrs.	• HTN: Used as additive therapy in resistant HTN when not responding to combination therapy. Initial dose 5 mg once daily. Maximum dose 10 mg once daily in 1 or 2 divided doses. • Altered Kidney Function: ♦ If CrCl 10 to 50 mL/min: Decrease normal dose by 50%. ♦ If CrCl ≤ 30 mL/min in adults ≥ 65 years: Use not recommended per the Beers Criteria. ♦ If CrCl < 10 mL/min: Avoid use.	• Administer with food or meals to avoid GI adverse effects.
Triamterene	• Onset of Action 2 to 4 hrs. • Peak Serum Level 3 hrs. • Duration 7 to 9 hrs.	• Edema: Initial dose 50 to 100 mg once daily. Maximum dose 300 mg once daily in divided doses. • Altered Kidney Function: If CrCl ≤ 50 mL/min: Avoid use.	• Administer after meals.
Eplerenone	• See Appendix 5 Reviewing MRAs. Also referred to as Potassium Sparing Diuretic.		
Finerenone	• See Appendix 5 Reviewing MRAs. Also referred to as Potassium Sparing Diuretic.		
Spironolactone	• See Appendix 5 Reviewing MRAs. Also referred to as Potassium Sparing Diuretic.		
Aquaretic Diuretics			
Tolvaptan Samsca Jynarque	• Onset of Action 2 to 4 hrs aquaretic and sodium effects (Samsca). • Peak Effect 4 to 8 hrs aquaretic and	Tolvaptan (*Samsca*) • Hyponatremia (euvolemic or hypervolemic): NOT recommended for ACUTE hyponatremia. Indicated to maintain serum sodium > 120 mEq/L or in those who continue to have neurologic symptoms despite therapy. Samsca should be initiated in the hospital where close and frequent monitoring of serum sodium can take place. Initial dose 15 mg orally once daily. May increase to	• May administer without regard to food. • Water should be readily available to the patient. If access

	sodium effects (Samsca). • Duration 60% of serum sodium increase is retained for 24 hrs (Samsca). • $T_{1/2}$ 15 mg dose 3 hrs; ≥120 mg doses ≈ 12 hrs.	30 mg once daily in 24 hrs. Maximum dose 60 mg once daily. Hospitalization should continue until serum sodium stable. Tolvaptan (*Jynarque*) • Autosomal Dominant Polycystic Kidney Disease (ADPKD): Use of this formulation of Tolvaptan is under the FDA REMS program and prescribers must be registered. Jynarque is included here to assure the reader understands there are two different forms of Tolvaptan that are used for two very different indications. Samsca may also be used for ADPKD and when used for that indication will fall under the REMS program. Jynarque is NOT indicated in the treatment for hyponatremia.	to water is interrupted, treatment should be stopped. • Grapefruit juice can increase serum tolvaptan concentrations. Avoid concurrent use.
Conivaptan	• $T_{1/2}$ 5.3 to 8.1 hrs.	• Hyponatremia (euvolemic or hypervolemic) in hospitalized patients: NOT recommended for ACUTE hyponatremia but may be considered in SIADH in combination with other therapies for severe symptomatic hyponatremia. Use in HF with persistent severe hypervolemic hyponatremia is off label. ♦ Initial IV Loading Dose: 20 mg IV over 30 mins. ♦ Continuous IV Infusion: Following loading dose with IV infusion of 20 mg over 24 hrs. Maximum dose of 40 mg over 24 hrs. Total duration of therapy not to exceed 4 days. • Altered Kidney Function: ♦ CrCl ≥ 30 mL/min: No adjustment recommended. ♦ CrCl < 30 mL/min: Use not recommended. Contraindicated in anuria.	• For IV use only. • Do not infuse with any other product in the same IV line.

Sympathomimetic Vasoactive Drugs (Appendix 10)			
Drug Name	**Drug Specific Pharmacokinetics**	**Dosing Information (<u>Note</u>: Dosing for select FDA labeled cardiovascular indications and key "off label" cardiovascular indications are covered below. Consult a drug reference manual for dosing recommendations for other FDA labeled and "off label" non-cardiac indications and for recommended dosing in patients receiving renal replacement therapy or for women who are pregnant or nursing).**	**Administration Information**

Dobutamine	• Onset of Action 1 to 10 mins.
	• Peak Effect 10 to 20 mins.
	• $T_{1/2}$ 2 mins.
		• Acute Decompensated HF: IV infusion initial dose 2 to 5 mcg/kg/min. Usual dosage range 2 to 10 mcg/kg/min. Maximum dose 20 mcg/kg/min.
		• Inotropic Support (off label): May be added to vasopressor therapy in shock states if not meeting hemodynamic goals on vasopressors alone. IV infusion initial dose 2 to 5 mcg/kg/min. Usual dosage range 2 to 10 mcg/kg/min. Maximum dose 20 mcg/kg/min.
		• Stress Echocardiography:
		  ♦ Dobutamine Stress Echocardiogram (off label): IV infusion initial dose 5 mcg/kg/min; increase at 3-min intervals to 20 mcg/kg/min, then 30 mcg/kg/min, and then 40 mcg/kg/min to achieve target heart rate.
		  ♦ Viability Assessment (off label): IV infusion initial dose 2.5 mcg/kg/min; increase at 5-min intervals in increments of 2.5 mcg/kg/min until contractile response is noted on echocardiogram.
			• Use large peripheral vein.
			• May be a Vesicant. Ensure proper needle or catheter placement prior to and during IV infusion to avoid extravasation.

Dopamine	• Onset of Action within 5 mins. • Duration < 10 mins. • $T_{1/2} \approx 2$ min	• Bradycardia / AV Block (symptomatic and unresponsive to atropine) (off label): Initial continuous IV dose 5 mcg/kg/min. Titrate every 2 mins in 5 mcg/kg/min increments to a maximum dose of 20 mcg/kg/min. • Cardiogenic Shock: Not typically preferred in cardiogenic shock secondary to increased risk of arrhythmia and possible mortality. IV infusion usual dose 0.5 to 20 mcg/kg/min. • Septic Shock / Vasodilatory Shock States: Not typically recommended for septic shock except as alternative to norepinephrine when bradycardia is present and the patient has a low risk for tachyarrhythmias. IV infusion initial dose 2 to 5 mcg/kg/min. Maximum dose 20 mcg/kg/min. • Post-Cardiac Arrest Shock: Not typically preferred agent in this population secondary to increased risk of tachyarrhythmias. IV infusion usual dose range 5 to 20 mcg/kg/min. • Inotropic Support: IV infusion usual dose range 5 to 15 mcg/kg/min. Lower end of dosage ranges provides inotropic support. Upper dosage range moves toward vasoconstriction with less inotropic effect (varies by patient). • Dosing in Obesity with BMI ≥ 30 kg/m^2: Recommended to use *ideal body weight* for dosing and titrate according to response.	• Central line preferred. Otherwise use large peripheral vein. • Duration of peripheral infusion should not exceed 72 hrs. • Vesicant. Ensure proper needle or catheter placement prior to and during IV infusion to avoid extravasation.

Epinephrine	• Onset of Action SQ 5 to 10 mins; IV < 5 mins.
	• Steady State Continuous IV
		• Hypotension / Shock:
		  ♦ Septic Shock / Vasodilatory Shock States: Adjunct therapy when MAP not achieved with initial vasopressor or inotropic support needed.
		    ▪ Weight-based Dosing: Initial dose 0.01 to 0.2 mcg/kg/min. Usual dose range 0.01 to 0.5 mcg/kg/min. Max infusion rate 0.5 to 2 mcg/kg/min.
			• Use central line for IV administration whenever possible.
			• Vesicant. Ensure proper needle or

	Infusion 5 to 10 mins. • $T_{1/2}$ IV Push < 5 mins.	▪ Non-weight-based Dosing: Initial dosing 1 to 15 mcg/min. Usual dose range 1 to 40 mcg/min. Max infusion rate 40 to 160 mcg/min. ♦ Cardiogenic Shock (off label): Not preferred agent in cardiogenic shock. ▪ Weight-based Dosing: Usual dose range 0.01 to 0.5 mcg/kg/min. ▪ Non-weight-based Dosing: Usual dose range 1 to 40 mcg/min. ♦ Post Cardiac Arrest Shock (off label): ▪ Weight-based Dosing: Usual dose range 0.01 to 1.0 mcg/kg/min. Maximum dose 2 mcg/kg/min. ▪ Non-weight-based Dosing: Usual dose range 1 to 80 mcg/min. Maximum dose 160 mcg/min. • Symptomatic Bradycardia / AV Block (unresponsive to atropine) (off label): Initial infusion 2 to 10 mcg/min. Usual dosage range 8 to 40 mcg/min. • Sudden Cardiac Arrest (pulseless) (off label): Initial dose 1 mg (0.1 mg/mL solution) IV or IO every 3 to 5 min or endotracheal 2 to 2.5 mg (1mg/mL solution) diluted in 5 to 10 mL NS or sterile water every 3 to 5 mins until return of spontaneous circulation.	catheter placement prior to and during IV infusion to avoid extravasation.
Isoproterenol	• Onset of Action immediate. • Duration 10 to 15 mins. • $T_{1/2}$ 2.5 to 5 mins.	• Symptomatic Bradycardia / AV Block unresponsive to atropine: IV infusion usual dose 1 to 20 mcg/min. Titrate to patient response. • Cardiogenic Shock due to Bradycardia (off label): IV infusion usual dose 2 to 20 mcg/min. Titrate to patient response. • Tilt table testing (provocation for syncope) (off label): IV infusion initial dose 1 mcg/min. Increase based on patient response up to 3 mcg/min. (Institutional procedural protocols may vary.) • Torsade de Pointes (off label): Used only for patients with bradycardia mediated TdP. IV infusion usual dose 2 to 10 mcg/min. Titrated to clinical response. Should only be managed by provider clinically experienced in the treatment of this situation. Avoid in long QT syndrome.	• Avoid combination of isoproterenol and epinephrine. Isoproterenol may enhance effect of systemic epinephrine.
Nor-epinephrine	• Onset of Action very rapid acting. • Steady state 5 mins. • Duration Vasopressor 1 to 2 mins. • $T_{1/2} \approx$ 2.4 mins.	• Cardiogenic Shock: ♦ Weight-based Dosing: Initial IV dose 0.05 mcg/kg/min. Usual dosage range 0.05 to 0.4 mcg/kg/min. ♦ Non-weight-based Dosing: Initial IV dose 5 mcg/min. Usual dose range 5 to 30 mcg/min. • Post Cardiac Arrest Shock: ♦ Weight-based Dosing: Initial IV dose 0.05 to 0.15 mcg/kg/min. Usual dosage range 0.05 to 1.0 mcg/kg/min. Maximum dosage range 1 to 3.3 mcg/kg/min. ♦ Non-weight-based Dosing: Initial IV dose 5 to 15 mcg/min. Usual dose range 5 to 80 mcg/min. Maximum dose 80 to 250 mcg/min. • Septic Shock / Vasodilatory Shock States: ♦ Weight-based Dosing: Initial IV dose 0.05 to 0.15 mcg/kg/min. Usual dosage range 0.025 to 1.0 mcg/kg/min. Maximum dosage range 1 to 3.3 mcg/kg/min. ♦ Non-weight-based Dosing: Initial IV dose 5 to 15 mcg/min. Usual dose range 2 to 80 mcg/min. Maximum dose 80 to 250 mcg/min.	• Central line recommended. Otherwise use large peripheral vein. • Duration of peripheral infusion should not exceed 72 hrs. • Vesicant. Ensure proper needle or catheter placement prior to and during IV infusion to avoid extravasation.

			• Do not infuse sodium bicarbonate or other alkaline solution in same IV line. Inactivation of norepinephrine can occur.
Phenylephrine	• Onset of Action IM/SQ 10 to 15 mins; IV immediate. • Duration IM 1 to 2 hrs; SQ 50 mins; IV 15 to 20 mins. • $T_{1/2}$ Alpha Phase ≈ 5 mins; terminal phase 2 to 3 hrs.	• Septic Shock / Vasodilatory Shock States: Not recommended 1st line agent for septic shock. Other recommended agents should be used prior to phenylephrine. ♦ Weight-based Dosing: IV infusion initial dose 0.5 to 2.0 mcg/kg/min. Usual dosage range 0.25 to 5.0 mcg/kg/min. Reports of dosage rates as high as 9.1 mcg/kg/min have been published. ♦ Non-weight-based Dosing (based on 80 kg patient): IV infusion initial dose 40 to 160 mcg/min. Reports of dosage rates as high as 730 mcg/min have been published. • Cardiogenic Shock due to aortic stenosis, mitral stenosis, or hypertrophic cardiomyopathy with left ventricular outflow tract obstruction: IV infusion initial dose 0.1 to 10 mcg/kg/min. • Hypotension During Anesthesia: ♦ IV Bolus: Initial dose 40 to 100 mcg/dose. Repeat as needed every 1 to 2 mins. Maximum total dose 200 mcg. ♦ IV Infusion: Initial dose 10 to 35 mcg/min. Maximum dose 200 mcg/min.	• Central line recommended. Otherwise use large peripheral vein. • Duration of peripheral infusion should not exceed 72 hrs. • Vesicant. Ensure proper needle or catheter placement prior to and during IV infusion to avoid extravasation.

Non-Sympathomimetic Vasoactive Drugs (Appendix 11)			
Drug Name	**Drug Specific Pharmacokinetics**	**Dosing Information (Note: Dosing for select FDA labeled cardiovascular indications and key "off label" cardiovascular indications are covered below. Consult a drug reference manual for dosing recommendations for other FDA labeled and "off label" non-cardiac indications and for recommended dosing in patients receiving renal replacement therapy or for women who are pregnant or nursing).**	**Administration Information**
Milrinone Phosphodiesterase-3 Enzyme Inhibitor	• Onset of Action 5 to 15 mins. • $T_{1/2}$ HF 2.3 to 2.4 hrs (prolonged in kidney impairment); 20.1 ± 3.3 hrs in severe HF with continuous CVVH.	• Acute Decompensated HF (short term use ≤ 48 hrs): IV infusion initial dose 0.125 to 0.25 mcg/kg/min. Usual dosage range 0.125 to 0.75 mcg/kg/min. IV bolus no longer recommended due to concerns for hypotension. There has been no demonstrated benefit for continuing infusion beyond 48 hrs and safety may be compromised with long term therapy (increased risk of death). • Postoperative Inotropic Support in Heart Transplant Recipients (off label): IV infusion usual dose range 0.375 to 0.75 mcg/kg/min. Titrate to lowest effective dose. • Altered Kidney Function: Drug clearance highly dependent on kidney function. Titrate cautiously based on clinical endpoints (systemic / end organ perfusion). ♦ CrCl 10 to 50 mL/min: IV infusion initial dose 0.0625 to 0.125 mcg/kg/min. Rates > 0.375 mcg/kg/min not recommended in severe kidney impairment. ♦ CrCl < 10 mL/min: Consider alternative therapy. • Obesity with BMI ≥ 30 kg/m^2: Recommended to use *ideal body weight* for dosing and titrate according to response.	• For IV use only.
Arginine Vasopressin Antidiuretic Hormone Analog	• Onset of Action Antidiuretic effect 1 to 2 hrs; vasopressor effect rapid. • Peak vasopressor effect within 15 mins of initiation of infusion. • Duration IV vasopressor effect eliminated within 20 mins of termination. • $T_{1/2}$ IV 10 to 20 mins.	• Septic Shock / Vasodilatory Shock States: Used as adjunct to primary vasopressor recommendations for vasodilatory shock states. IV infusion with initial fixed dose (not titrated) of 0.03 units/min added as adjunct to IV norepinephrine therapy. Usual dosage range of 0.01 to 0.04 units/min. Doses > 0.04 units/min carry a potential risk of inducing ischemia and are therefore reserved for salvage therapy. • Diabetes Insipidus (central) (off label): Used short-term in postoperative period after transsphenoidal surgery (in neurocritical care). Continuous IV infusion with wide variety of dosing ranges defined by individual institutional protocols. Minimum effective dose should be used with the goal to control polyuria. Close monitoring of urine output is essential. • Deceased Organ Donor Management (off label): Considered if remains hypotensive after appropriate fluid resuscitation, LVEF < 45%, low SVR, or in the presence of diabetes insipidus. Usual dosage range of 0.01 to 0.04 units/min. Recommended SVR goal of 800 to 1,200 dynes•second/cm^5.	• Use large peripheral veins. • Vesicant. Ensure proper needle or catheter placement prior to and during IV infusion to avoid extravasation.
Nitroglycerin IV	• Onset of Action IV immediate.	• Acute Decompensated HF / Acute Angina (unrelieved by other forms of NTG): IV infusion initial dose 5 to 10 mcg/min. Titrate by increments of 5 mcg/min every 3 to 5 mins to 20	• IV NTG should be in glass bottle (avoid

	• Peak Effect IV immediate. • Duration IV 3 to 5 mins. • $T_{1/2}$ 1 to 4 mins.	mcg/min. If no response at 20 mcg/min then increase by 10 mcg/min every 3 to 5 mins, up to 200 mcg/min. • Hypertensive Emergency (off label): IV infusion initial dose 5 mcg/min. Titrate by increments of 5 mcg/min every 3 to 5 mins to 20 mcg/min. If no response at 20 mcg/min then increase by 10 mcg/min every 3 to 5 mins, up to 200 mcg/min.	containers with PCV plastic). • Avoid use of PVC administration sets that absorb NTG into the tubing. • Use special non-absorptive (non-PVC) IV tubing.
Nitroglycerin Sublingual Tablets (SL) Lingual Spray (LS)	• Onset of Action SL / LS 1 to 3 mins. • Peak Effect SL 5 mins; LS 4 to 15 mins. • Duration SL / LS at least 25 mins. • $T_{1/2}$ 1 to 4 mins.	• Acute Angina: ◆ SL: Initial dose SL tablet 0.3 or 0.4 mg dissolved under the tongue at onset. May repeat every 5 mins up to 3 total doses in 15 mins. ◆ LS: Initial dose of 1 to 2 sprays (400 mcg per spray) on or under the tongue. May repeat every 5 mins up to 3 total doses in 15 mins. ◆ SL and LS: ▪ Stable Coronary Artery Disease / Stable Angina: Patients are usually instructed to seek medical treatment if there is no improvement in symptoms after 15 mins (3 dose) unless otherwise advised by their provider. Some with stable coronary artery disease / stable angina may be instructed to use these preparations prophylactically 5 to 10 mins prior to activities which are known to provoke an anginal attack to prevent the onset of symptoms. ▪ Post Successful Treatment of Coronary Artery Disease: Patients who have been successfully treated with coronary bypass grafting or intracoronary stenting are advised to access the emergency medical system if there is no improvement after 1 dose. Once 911 is activated the patient should continue with treatment every 5 minutes until emergency personnel arrive.	• SL: May moisten mouth with water prior to use to assist with dissolving tablet. • LS: Close mouth after administration. Do not inhale spray. Do not drink fluid or expectorate for 5 to 10 mins after use.
Nitroglycerin Topical Paste (PST) Transdermal Patch (TP)	• Onset of Action PST 15 to 30 mins.; TP ≈ 30 mins. • Peak Effect PST 60 mins.; TP 120 mins. • Duration PST 7 hrs; TP 10 to 12 hrs. • $T_{1/2}$ 1 to 4 mins.	• Angina: For the prevention of angina pectoris due to stable coronary artery disease. Onset of action not fast enough to use for acute anginal attacks. ◆ PST: Initial dose ½ inch of paste applied 2 times daily. First dose is usually applied upon rising and again in 6 hrs. Second dose is removed after 6 hrs to allow for a nitrate free period. Dose may be increased if lower dose is not effective in preventing angina by doubling the dose with each increase to a maximum dose of 2 inches per application 2 times daily. ◆ TP: Initial dose 0.2 to 0.4 mg/hr patch. Increase dose based on response to a maximum dose of 0.8 mg/patch. Patch should be applied upon rising and removed after 12-14 hrs to provide nitrate free period of 10 to 12 hrs.	• Apply to clean, dry, hair free surface – usually arms or chest wall. • Rotate sites with each application. • PST: Touching the paste can cause headaches.
Isosorbide Dinitrate	• Onset of Action 1 hr. • Peak Effect 8 hrs. • Duration 1 hr. • $T_{1/2}$ 1 hr.	• Angina Prevention: Initial dose 5 to 20 mg 2 to 3 times daily. Suggested times to allow for an approximately 14-hr nitrate free period for twice daily dosing are 8 AM and 1 PM and for 3 times daily dosing 8 AM, 1 PM and 6 PM. • HFrEF (off label): ◆ Must be in combination with hydralazine to improve outcomes in HFrEF.	• In angina prevention to prevent nitrate tachyphylaxis do not administer around the clock.

		♦ Initial dose 20 mg 3 times daily. Titrate to a target dose of 40 mg 3 times daily. ♦ No need for a nitrate free period when given with hydralazine as nitrate tachyphylaxis is prevented when co-administered with hydralazine. • Altered Kidney Function: No dosage adjustment for altered kidney function	
Isosorbide Mononitrate Immediate Release (IR) Extended Release (ER)	• Onset of Action IR 30-40 mins; ER 30-45 mins. • Peak Effect IR 30-60 mins; ER 30-60 mins. • Duration IR $\geq$ 6 hrs; ER $\geq$ 12-24 hrs. • $T_{1/2}$ IR 5 hrs; ER 5.5 hrs.	• Angina Prevention: ♦ IR: Initial dose 20 mg 2 times daily. Second dose should be administered 7 hrs after 1st dose to ensure nitrate free period (8 AM and 3 PM). Can be initiated at 5 mg 2 times daily and up titrated every 2 to 3 days if concerned about hypotension. ♦ ER: Initial dose 30 to 60 mg every morning. Maximum daily dose 240 mg once daily. • Altered Kidney Function: No dosage adjustment for altered kidney function.	• To prevent nitrate tachyphylaxis do not administer around the clock.
Nitroprusside Vasodilator	• Onset of Action < 2 mins. • Duration 1 to 10 mins. • $T_{1/2}$ Parent drug ≈ 2 mins; Thiocyanate elimination ≈ 3 days (may be prolong in renal failure).	• Acute Aortic Syndrome / Acute Aortic Dissection (off label): Control pain and manage HR (target HR 60-80 bmp) prior to addressing SBP (target SBP < 120 mm Hg without hypoperfusion). Initial continuous IV dose 0.25 to 0.5 mcg/kg/min. Titrate as needed every 5 mins in increments of 0.5 mcg/kg/min. Maximum dose 10 mcg/kg/min. To avoid toxicity doses $\geq$ 8 to 10 mcg/kg/min should only be used for a maximum of 10 mins. • Acute Decompensated HF (without symptomatic hypotension): IV infusion initial dose 0.1 to 0.3 mcg/kg/min. Titrate at 5 to 15 min intervals to desired hemodynamic effect. Usual dose 1 to 3 mcg/kg/min. Maximum dose 5 mcg/kg/min (for average 80 kg patient). • Acute Ischemic Stroke – BP Management with Reperfusion Strategy (off label): Prior to initiating reperfusion strategy BP should be maintained at $\leq$ 185/110 mm Hg. Nitroprusside reserved for refractory HTN. Initial continuous IV dose 0.25 to 0.5 mcg/kg/min. Titrate as needed in increments of 0.5 mcg/kg/min in 5 min intervals. Maximum dose of 10 mcg/kg/min. Do not infuse at $\geq$ 8 - 10 mcg/kg/min for more than 10 mins to avoid toxicity. • Hypertensive Emergency: IV infusion initial dose 0.25 to 0.5 mcg/kg/min. Titrate as needed in increments of 0.5 mcg/kg/min in 5 min intervals. Preferred (to avoid toxicity) usual dose $\leq$ 2 mcg/kg/min. Maximum dose 10 mcg/kg/min. Do not infuse at 10 mcg/kg/min for more than 10 mins to avoid toxicity. • Kidney impairment may lead to toxicity from thiocyanate accumulation. ♦ eGFR < 30 mL/min/1.73 m^2: Limit infusion rate to < 3 mcg/kg/min. ♦ Anuric Patients: Limit infusion rate to < 1 mcg/kg/min.	• Light sensitive solution: IV bag must always be wrapped to protect from light. • Risk of cyanide or thiocyanate toxicity increased with higher doses (> 3 mcg/kg/min), prolonged infusions (> 3 days) or in renal failure.

Direct Smooth Muscle Relaxants			
Hydralazine	• Onset of Action IV 10-80 mins. • Peak Effect Oral 1 to 2 hrs. • Duration IM/IV up to 12 hrs. • $T_{1/2}$ 3 to 7 hrs.	• Heart Failure with Reduced Ejection Fraction with persistent NYHA Class III or IV (off label): For individuals who are intolerant of Entresto, ACE inhibitors, or ARBs, or as an adjunctive therapy for those with residual symptoms despite optimal medical treatment. Initial oral dose 25 mg 3 times daily in combination with isosorbide dinitrate. Titrate every 1 to 2 weeks. Maximum dose 75 to 100 mg 3 times daily. • Chronic HTN: Used as an additional treatment strategy for resistant HTN when combination therapy fails. Not recommended for initial treatment. Combining beta-blockers and/or diuretics with hydralazine can mitigate reflex tachycardia and fluid retention associated with hydralazine use. Alternative agent for severe asymptomatic HTN as a short-term solution (other agents carry higher recommendations). Initial dose 10 mg 4 times daily for 2 to 4 days. • Hypertensive Emergency (alternative agent): Hydralazine is not commonly used due to its unpredictable and delayed antihypertensive effects. IM or IV dose 10 to 20 mg every 4 to 6 hrs as necessary. Maximum dose: 40 mg/dose. It is advisable to consider the concurrent administration of a beta-blocker to reduce the likelihood of reflex tachycardia. • Perioperative HTN (alternative agent): Suggested for those with chronic HTN prior to surgery. Once hemodynamically stable return to oral therapies. Administered IV 5 to 20 mg every 4 hrs as needed. • Altered Kidney Function: ♦ If eGFR ≥ 10 mL/min/1.73 m^2: No adjustment recommended. ♦ If eGFR < 10 mL/min/1.73 m^2: No adjustment recommended if used sort-term. However, encouraged to use with caution. Oral dose administered every 8 to 12 hrs. ♦ Hemodialysis / Peritoneal Dialysis: Not likely to be significantly dialyzed. Administer post dialysis to avoid intra-dialytic hypotension. • Liver Impairment: Hydralazine undergoes significant hepatic metabolism, however, there are no dosage adjustments recommended.	• May administer without regard to food. But administration related to meals should be consistent.
Minoxidil	• Onset of Action ≈ 30 min. • Peak Effect 2-3 hrs. • Duration 2 to 5 days. • $T_{1/2}$ 3.5 to 4.2 hrs.	• HTN (alternative agent): Reserved for patients who do not respond to a 3 or 4 drug regimen including a diuretic with optimized dosing. Consider referral to Hypertensive Specialist if not already involved in treatment of hypertensive. Often used with beta blockers or other agents with HR control properties (verapamil or diltiazem) to prevent reflex tachycardia. These agents should be on board prior to the initiation of minoxidil. Initial dose 5 mg once daily. Increase dose every 3 or more days. Average dose: 10 to 40 mg/day in 1 to 3 divided doses. Maximum dose: 100 mg/day in 1 to 3 divided doses. • No recommended adjustments for kidney impairment. The manufacturer notes that reduction in dosing may be needed in those with renal failure or receiving dialysis. • No manufacturer recommendations for dosage adjustments related to liver disease. However, clearance is expected to decrease with mild cirrhosis.	• May be administered without regard to food.

Selective $Alpha_1$ Adrenergic Receptor Antagonists			
Doxazosin Immediate Release (IR) Extended Release (ER)	• Peak Effect IR 2 to 3 hrs. ER ≈ 8 to 9 hrs. • Duration > 24 hrs. • $T_{1/2}$ IR ≈ 22 hrs; ER 15 to 19 hrs. May be extended in elderly and mild hepatic function.	• HTN: Not recommended for initial therapy. Consider as additional therapy in resistant HTN when combination therapy is not effective. IR initial dose 1 mg/day. Titrate as needed gradually. Maximum dose 16 mg once daily. • BPH: Should be used in combination with beta-3 agonist or anticholinergic agent with moderate to severe symptoms or in combination with a 5-alpha reductase inhibitor with significant prostate enlargement. IR oral 1 mg once daily. Titrate by doubling dose every 1 to 2 weeks. Maximum dose 8 mg once daily. • Ureteral Stone Expulsion (off label): IR 4 mg once daily in the evening. Continue for up to 4 weeks or until the stone is passed, whichever occurs first. ER 4 mg once daily in morning. Titration every 3 to 4 weeks. Maximum dose 8 mg/day.	• IR can be taken without regard to meals.
Prazosin	• Onset of Action antihypertensive effect within 2 hrs. • Peak Effect 2 to 4 hrs. • Duration 10 to 24 hrs. • $T_{1/2}$ 2 to 3 hrs. Prolonged in CHF.	• Hypertensive (chronic): Consider as additional therapy in resistant HTN when combination therapy with preferred therapy has not been effective. Initial dose 1 mg 2 or 3 times daily. Titrate to a maximum dose of 20 mg/day in 2 or 3 divided doses. • Posttraumatic Stress Disorder Related Nightmares / Sleep Disturbances (off label): Initial dose 1 mg/day at bedtime. Titrate to 2 mg at bedtime after 2 to 3 days. Further titration based on tolerance to maximum dose to 15 mg/day. Usual range: 3 to 15 mg/day.	• Can be taken without regard to meals.
Terazosin	• Onset of Action antihypertensive effect within 15 mins. • Peak Effect 2 to 3 hrs. • Duration 24 hrs. • $T_{1/2}$ ≈ 12 hrs. Prolonged to 14 hrs in patients ≥ 70 years.	• HTN: Not recommended for initial therapy. Consider as additional therapy in resistant HTN when combination therapy is not effective. Initiation 1 mg/day. Titrate as needed with maximum daily dose of 20 mg/day in 1 or 2 divided doses. • BPH: Should be used in combination with beta-3 agonist or anticholinergic agent with moderate to severe symptoms or in combination with a 5-alpha reductase inhibitor with significant prostate enlargement. Initiation 1 mg/day. Slow titration every few weeks. Manufacture suggestion 2 mg, 5 mg, 10 mg titration plan. Maximum dose 20 mg once daily. • Ureteral Stone Expulsion (off label): 2 to 5 mg once daily at bedtime. Continue for up to 4 weeks or until the stone is passed, whichever occurs first.	• Administration time of day should be consistent.
$Alpha_2$ Adrenergic Agonist			
Clonidine Oral Immediate Release (IR)	• Onset of Action antihypertensive effect Oral: 0.5 to 1 hr; TP 2 to 3 days;	• HTN Chronic: ◆ Oral IR: Initial dose of 0.1 mg 2 times daily with initiation and dose increases started at bedtime. Increase dosage in increments of 0.1 mg/day at weekly intervals. Usual range is 0.2 to 0.6 mg/day in divided doses taken 2 to 3 times a day. Maximum recommended dose of 2.4 mg but is rarely used in practice.	• Administration time of day should be consistent. • ER tablets should not be crushed due

Extended Release (ER) Transdermal Patch (TP)	• Peak Effect 2 to 4 hrs oral; TP steady state 3 days. • $T_{1/2}$ Oral 12 to 16 hrs; oral ≤ 41 hrs with renal impairment; TD after removal ≈ 20 hrs.	♦ Oral ER: 0.17 mg once daily. Usually at bedtime. Increase dosage in increments of 0.09 mg/day at weekly intervals. Usual range is 0.17 to 0.52 mg/day once daily. Maximum recommended dose is 0.52 mg/day. ♦ TP: Initial dose of 0.1 mg per 24-hr patch applied once weekly. Increase dosage in increments of 0.1 mg at 1-to-2-week intervals. Usual range is 0.1 to 0.3 mg per 24-hr patch applied once a week. Maximum dose available is 0.3 mg per 24-hr patch. • Altered Kidney Function: ♦ If eGFR ≥ 30 mL/min/1.73 m^2: No adjustment recommended. ♦ If eGFR < 30 mL/min/1.73 m^2: Recommend starting with lower dose and titrate slowly.	to alteration in delivery. • Apply TP to clean, dry, hair free surface – usually arms or chest wall. • Rotate sites with each TP application.
Guanfacine Immediate Release (IR)	• Peak Effect 1 to 4 hrs. Average 2.6 hrs. • Duration 24 hrs. • $T_{1/2}$ ≈ 17 hrs. Range from 10 to 30 hrs.	• HTN: Reserved for last-line therapy. Initial dose 0.5 to 1.0 mg once daily at bedtime. May gradually increase after 3 to 4 weeks if BP goals not met. Recommended maximum dose 2 mg once daily at bedtime. Adverse effects increase as doses increase and become more noticeable at dose > 3 mg/day. • Altered Kidney Function: No dosage adjustment for altered kidney function.	• Recommended to be administered at bedtime to minimize impact of side effects.
Methyldopa	• Peak Effect 2 to 4 hrs. • Duration Single dose 12 to 24 hrs. Multiple doses 24 to 48 hrs. • $T_{1/2}$ 1.5 to 2 hrs. Prolong in end stage renal disease.	• HTN (alternative agent): ♦ Initial dose 250 mg 2 to 3 times daily. Titrate every 2 to 3 days. Usual dosage 250 mg 1 gram divided into 2 to 4 doses per day. Maximum dose 3 grams per day in 2 to 4 divided doses. ♦ If prescribed with other antihypertensives (except thiazide diuretics) initial daily dose should be limited to 500 mg/day in divided doses. • Altered Kidney Function: No dosage adjustment for altered kidney function. ♦ If eGFR > 50 mL/min/1.73 m^2: Administer every 8 hrs. ♦ If eGFR 10 to 50 mL/min/1.73 m^2: Administer every 8 to 12 hrs. ♦ If eGFR < 10 mL/min/1.73 m^2: Administer every 12 to 24 hrs.	• Recommended to be administered at bedtime to minimize impact of side effects.

Table abbreviations: ACE I (Angiotensin Converting Enzyme Inhibitor), ACS (Acute Coronary Syndromes), ADPKD (Autosomal Dominant Polycystic Kidney Disease), ≈ (approximately), A Fib/Flutter (Atrial Fibrillation / Atrial Flutter); ARB (Angiotensin Receptor Blocker), ARNI (Angiotensin Receptor Blocker / Neprilysin Inhibitor), ASCVD (Atherosclerotic Cardiovascular Disease), BP (Blood Pressure), BPH (Benign Prostatic Hypertrophy), bpm (beats per minute); CAD (Coronary Artery Disease), CHF (congestive heart failure), CKD (Chronic Kidney Disease), CrCl (Creatinine Clearance), CV (Cardiovascular), DMT2 (Diabetes Mellitus Type II), eGFR (estimated glomerular filtration rate), ER: Extended Release; FDA (Federal Drug Administration), G (grams), HF (heart failure), HFmrEF (Heart Failure with mildly reduced Ejection Fraction);HFpEF (Heart Failure with preserved Ejection Fraction), HFrEF (Heart Failure with reduced Ejection Fraction), HR (heart rate), HTN (hypertension), hour (hr); hours (hrs); IM (intramuscular); IR: Immediate Release; ISA (Intrinsic Sympathetic Activity); IV (intravenous), IR: Immediate Release; kg (kilograms), LV (Left Ventricular), LVEF (Left Ventricular Ejection Fraction), MAP (men arterial pressure), mcg (micrograms), mg (milligrams), MI (myocardial infarction), minute (min); minutes (mins), NSTEMI (NonST Elevation Myocardial Infarction), NYHA (New York Heart Association), PVC (Premature Ventricular Contraction), REMS (Risk Evaluation and Mitigation Strategies), SIADH (Syndrome of Inappropriate Antidiuretic Hormone); SBP (systolic BP); SL (sublingual), STEMI (ST Segment Myocardial Infarction), SVT (Supraventricular Tachycardia), $T_{1/2}$ (Terminal half-life), VT (Ventricular Tachycardia

Abbreviation List

α: alpha

α1: $alpha_1$

α2: $alpha_2$

A1c: Hemoglobin A1c

ACC: American College of Cardiology

ACE: angiotensin converting enzyme

ACEI: angiotensin converting enzyme inhibitor

ACTH: adrenocorticotropic hormone

ACS: acute coronary syndrome

ADA: American Diabetes Association

AHA: American Heart Association

AKI: acute kidney injury

ALT: alanine aminotransferase

APRN: advanced practice registered nurse

ARB: angiotensin receptor blocker

ARNI: angiotensin II receptor blocker and neprilysin inhibitor

AST: aspartate aminotransferase

AUC: area under the curve

AV: atrioventricular

AVNRT: AV nodal reentrant tachycardia

AVRT: AV reentrant tachycardia

ß: beta

ß1: $beta_1$

ß2: $beta_2$

BNP: brain natriuretic peptide

BP: blood pressure

BPH: benign prostatic hypertrophy

CAD: coronary artery disease

cAMP: cyclic adenosine monophosphate

CCBs: calcium channel blockers

cGMP: cyclic guanosine monophosphate

CNS: central nervous system

CO: cardiac output

CO_2: carbon dioxide

CKD: chronic kidney disease

CrCl: creatinine clearance

CV: cardiovascular

DI: diabetes insipidus

dL: deciliter

DPP-4: dipeptidyl peptidase-4

DKA: diabetic ketoacidosis

DKD: diabetic kidney disease

DMT1: Diabetes mellitus type 1

DMT2: Diabetes mellitus type 2

eDKA: euglycemic DKA

EF: ejection fraction

eGFR: estimated measured glomerular filtration rate

ER: extended release

ESKD: end stage kidney disease

FDA: Food and Drug Administration

g: gram(s)

GFR: glomerular filtration rate

H^+: hydrogen

H/A, H/As: headache, headaches

HCM: hypertrophic cardiomyopathy

HCO_3: bicarbonate

HES: hydroxyethyl starch (hetastarch)

HF: heart failure

HFrEF: heart failure with reduced ejection fraction

HFpEF: heart failure with preserved ejection fraction

HFmrEF: heart failure with mildly reduced ejection fraction

HFSA: Heart Failure Society of America

HOCM: hypertrophic obstructive cardiomyopathy

HR: heart rate

Hr / hrs: hour(s)

HTN: hypertension

ICU: intensive care unit

IR: immediate release

IV: Intravenous

ISA: intrinsic sympathomimetic activity

Kg: kilogram

KDIGO: Kidney Disease: Improving Global Outcomes

LOS: length of stay

LR: lactated Ringer's / Ringer's lactate

LV: left ventricle; left ventricular

LVAD: left ventricular assist device

LVEF: left ventricular ejection fraction

LVSWI: left ventricular stroke work index

MAO: monoamine oxidase

MAP: mean arterial pressure

mg(s): milligram (s)

mEq: milliequivalent(s)

mEq/L: milliequivalents per liter

MI: myocardial infarction

Min / mins: minute(s)

mL(s): milliliter (s)

mmHg: millimeters of mercury

mOsm: milliosmole

MRA: mineralocorticoid receptor antagonists

MVO_2: myocardial oxygen consumption

$NaHCO_3$: sodium bicarbonate

NPO: Nothing by mouth

NS: normal saline

NSAIDs: nonsteroidal anti-inflammatory drugs

NSTE-ACS: non-ST segment elevation ACS

N&V: nausea and vomiting

O_2: oxygen

PAD: peripheral arterial disease

PAOP: Pulmonary artery occlusion pressure

PEEP: Positive end expiratory pressure

PDE: phosphodiesterase

PVC: premature ventricular contraction

PVR: pulmonary vascular resistance

RAAS: renin-angiotensin-aldosterone-system

RAP: right atrial pressure

REMS: FDA approved Risk Evaluation and Mitigation Strategy

RN: registered nurse

RRT: renal replacement therapy

RV: right ventricle; right ventricular

S&S: Signs and symptoms

SCLE: subacute cutaneous lupus erythematosus

SGLT2I: sodium-glucose cotransporter 2 inhibitor

SIADH: syndrome of inappropriate antidiuretic hormone

SIRS: systemic inflammatory response syndrome

SL: sublingual

SLE: systemic lupus erythematosus

SNS: sympathetic nervous system

SOFA: sequential organ failure assessment

SQ: subcutaneous

STEMI: ST segment elevation myocardial infarction

SV: stroke volume

SVR: systemic vascular resistance

SVT: supraventricular tachycardia

TIA: transient ischemic attack

US: United States

UTI(s): urinary tract infection(s)

VT: ventricular tachycardia

References

2023 American Geriatrics Society Beers Criteria® Update Expert Panel. (2023). American Geriatrics Society 2023 updated AGS Beers Criteria® for potentially inappropriate medication use in older adults. *Journal of the American Geriatrics Society*, *71*(7), 2052-2081.

Abbott Laboratories (2009). Terazosin Prescribing Information.

Abosamak NER & Shahin MH. Beta2 Receptor Agonists and Antagonists. [Updated 2023 Jul 3]. In: StatPearls [Internet]. Treasure Island (FL):StatPearls Publishing; 2023 Jan.

Abrams, J. (1985). Hemodynamic effects of nitroglycerin and long-acting nitrates. American heart journal, 110(1), 217-224.

Achim, A., Johnson, N. P., Liblik, K., Burckhardt, A., Krivoshei, L., & Leibundgut, G. (2023). Coronary steal: how many thieves are out there?. *European Heart Journal*, *44*(30), 2805-2814.

Actavis Pharma, Inc. (2023). Clonidine Transdermal System Prescribing Information.

Adamopoulos, C., Ahmed, A., Fay, R., Angioi, M., Filippatos, G., Vincent, J., ... & EPHESUS Investigators. (2009). Timing of eplerenone initiation and outcomes in patients with heart failure after acute myocardial infarction complicated by left ventricular systolic dysfunction: insights from the EPHESUS trial. *European Journal of Heart Failure*, *11*(11), 1099-1105.

Adams, C., Tucker, C., Allen, B., McRae, A., Balazh, J., Horst, S., ... & Ferreira, J. (2017). Disparities in hemodynamic resuscitation of the obese critically ill septic shock patient. *Journal of critical care*, *37*, 219-223.

Afsar, B., Afsar, R. E., Demiray, A., Altay, S., Korkmaz, H., Yildiz, A., ... & Kanbay, M. (2022). Sodium–glucose cotransporter inhibition in polycystic kidney disease: fact or fiction. *Clinical kidney journal*, *15*(7), 1275-1283.

Agarwal, R., Anker, S. D., Bakris, G., Filippatos, G., Pitt, B., Rossing, P., ... & FIDELIO-DKD and FIGARO-DKD Investigators. (2022). Investigating new treatment opportunities for patients with chronic kidney disease in type 2 diabetes: the role of finerenone. *Nephrology Dialysis Transplantation*, *37*(6), 1014-1023.

Agarwal, R., Sinha, A. D., Cramer, A. E., Balmes-Fenwick, M., Dickinson, J. H., Ouyang, F., & Tu, W. (2021). Chlorthalidone for hypertension in advanced chronic kidney disease. *New England Journal of Medicine*, *385*(27), 2507-2519.

Ahmad Mann, J. F. E., Hilgers, K. (2017). Renal effects of ACE inhibitors in hypertension. In J.P. Forman (Ed.), *UpToDate*.

Ahmad, T., Butler, J., Borlaug, B. (2017). The diagnosis and management of chronic heart failure. In V. Fuster, R.A. Harrington, J. Narula, Z.J. Eapen (Eds.), Hurst's The Heart (14th ed., pp. 1690-1725). New York: McGraw Hill.

Ahmed, A., Fay, R., Angioi, M., Filippatos, G., Vincent, J., ... & EPHESUS Investigators. (2009). Timing of eplerenone initiation and outcomes in patients with heart failure after acute myocardial infarction complicated by left ventricular systolic dysfunction: insights from the EPHESUS trial. *European Journal of Heart Failure*, *11*(11), 1099-1105.

Alhayek, S. & Preuss, C.V. (2023). Beta 1 Receptors. [Updated 2023 Aug 14]. In: StatPearls [Internet]. Treasure Island (FL). StatPearls Publishing.

Alkazemi, A., Almoosawy, S. A., Murad, A., & Alfares, A. (2024). Methylene Blue for Septic Shock: A Systematic Review and Meta-analysis of Randomized and Prospective Observational Studies. *Journal of Intensive Care Medicine*, 08850666241300312.

Al-Khatib, S.M., Stevenson, W.G., Ackerman, M.J., Bryant, W.J., Callans, D.J., Curtis, A.B., Deal, B.J.,. . . Page, R.L. (2018). 2017 AHA/ACC/HRS guideline for management of patients with ventricular arrhythmias and the prevention of sudden cardiac death. Heart Rhythm, 15, e75-e189.

American Diabetes Association (2023). Standards of care in diabetes – 2023. Diabetes Care, 46 (suppl 1), S1-S291.

American Heart Association. (2025). Adult cardiac arrest circular algorithm. Retrieved from https://cpr.heart.org/en/resuscitation-science/cpr-and-ecc-guidelines/algorithm.

American Regent, Inc (2021). Nitroglycerin Injection Prescribing Information.

Amsterdam, E. A., Wenger, N. K., Brindis, R. G., Casey, D. E., Ganiats, T. G., Holmes, D. R., ... & Zieman, S. J. (2014). 2014 AHA/ACC guideline for the management of patients with non–ST-elevation acute coronary syndromes: a report of the American College of Cardiology/American Heart Association Task Force on Practice Guidelines. *Journal of the American College of Cardiology*, *64*(24), e139-e228.

Anker, S. D., Butler, J., Filippatos, G., Ferreira, J. P., Bocchi, E., Böhm, M., ... & Packer, M. (2021). Empagliflozin in heart failure with a preserved ejection fraction. New England Journal of Medicine.

Annane, D., Siami, S., Jaber, S., Martin, C., Elatrous, S., Declère, A. D., ... & CRISTAL Investigators. (2013). Effects of fluid resuscitation with colloids vs crystalloids on mortality in critically ill patients presenting with hypovolemic shock: the CRISTAL randomized trial. *Jama*, *310*(17), 1809-1817.

Arias-Ortiz, J., & Vincent, J. L. (2024). Administration of methylene blue in septic shock: pros and cons. *Critical Care*, *28*(1), 46.

Arshad, M., Farooq, S., Majeed, K., Khalid, U., Afsheen, A., & Artemis, P. (2024). Labetalol versus Methyldopa for Treatment of Pregnancy Induced Hypertension. *Pakistan Armed Forces Medical Journal*, *74*(4), 1024.

AstraZeneca Pharmaceuticals (2024). Dapagliflozin (Farxiga) Prescribing Information.

Athena Bioscience, LLC. and Tris Pharma, Inc. (2021). Clonidine (Nexiclon™ XR) Prescribing Information.

August, P. (2025). Treatment of Hypertension in Pregnant and Postpartum Patients. In K. Eckler (ED), *UptoDate.*
Bailey, C. J., Day, C., & Bellary, S. (2022). Renal protection with SGLT2 inhibitors: effects in acute and chronic kidney disease. *Current diabetes reports*, *22*(1), 39-52.
Ballarin, R. S., Lazzarin, T., Zornoff, L., Azevedo, P. S., Pereira, F. W. L., Tanni, S. E., & Minicucci, M. F. (2024). Methylene blue in sepsis and septic shock: a systematic review and meta-analysis. *Frontiers in Medicine*, *11*, 1366062.
Bamgboye, A. O., Oni, I. O., & Collier, A. (2021). Predisposing factors for the development of diabetic ketoacidosis with lower than anticipated glucose levels in type 2 diabetes patients on SGLT2-inhibitors: a review. *European Journal of Clinical Pharmacology*, *77*(5), 651-657.
Barbieri, R.L. & Ehrmann, D.A. (2023). Pathophysiology and causes of hirsutism. In K.A. Martin (Ed.) *UpToDate.*
Barold, S. S., De Wilde, H. E., Timmers, L., Van Heuverswyn, F. E., & Stroobandt, R. X. (2015). Atrioventricular block precipitated by isoproterenol. *Annals of Noninvasive Electrocardiology*, *20*(4), 397-401.
Basquez, R., & Pippin, M. M. (2023). Prazosin. In *StatPearls [Internet]*. StatPearls Publishing.
Bauer, J. A., & Fung, H. L. (1993). Effect of apparent elimination half-life on nitroglycerin-induced hemodynamic rebound in experimental heart failure. *Pharmaceutical research*, *10*, 1341-1345.
Bauer, S. R., Aloi, J. J., Ahrens, C. L., Yeh, J. Y., Culver, D. A., & Reddy, A. J. (2010). Discontinuation of vasopressin before norepinephrine increases the incidence of hypotension in patients recovering from septic shock: a retrospective cohort study. *Journal of critical care*, *25*(2), 362-e7.
Bauer, S. R., Sacha, G. L., Siuba, M. T., Wang, L., Wang, X., Scheraga, R. G., & Vachharajani, V. (2023). Vasopressin response and clinical trajectory in septic shock patients. *Journal of intensive care medicine*, *38*(3), 273-279.
Baxter (2007). Plasma-Lyte A prescribing information.
Baxter (2019). Lactated Ringer's prescribing information.
Baxter Health Corporation (2016). Nitroglycerine Prescribing Information.
Bayer HealthCare Pharmaceuticals Inc. (2021). Finerenone Prescribing Information.
Becker, C. D., Sabang, R. L., Cordeiro, M. F. N., Hassan, I. F., Goldberg, M. D., & Scurlock, C. S. (2020). Hyperglycemia in medically critically ill patients: risk factors and clinical outcomes. *The American journal of medicine*, *133*(10), e568-e574.
Becker, R. C., Corrao, J. M., Bovill, E. G., Gore, J. M., Baker, S. P., Miller, M. L., ... & Alpert, J. A. Intravenous nitroglycerin-induced heparin resistance: a qualitative antithrombin III abnormality. *American Heart Journal*, *119*(6), 1254-1261.
Bellomo, R. G. (2022). Function and mechanism of action of alpha-methyldopa: An update. *European Journal of Neurodegenerative Diseases*, *11*(S1), S10-S14.
Bellomo, R., Hegarty, C., Story, D., Ho, L., & Bailey, M. (2012). Association between a chloride-liberal vs chloride-restrictive intravenous fluid administration strategy and kidney injury in critically ill adults. *Jama*, *308*(15), 1566-1572.
Berk, S. I., Grunwald, A., Pal, S., & Bodenheimer, M. M. (1993). Effect of intravenous nitroglycerin on heparin dosage requirements in coronary artery disease. *The American journal of cardiology*, *72*(5), 393-396.
Bhandari, S., Mehta, S., Khwaja, A., Cleland, J., Ives, N., Brettell, E., ... & STOP-ACEi Trial Investigators. (2024). Withdrawal of renin-angiotensin system inhibitors' effect on estimated glomerular filtration rate in adults with advanced kidney disease: the STOP-ACEi RCT.
Bhatt, D. L., Szarek, M., Pitt, B., Cannon, C. P., Leiter, L. A., McGuire, D. K., ... & Steg, P. G. (2021a). Sotagliflozin in patients with diabetes and chronic kidney disease. *New England Journal of Medicine*, *384*(2), 129-139.
Bhatt D..L, Szarek M., Steg P.G., Cannon C.P., Leiter L.A,. McGuire D.K.,….& Lund L.H. (2021b). Sotagliflozin in patients with diabetes and recent worsening heart failure. New England Journal of Medicine. *384*(2):117-28.
Bhattacharjee, S., & Maitra, S. (2023). Vasopressor weaning in sepsis: Debate is being continued!. *Journal of Anaesthesiology Clinical Pharmacology*, *39*(3), 497-498.
Bilo, G., Grillo, A., Guida, V., & Parati, G. (2018). Morning blood pressure surge: pathophysiology, clinical relevance and therapeutic aspects. *Integrated blood pressure control*, 47-56.
Bissell, B. D., Magee, C., Moran, P., Bastin, M. L. T., & Flannery, A. H. (2019). Hemodynamic instability secondary to vasopressin withdrawal in septic shock. *Journal of intensive care medicine*, *34*(9), 761-765.
Black, J.H. & Burke, C.R. (2022). Management of acute type A aortic dissection. In G.S. Aldea, E. Verrier, & K.A.Collis (Eds.), *Uptodate.*
Bloomgarden, Z., Einhorn, D., Grunberger, G., & Handelsman, Y. (2019). Fournier's gangrene and sodium–glucose cotransporter 2 inhibitors: is there a causal association? *Journal of Diabetes*, *11*(5).
Blumberg, N., Cholette, J. M., Pietropaoli, A. P., Phipps, R., Spinelli, S. L., Eaton, M. P., ... & Refaai, M. A. (2018). 0.9% NaCl (normal saline)–perhaps not so normal after all?. *Transfusion and Apheresis Science*, *57*(1), 127-131.
Boehringer Ingelheim. (2021, August 18). Jardiance® (empagliflozin) to treat adults living with heart failure with reduced ejection fraction. Retrieved December 9, 2021 from https://www.boehringer-ingelheim.us/press-release/us-fda-approves-jardiance-empagliflozin-treat-adults-living-heart-failure-reduced.

Boehringer Ingelheim. (2021, September 9). FDA grants Jardiance® Breakthrough Therapy designation for heart failure with preserved ejection fraction. Retrieved on December 12, 2022 from: https://investor.lilly.com/news-releases/news-release-details/fda-grants-jardiancer-breakthrough-therapy-designation-heart

Boehringer Ingelheim International (2009). Clonidine Hydrochloride Immediate Release Prescribing Information.

Boehringer Ingelheim International (2023). Clonidine Transdermal System Prescribing Information.

Boehringer Ingelheim International (2023). Empagliflozin (Jardiance) Prescribing Information.

Bohula, E.A.& Morrow, D.A. (2019). ST-elevation myocardial infarction: management. In D.P. Zipes, P. Libby, R.O. Bonow, D.L. Mann, G.F. Tomaselli (Eds.), Braunwald's Heart Disease: A Textbook of Cardiovascular Medicine (11th ed., pp. 1123-1180). Philadelphia: Elsevier.

Bojar, R. M., Rastegar, H., Payne, D. D., Harkness, S. H., England, M. R., Stetz, J. J., ... & Cleveland, R. J. (1987). Methemoglobinemia from intravenous nitroglycerin: a word of caution. *The Annals of thoracic surgery*, *43*(3), 332-334.

Bonora, B. M., Avogaro, A., & Fadini, G. P. (2020). Extraglycemic effects of SGLT2 inhibitors: a review of the evidence. *Diabetes, Metabolic Syndrome and Obesity*, 161-174.

Bouchard, J., Soroko, S. B., Chertow, G. M., Himmelfarb, J., Ikizler, T. A., Paganini, E. P., & Mehta, R. L. (2009). Fluid accumulation, survival and recovery of kidney function in critically ill patients with acute kidney injury. *Kidney international*, *76*(4), 422-427.

Brask, A. L., Shemanski, S. M., Barnes, T. E., & Holmes, A. K. (2023). Timing of vasopressin addition to norepinephrine and efficacy outcomes in patients with septic shock. *Annals of Pharmacotherapy*, *57*(5), 521-526.

Brater, D.C. & Ellison, D.H. (2023). Mechanism of action of diuretics. In J.P. Forman (Ed.), *UptoDate.*

Braunwald, E., Antman, E. M., Beasley, J. W., Califf, R. M., Cheitlin, M. D., Hochman, J. S., ... & Smith, S. C. (2002). ACC/AHA 2002 guideline update for the management of patients with unstable angina and non–ST-segment elevation myocardial infarction—summary article: a report of the American College of Cardiology/American Heart Association task force on practice guidelines (Committee on the Management of Patients With Unstable Angina). *Journal of the American College of Cardiology*, *40*(7), 1366-1374.

Braunwald, E., Oldham Jr, H. N., Ross, JR, J. O., Linhart, J. W., Mason, D. T., & Fort III, L. Y. (1964). The circulatory response of patients with idiopathic hypertrophic subaortic stenosis to nitroglycerin and to the Valsalva maneuver. *Circulation*, *29*(3), 422-431.

Brisco-Bacik, M. A., Ter Maaten, J. M., Houser, S. R., Vedage, N. A., Rao, V., Ahmad, T., ... & Testani, J. M. (2018). Outcomes associated with a strategy of adjuvant metolazone or high-dose loop diuretics in acute decompensated heart failure: a propensity analysis. *Journal of the American Heart Association*, *7*(18), e009149.

Brooks, M. (2023). FDA Expands Use of Dapagliflozin to Broader Range of HF. *Medscape.*

Brown, N. J., & Vaughan, D. E. (1998). Angiotensin-converting enzyme inhibitors. *Circulation*, *97*(14), 1411-1420.

Brunkhorst, F. M., Engel, C., Bloos, F., Meier-Hellmann, A., Ragaller, M., Weiler, N., ... & Reinhart, K. (2008). Intensive insulin therapy and pentastarch resuscitation in severe sepsis. *New England Journal of Medicine*, *358*(2), 125-139.

Bundhun, P. K., & Huang, F. (2018). Adverse drug events associated with sitagliptin versus canagliflozin for the treatment of patients with type 2 diabetes mellitus: a systematic comparison through a meta-analysis. *Diabetes Therapy*, *9*(5), 1883-1895.

Burnstock, G. (2018). Purine and purinergic receptors. *Brain and neuroscience advances*, *2*, 2398212818817494.

Buter, J., Steele, K. T., Chung, K. C., Elzinga, K. (2024). Extravasation injury from cytotoxic and other noncytotoxic vesicants in adults. In K.A. Collins (Ed.), *UptoDate*.

Byrne, R. A., Rossello, X., Coughlan, J. J., Barbato, E., Berry, C., Chieffo, A., ... & Ibanez, B. (2024). 2023 ESC guidelines for the management of acute coronary syndromes: developed by the task force on the management of acute coronary syndromes of the European Society of Cardiology (ESC). *European Heart Journal: Acute Cardiovascular Care*, *13*(1), 55-161.

Caironi, P., Tognoni, G., Masson, S., Fumagalli, R., Pesenti, A., Romero, M., ... & Gattinoni, L. (2014). Albumin replacement in patients with severe sepsis or septic shock. *New England Journal of Medicine*, *370*(15), 1412-1421.

Campbell, P., Baker, W. L., Bendel, S. D., & White, W. B. (2011). Intravenous hydralazine for blood pressure management in the hospitalized patient: its use is often unjustified. *Journal of the American Society of Hypertension*, *5*(6), 473-477.

Cantrell, M. A., Bream-Rouwenhorst, H. R., Steffensmeier, A., Hemerson, P., Rogers, M., & Stamper, B. (2008). Intraoperative floppy iris syndrome associated with alpha1-adrenergic receptor antagonists. *The Annals of pharmacotherapy*, *42*(4), 558–563.

Caparrotta, T. M., Greenhalgh, A. M., Rosinsky, K., Gifford, R. M., Moser, S., Wild, S. H., ... & Colhoun, H. M. (2021). Sodium–Glucose Co-Transporter 2 Inhibitors (SGLT2i) Exposure and Outcomes in Type 2 Diabetes: A Systematic Review of Population-Based Observational Studies. *Diabetes Therapy*, 1-38.

Carstairs, K. C., Breckenridge, A., Dollery, C. T., & Worlledge, S. (1966). Incidence of a positive direct Coombs test in patients on α-methyldopa. *The Lancet*, *288*(7455), 133-135.

Cefalu, W. T., Kaul, S., Gerstein, H. C., Holman, R. R., Zinman, B., Skyler, J. S., ... & Riddle, M. C. (2018). Cardiovascular outcomes trials in type 2 diabetes: where do we go from here? Reflections from a diabetes care editors' expert forum. *Diabetes care*, *41*(1), 14-31.

Chartwell RX, LLC. (2024). Guanfacine Hydrochloride Immediate Release Prescribing Information.
Chartwell RX, LLC. (2025). Methyldopa Prescribing Information.
Charytan, D. M., Himmelfarb, J., Ikizler, T. A., Raj, D. S., Hsu, J. Y., Landis, J. R., ... & Kusek, J. (2019). Safety and cardiovascular efficacy of spironolactone in dialysis-dependent ESRD (SPin-D): a randomized, placebo-controlled, multiple dosage trial. *Kidney International*, *95*(4), 973-982.
Chatterjee, K., Parmley, W. W., Swan, H. J. C., Berman, G., Forrester, J., & Marcus, H. S. (1973). Beneficial effects of vasodilator agents in severe mitral regurgitation due to dysfunction of subvalvar apparatus. *Circulation*, *48*(4), 684-690.
Chen, H. H., Anstrom, K. J., Givertz, M. M., Stevenson, L. W., Semigran, M. J., Goldsmith, S. R., ... & NHLBI Heart Failure Clinical Research Network. (2013). Low-dose dopamine or low-dose nesiritide in acute heart failure with renal dysfunction: the ROSE acute heart failure randomized trial. *Jama*, *310*(23), 2533-2543.
Cheung, A. K., Chang, T. I., Cushman, W. C., Furth, S. L., Hou, F. F., Ix, J. H., ... & Mann, J. F. (2021). KDIGO 2021 clinical practice guideline for the management of blood pressure in chronic kidney disease. *Kidney International*, *99*(3), S1-S87.
Chimura, M., Petrie, M. C., Schou, M., Martinez, F. A., Henderson, A. D., Claggett, B. L., ... & McMurray, J. J. (2024). Finerenone Improves Outcomes in Patients with Heart Failure with Mildly Reduced or Preserved Ejection Fraction Irrespective of Age: A Prespecified Analysis of FINEARTS-HF. *Circulation: Heart Failure*, *17*(0).
China, L., Freemantle, N., Forrest, E., Kallis, Y., Ryder, S. D., Wright, G., ... & O'Brien, A. (2021). A randomized trial of albumin infusions in hospitalized patients with cirrhosis. *New England Journal of Medicine*, *384*(9), 808-817.
Chong, L. Y. Z., Satya, K., Kim, B., & Berkowitz, R. (2018). Milrinone dosing and a culture of caution in clinical practice. *Cardiology in review*, *26*(1), 35-42.
Christou, C. D., Tsinopoulos, I., Ziakas, N., & Tzamalis, A. (2020). Intraoperative floppy iris syndrome: updated perspectives. *Clinical Ophthalmology*, 463-471.
Clark, A., Mohammed, A. S., Raut, A., Moore, S., Houlden, R., & Awad, S. (2021). Prevalence and clinical characteristics of adults presenting with sodium-glucose cotransporter-2 inhibitor-associated diabetic ketoacidosis at a Canadian Academic Tertiary Care Hospital. *Canadian Journal of Diabetes*, *45*(3), 214-219.
Clark, K. A., & McNamara, R. L. (2020). Is Left Ventricular Stroke Work Index Useful in the Cardiac Intensive Care Unit?
Collins, K. S., Raviele, A. L., Elchynski, A. L., Woodcock, A. M., Zhao, Y., Cooper-DeHoff, R. M., & Eadon, M. T. (2020). Genotype-guided hydralazine therapy. *American journal of nephrology*, *51*(10), 764-776.
Colucci, W.S. (2024). Renal effects of ACE inhibitors in heart failure. In J.P. Forman (Ed.), *UpToDate*.
Colucci, W.S. & Pfeffer, M.A. (2022). Secondary pharmacologic therapy in heart failure with reduced ejection fraction (HFrEF) in adults. In T.F Dardas (Ed.), *UpToDate*.
Colucci, W.S. & Sterns, R. H. (2022). Use of diuretics in patients with HF. In T.F Dardas (Ed.), *UpToDate*.
Colucci, W.S. & Sterns, R. H. (2025). Use of diuretics in patients with HF. In H.Li & N.F. Botkin (Eds.), *UpToDate*.
Cuffe, M. S., Califf, R. M., Adams Jr, K. F., Benza, R., Bourge, R., Colucci, W. S., ... & Outcomes of a Prospective Trial of Intravenous Milrinone for Exacerbations of Chronic Heart Failure (OPTIME-CHF) Investigators. (2002). Short-term intravenous milrinone for acute exacerbation of chronic heart failure: a randomized controlled trial. *Jama*, *287*(12), 1541-1547.
Dalal R, Grujic D. Epinephrine. [Updated 2023 May 1]. In: StatPearls [Internet]. Treasure Island (FL): StatPearls Publishing; 2024 Jan-. Available from: https://www.ncbi.nlm.nih.gov/books/NBK482160/
Dean II, J.S. & Reddivari, A.K.R. (2023) Alpha-1 Receptor Agonists. In: StatPearls [Internet]. Treasure Island (FL): StatPearls Publishing.
De Backer, D., Aldecoa, C., Njimi, H., & Vincent, J. L. (2012). Dopamine versus norepinephrine in the treatment of septic shock: a meta-analysis. *Critical care medicine*, *40*(3), 725-730.
De Backer, D., Biston, P., Devriendt, J., Madl, C., Chochrad, D., Aldecoa, C., ... & Vincent, J. L. (2010). Comparison of dopamine and norepinephrine in the treatment of shock. *New England Journal of Medicine*, *362*(9), 779-789.
de Boer, I. H., Khunti, K., Sadusky, T., Tuttle, K. R., Neumiller, J. J., Rhee, C. M., ... & Bakris, G. (2022). Diabetes management in chronic kidney disease: a consensus report by the American Diabetes Association (ADA) and Kidney Disease: Improving Global Outcomes (KDIGO). *Diabetes care*, *45*(12), 3075-3090.
D'Elia, S., Franzese, R., Gentile, C., Solimene, A., Luisi, E., Caiazzo, A., ... & Cimmino, G. (2024). Sodium Nitroprusside: The Forgotten Vasodilator? A Brief Guide for Informed and Safe Use from Heart Failure to Hypertensive Crisis and Aortic Dissection. *Future Pharmacology*, *5*(1), 1.
Desai, S., & Su, M.K. (2024). Cyanide poisoning. In M. Ganetsky (Ed.), *UpToDate*.
DeSantis A. SGLT2 Inhibitors for the Treatment of Hyperglycemia in Type 2 Diabetes Mellitus. In K. Rubinow (Ed.), *UpToDate*.
Desouza, C. V., Gupta, N., & Patel, A. (2015). Cardiometabolic effects of a new class of antidiabetic agents. *Clinical therapeutics*, *37*(6), 1178-1194.
Devi, R., Mali, G., Chakraborty, I., Unnikrishnan, M. K., & Abdulsalim, S. (2017). Efficacy and safety of empagliflozin in type 2 diabetes mellitus: a meta-analysis of randomized controlled trials. *Postgraduate medicine*, *129*(3), 382-392.
Dineva, S., Uzunova, K., Pavlova, V., Filipova, E., Kalinov, K., & Vekov, T. (2019). Comparative efficacy and safety of chlorthalidone and hydrochlorothiazide—meta-analysis. *Journal of human hypertension*, *33*(11), 766-774.

Dive, A., Foret, F., Jamart, J., Bulpa, P., & Installé, E. (2000). Effect of dopamine on gastrointestinal motility during critical illness. *Intensive care medicine*, *26*, 901-907.

Dorsch, M. P., Gillespie, B. W., Erickson, S. R., Bleske, B. E., & Weder, A. B. (2011). Chlorthalidone reduces cardiovascular events compared with hydrochlorothiazide: a retrospective cohort analysis. *Hypertension*, *57*(4), 689-694.

Duenser, M. W., Bouvet, O., Knotzer, H., Arulkumaran, N., Hajjar, L. A., Ulmer, H., & Hasibeder, W. R. (2018). Vasopressin in cardiac surgery: a meta-analysis of randomized controlled trials. *Journal of cardiothoracic and vascular anesthesia*, *32*(5), 2225-2232.

Duong, H., Masarweh, O. M., Campbell, G., Win, T. T., & Joolhar, F. (2020). Isoproterenol causing coronary vasospasm and ST elevations during tilt table testing. *Journal of Investigative Medicine High Impact Case Reports*, *8*, 2324709620966862.

Edenbridge Pharmaceuticals, LLC. (2025). Isosorbide mononitrate prescribing information.

Edmonds, M., Manu, C., & Vas, P. (2021). The current burden of diabetic foot disease. *Journal of clinical orthopaedics and trauma*, *17*, 88-93.

Eid, P. S., Ibrahim, D. A., Zayan, A. H., Abd Elrahman, M. M., Shehata, M. A. A., Kandil, H., ... & Huy, N. T. (2021). Comparative effects of furosemide and other diuretics in the treatment of heart failure: a systematic review and combined meta-analysis of randomized controlled trials. *Heart Failure Reviews*, *26*(1), 127-136.

El Hage, L., Kashyap, S. R., & Rao, P. (2019). Use of SGLT-2 inhibitors in patients with type 1 diabetes mellitus. *Journal of Primary Care & Community Health*, *10*, 2150132719895188.

Elliott, P.M., Anastasakis, A., Borger, M.A., Borggrefe, M., Cecchi, F. Charon, P., Hagege, A.A., . . . Watkins, H. (2014). 2014 ESC guidelines on diagnosis and management of hypertrophic cardiomyopathy. European Heart Journal, 35, 2733-2779.

Elliott, W. (2025). Tapering and discontinuing antihypertensive medications. In K. Law (Ed.), *UpToDate*.

Elliott, W. J., & Ram, C. V. S. (2011). Calcium channel blockers. *The Journal of Clinical Hypertension*, *13*(9), 687.

EMPA-Kidney Collaborative Group. (2023). Empagliflozin in patients with chronic kidney disease. *New England Journal of Medicine*, *388*(2), 117-127.

Engelhardt, K., Ferguson, M., & Rosselli, J. L. (2021). Prevention and Management of Genital Mycotic Infections in the Setting of Sodium-Glucose Cotransporter 2 Inhibitors. *Annals of Pharmacotherapy*, *55*(4), 543-548.

Ernst, M. E., Neaton, J. D., Grimm Jr, R. H., Collins, G., Thomas, W., Soliman, E. Z., & Prineas, R. J. (2011). Long-term effects of chlorthalidone versus hydrochlorothiazide on electrocardiographic left ventricular hypertrophy in the multiple risk factor intervention trial. *Hypertension*, *58*(6), 1001-1007.

Eschenhagen, T. (2018). Treatment of ischemic heart disease. In L.L. Brunton, R. Hilal-Dandan, B.C. Knollmann (Eds.), Goodman & Gilman's The Pharmacological Basis of Therapeutics (13th Ed., pp 489-506). New York: McGraw Hill.

Espero Pharmaceuticals, Inc. (2018). Nitrolingual® Pumpspray Prescribing Information

Evans, L., Rhodes, A., Alhazzani, W., Antonelli, M., Coopersmith, C. M., French, C., ... & Levy, M. (2021). Surviving sepsis campaign: international guidelines for management of sepsis and septic shock 2021. *Critical care medicine*, *49*(11), e1063-e1143.

Exela Pharma Sciences, LLC. (2017). Sodium Nitroprusside Prescribing Information.

Faselis, C., Arundel, C., Patel, S., Lam, P. H., Gottlieb, S. S., Zile, M. R., ... & Ahmed, A. (2020). Loop diuretic prescription and 30-day outcomes in older patients with heart failure. *Journal of the American College of Cardiology*, *76*(6), 669-679.

FDA. (2012, April 20). FDA Drug Safety Communication: New Warning and Contraindication for blood pressure medicines containing aliskiren (Tekturna)

FDA (2013, June 24). FDA Safety Communication: Boxed Warning on increased mortality and severe renal injury, and additional warning on risk of bleeding, for use of hydroxyethyl starch solutions in some settings.

FDA. (2013, July 3). FDA approves label changes to include intestinal problems (sprue-like enteropathy) linked to blood pressure medicine olmesartan medoxomil.

FDA. (2015, May 15). FDA Drug Safety Communication: FDA warns that SGLT2 inhibitors for diabetes may result in a serious condition of too much acid in the blood.

FDA. (2015, December 5). FDA Drug Safety Communication: FDA warns that SGLT2 inhibitors for diabetes may result in a serious condition of too much acid in the blood.

FDA. (2016, December 2). FDA approves Jardiance to reduce cardiovascular death in adults with type 2 diabetes.

FDA. (2018, August 28). FDA warns about rare occurrences of a serious infection of the genital area with SGLT2 inhibitors for diabetes.

FDA. (2020a, May 5). FDA approves new treatment for a type of heart failure.

FDA. (2020b, August 6). FDA removes Boxed Warning about risk of leg and foot amputations for the diabetes medicine canagliflozin (Invokana, Invokamet, Invokamet XR). FDA drug safety communication.

FDA (2021, July 7). Labeling Changes on mortality, kidney injury, and excess bleeding with hydroxyethyl starch products.

FDA. (2022, February 24) FDA Approves Treatment for Wider Range of Patients with Heart Failure.

FDA. (2022, March 15). FDA revises labels of SGLT2 inhibitors for diabetes to include warnings about too much acid in the blood and serious urinary tract infections.

FDA. (2023, May 26) FDA NDA Approval Sotagliflozin.

FDA. (2024, May 31). FDA Roundup: The FDA approved first generics of Entresto (sacubitril and valsartan) tablets, indicated to reduce the risk of cardiovascular death and hospitalization for heart failure in adult patients with chronic heart failure, and for the treatment of symptomatic heart failure with systemic left ventricular systolic dysfunction in pediatric patients aged one year and older.

Feneck, R. O., Sherry, K. M., Withington, P. S., Oduro-Dominah, A., & European Milrinone Multicenter Trial Group. (2001). Comparison of the hemodynamic effects of milrinone with dobutamine in patients after cardiac surgery. *Journal of cardiothoracic and vascular anesthesia*, *15*(3), 306-315.

Feng, M., Lv, H., Xu, X., Wang, J., Lyu, W., & Fu, S. (2019). Efficacy and safety of dapagliflozin as monotherapy in patients with type 2 diabetes mellitus: a meta-analysis of randomized controlled trials. *Medicine*, *98*(30).

Feng, Z., Wang, X., Zhang, L., Apaer, R., Xu, L., Ma, J., ... & Liu, S. (2022). Pharmacokinetics and pharmacodynamics of sacubitril/valsartan in maintenance hemodialysis patients with heart failure. *Blood Purification*, *51*(3), 270-279.

Fernando, S. M., Tran, A., Soliman, K., Flynn, B., Oommen, T., Wenzhe, L., ... & Rochwerg, B. (2024). Methylene blue in septic shock: a systematic review and meta-analysis. *Critical Care Explorations*, *6*(7), e1110.

Fihn, S.D., Gardin, J.M., Abrams, J., Berra, K., Blankenship, J.C., Dallas, A.P., Douglas, P.S., . . . Williams, S.V. (2012). 2012 ACCF/AHA/ACP/AATS/PCNA/SCAI/STS Guideline for the Diagnosis and Management of Patients With Stable Ischemic

Filippatos, G., Anker, S. D., Agarwal, R., Ruilope, L. M., Rossing, P., Bakris, G. L., ... & FIGARO-DKD Investigators. (2022). Finerenone reduces risk of incident heart failure in patients with chronic kidney disease and type 2 diabetes: analyses from the FIGARO-DKD trial. *Circulation*, *145*(6), 437-447.Heart Disease. Circulation, 126, e354-e471.

Fleming, G. A., Murray, K. T., Yu, C., Byrne, J. G., Greelish, J. P., Petracek, M. R., ... & Pretorius, M. (2008). Milrinone use is associated with postoperative atrial fibrillation after cardiac surgery. *Circulation*, *118*(16), 1619-1625.

Frishman, W. H. (1992). Tolerance, rebound, and time-zero effect of nitrate therapy. *The American journal of cardiology*, *70*(17), G43-G48.

Futier, E., Garot, M., Godet, T., Biais, M., Verzilli, D., Ouattara, A., ... & FLASH Trial Group. (2020). Effect of hydroxyethyl starch vs saline for volume replacement therapy on death or postoperative complications among high-risk patients undergoing major abdominal surgery: the FLASH randomized clinical trial. *Jama*, *323*(3), 225-236.

Garber, A. J., Handelsman, Y., Grunberger, G., Einhorn, D., Abrahamson, M. J., Barzilay, J. I., ... & Umpierrez, G. E. (2020). Consensus statement by the American Association of Clinical Endocrinologists and American College of Endocrinology on the comprehensive type 2 diabetes management algorithm–2020 executive summary. *Endocrine Practice*, *26*(1), 107-139.

García-Álvarez, R., & Arboleda-Salazar, R. (2023). Vasopressin in Sepsis and other Shock States: state of the art. *Journal of Personalized Medicine*, *13*(11), 1548.

Garg, S. K., Peters, A. L., Buse, J. B., & Danne, T. (2018). Strategy for mitigating DKA risk in patients with type 1 diabetes on adjunctive treatment with SGLT inhibitors: a STICH protocol. *Diabetes technology & therapeutics*, *20*(9), 571-575.

Garimella, B., Lehr, A., Elnadoury, O., & Lubinsky, A. (2020). EFFECTS OF DISCONTINUING VS TAPERING VASOPRESSIN INFUSION ON HEMODYNAMIC RECOVERY IN VASODILATORY SHOCK. *Chest*, *158*(4), A619.

Geerlings, S., Fonseca, V., Castro-Diaz, D., List, J., & Parikh, S. (2014). Genital and urinary tract infections in diabetes: impact of pharmacologically induced glucosuria. *Diabetes research and clinical practice*, *103*(3), 373-381.

Geyskes, G. G., Boer, P., & Mees, D. E. (1979). Clonidine withdrawal. Mechanism and frequency of rebound hypertension. *British journal of clinical pharmacology*, *7*(1), 55-62.

Gibbons, R. J., Chatterjee, K., Daley, J., Douglas, J. S., Fihn, S. D., Gardin, J. M., ... & Smith, S. C. (1999). ACC/AHA/ACP-ASIM guidelines for the management of patients with chronic stable angina: a report of the American College of Cardiology/American Heart Association Task Force on Practice Guidelines (Committee on Management of Patients With Chronic Stable Angina). *Journal of the American College of Cardiology*, *33*(7), 2092-2197.

Gilani, R. (2024). Acute mesenteric arterial occlusion. In K.A. Collins (Ed.), *UpToDate*.

Giovannitti Jr, J. A., Thoms, S. M., & Crawford, J. J. (2015). Alpha-2 adrenergic receptor agonists: a review of current clinical applications. *Anesthesia progress*, *62*(1), 31.

Giugliano, R.P. & Braunwald, E. (2019). Non-ST-elevation acute coronary syndromes. In D.P. Zipes, P. Libby, R.O. Bonow, D.L. Mann, G.F. Tomaselli (Eds.), Braunwald's Heart Disease: A Textbook of Cardiovascular Medicine (11th ed., pp. 1181-1208). Philadelphia: Elsevier.

Gogia, H., Mehra, A., Parikh, S., Raman, M., Ajit-Uppal, J., Johnson, J. V., & Elkayam, U. (1995). Prevention of tolerance to hemodynamic effects of nitrates with concomitant use of hydralazine in patients with chronic heart failure. *Journal of the American College of Cardiology*, *26*(7), 1575-1580.

Goldenberg, R. M., Berard, L. D., Cheng, A. Y., Gilbert, J. D., Verma, S., Woo, V. C., & Yale, J. F. (2016). SGLT2 inhibitor–associated diabetic ketoacidosis: clinical review and recommendations for prevention and diagnosis. *Clinical Therapeutics*, *38*(12), 2654-2664.

Gomez-Peralta, F., Abreu, C., Lecube, A. *et al.* Practical Approach to Initiating SGLT2 Inhibitors in Type 2 Diabetes. *Diabetes Ther* 8, 953–962 (2017).

Gonzalez, E. R., Jones, H. D., Graham, S., & Elswick, R. K. (1992). Assessment of the drug interaction between intravenous nitroglycerin and heparin.
Gordon, A. C., Mason, A. J., Thirunavukkarasu, N., Perkins, G. D., Cecconi, M., Cepkova, M., ... & VANISH Investigators. (2016). Effect of early vasopressin vs norepinephrine on kidney failure in patients with septic shock: the VANISH randomized clinical trial. *Jama*, *316*(5), 509-518.
Gordon, A. C., Wang, N., Walley, K. R., Ashby, D., & Russell, J. A. (2012). The cardiopulmonary effects of vasopressin compared with norepinephrine in septic shock. *Chest*, *142*(3), 593-605.
Goyer, I., Lakbar, I., Freund, Y., Lévy, B., & Leone, M. (2024). Norepinephrine dosing in France: time to move forward!. *Anaesthesia Critical Care & Pain Medicine*, *43*(4), 101397.
Graves, L. E., & Donaghue, K. C. (2019). Management of diabetes complications in youth. *Therapeutic Advances in Endocrinology and Metabolism*, *10*, 2042018819863226.
Grossman, E. & Messerli, F. H. (2007). Hypertensive Urgencies and Emergencies, In G.Y.H. Lip & J.E. Hall (Eds.). *Comprehensive Hypertension* (pp. 761-774). Mosby.
Guarracino, F., Habicher, M., Treskatsch, S., Sander, M., Szekely, A., Paternoster, G., ... & Heringlake, M. (2021). Vasopressor therapy in cardiac surgery—an experts' consensus statement. *Journal of Cardiothoracic and Vascular Anesthesia*, *35*(4), 1018-1029.
Gupta, M, & Al Khalili, Y. (2023). Methyldopa. [Updated 2023 Jul 10]. In: StatPearls [Internet]. Treasure Island (FL): StatPearls Publishing.
Gupta, P. K., Natarajan, B., Gupta, H., Fang, X., & Fitzgibbons Jr, R. J. (2011). Morbidity and mortality after bowel resection for acute mesenteric ischemia. *Surgery*, *150*(4), 779-787.
Guyer, A.C. & Banerji, A. (2022). ACE inhibitor-induced angioedema. In A. M. Feldweg (Ed.), *UpToDate*.
Haber, H. L., Simek, C. L., Bergin, J. D., Sadun, A., Gimple, L. W., Powers, E. R., & Feldman, M. D. (1993). Bolus intravenous nitroglycerin predominantly reduces afterload in patients with excessive arterial elastance. *Journal of the American College of Cardiology*, *22*(1), 251-257.
Hajjar, L. A., Vincent, J. L., Barbosa Gomes Galas, F. R., Rhodes, A., Landoni, G., Osawa, E. A., ... & Costa Auler, J. O. (2017). Vasopressin versus norepinephrine in patients with vasoplegic shock after cardiac surgery. *Anesthesiology*, *126*(1), 85-93.
Hammer, F., Malzahn, U., Donhauser, J., Betz, C., Schneider, M. P., Grupp, C., ... & Zimmermann, J. (2019). A randomized controlled trial of the effect of spironolactone on left ventricular mass in hemodialysis patients. *Kidney international*, *95*(4), 983-991.
Hammond, D. A., Cullen, J., Painter, J. T., McCain, K., Clem, O. A., Brotherton, A. L., ... & Meena, N. (2019). Efficacy and safety of the early addition of vasopressin to norepinephrine in septic shock. *Journal of intensive care medicine*, *34*(11-12), 910-916.
Hammond, D. A., Sacha, G. L., Bissell, B. D., Musallam, N., Altshuler, D., Flannery, A. H., ... & Bauer, S. R. (2019). Effects of norepinephrine and vasopressin discontinuation order in the recovery phase of septic shock: a systematic review and individual patient data meta-analysis. *Pharmacotherapy: The Journal of Human Pharmacology and Drug Therapy*, *39*(5), 544-552.
Hamzaoui, O., Goury, A., & Teboul, J. L. (2023). The eight unanswered and answered questions about the use of vasopressors in septic shock. *Journal of Clinical Medicine*, *12*(14), 4589.
Harshaw, C. W., Gossman, W., Munro, A. B., & McLaurin, L. P. (1975). Reduced systemic vascular resistance as therapy for severe mitral regurgitation of valvular origin. *Annals of internal medicine*, *83*(3), 312-316.
Hart, G. R., & Anderson, R. J. (1981). Withdrawal syndromes and the cessation of antihypertensive therapy. *Archives of Internal Medicine*, *141*(9), 1125-1127.
Hawn, J. M., Bauer, S. R., Yerke, J., Li, M., Wang, X., Reddy, A. J., ... & Sacha, G. L. (2021). Effect of phenylephrine push before continuous infusion norepinephrine in patients with septic shock. *Chest*, *159*(5), 1875-1883.
Haymore, B. R., Yoon, J., Mikita, C. P., Klote, M. M., & DeZee, K. J. (2008). Risk of angioedema with angiotensin receptor blockers in patients with prior angioedema associated with angiotensin-converting enzyme inhibitors: a meta-analysis. *Annals of Allergy, Asthma & Immunology*, *101*(5), 495-499.
Heerspink, H. J., Stefánsson, B. V., Correa-Rotter, R., Chertow, G. M., Greene, T., Hou, F. F., ... & Wheeler, D. C. (2020). Dapagliflozin in patients with chronic kidney disease. *New England Journal of Medicine*, *383*(15), 1436-1446.
Heidenreich, P. A., Bozkurt, B., Aguilar, D., Allen, L. A., Byun, J. J., Colvin, M. M., ... & Yancy, C. W. (2022). 2022 AHA/ACC/HFSA guideline for the management of heart failure: a report of the American College of Cardiology/American Heart Association Joint Committee on Clinical Practice Guidelines. *Journal of the American College of Cardiology*, *79*(17), e263-e421.
Heradstveit, B. E., Sunde, G. A., Asbjørnsen, H., Aalvik, R., Wentzel-Larsen, T., & Heltne, J. K. (2023). Pharmacokinetics of epinephrine during cardiac arrest: A pilot study. *Resuscitation*, *193*, 110025.
Heritage Pharmaceuticals Inc., 2021. Isosorbide mononitrate Extended-Release Prescribing Information.
Herman, L.L., Bruss, Z.S., & Tivakaran V.S. (2023). Hydralazine. In: StatPearls. StatPearls Publishing, Treasure Island (FL).
Hikma Pharmaceuticals USA Inc. (2025) Isosorbide Dinitrate Prescribing information.

Hilal-Dandan R. (2018). Renin and Angiotensin. In L.L. Brunton, R. Hilal-Dandan, B.C. Knollmann (Eds.), Goodman & Gilman's The Pharmacological Basis of Therapeutics (13th Ed., pp 471-488). New York: McGraw Hill.

Hintze, T. H., Kaley, G., & Panzenbeck, M. J. (1984). Mechanisms of reflex bradycardia and hypotension by metabolites of arachidonic acid in the cat. *British journal of pharmacology*, *82*(1), 117.

Hoff, R., & Koh, C. K. (2018). Isoproterenol induced insulin resistance leading to diabetic ketoacidosis in type 1 diabetes mellitus. *Case reports in endocrinology*.

Hollenberg, S. M., Warner Stevenson, L., Ahmad, T., Amin, V. J., Bozkurt, B., Butler, J., ... & Storrow, A. B. (2019). 2019 ACC expert consensus decision pathway on risk assessment, management, and clinical trajectory of patients hospitalized with heart failure: a report of the American College of Cardiology Solution Set Oversight Committee. *Journal of the American College of Cardiology*, *74*(15), 1966-2011.

Holmes, C. L., Patel, B. M., Russell, J. A., & Walley, K. R. (2001). Physiology of vasopressin relevant to management of septic shock. *Chest*, *120*(3), 989-1002.

Holme, M. R., & Sharman, T. (2020). Sodium nitroprusside. [Updated 2023 May 22]. In *StatPearls* [Internet]. StatPearls Publishing, Treasure Island, FL. Retrieved Jan 23, 2025 from: https://europepmc.org/article/NBK/nbk557487.

Hospira, Inc. (2016). Dobutamine prescribing information.

Hospira, Inc. (2018a). Dextran prescribing information

Hospira, Inc. (2018b). Isoproterenol prescribing information.

Hospira, Inc. (2019). Epinephrine prescribing information.

Hottinger, D. G., Beebe, D. S., Kozhimannil, T., Prielipp, R. C., & Belani, K. G. (2014). Sodium nitroprusside in 2014: A clinical concepts review. *Journal of anaesthesiology clinical pharmacology*, *30*(4), 462-471.

Hripcsak, G., Suchard, M. A., Shea, S., Chen, R., You, S. C., Pratt, N., ... & Schuemie, M. J. (2020). Comparison of cardiovascular and safety outcomes of chlorthalidone vs hydrochlorothiazide to treat hypertension. *JAMA internal medicine*, *180*(4), 542-551.

Hu, Y., Bai, Z., Tang, Y., Liu, R., Zhao, B., Gong, J., & Mei, D. (2020). Fournier gangrene associated with sodium-glucose cotransporter-2 inhibitors: a pharmacovigilance study with data from the US FDA Adverse Event Reporting System. *Journal of Diabetes Research, 2020.*

Huang, H., Wu, C., Shen, Q., Xu, H., Fang, Y., & Mao, W. (2021). The effect of early vasopressin use on patients with septic shock: A systematic review and meta-analysis. *The American journal of emergency medicine*, *48*, 203-208.

Huang, P., Guo, Y., Li, B., & Liu, Q. (2019). Terlipressin versus norepinephrine for septic shock: a systematic review and meta-analysis. *Frontiers in pharmacology*, *10*, 1492.

Huayllani, M. T., Cheema, A. S., McGuire, M. J., & Janis, J. E. (2022). Practical review of the current management of Fournier's gangrene. *Plastic and Reconstructive Surgery–Global Open*, *10*(3), e4191.

Hunyor, S. N., Hansson, L., Harrison, T. S., & Hoobler, S. W. (1973). Effects of clonidine withdrawal: possible mechanisms and suggestions for management. *Br Med J*, *2*(5860), 209-211.

Hussien, R. M., El-Gendy, H. A., Elsaidy, M. I., Abdelhamid, M. S., & Shabana, T. S. (2021). Comparison between norepinephrine alone versus norepinephrine/vasopressin combination for resuscitation in septic shock: a randomized clinical trial. *Egyptian Journal of Critical Care Medicine*, *8*(3), 58-65.

Ibarra-Estrada, M., Kattan, E., Aguilera-González, P., Sandoval-Plascencia, L., Rico-Jauregui, U., Gómez-Partida, C. A., ... & Hernández, G. (2023). Early adjunctive methylene blue in patients with septic shock: a randomized controlled trial. *Critical Care*, *27*(1), 110.

Ikram, H., Low, C. J., Crozier, I. G., & Shirlaw, T. (1992). Hemodynamic effects of nitroprusside on valvular aortic stenosis. *The American journal of cardiology*, *69*(4), 361-366.

Ishani, A., Cushman, W. C., Leatherman, S. M., Lew, R. A., Woods, P., Glassman, P. A., ... & Ferguson, R. E. (2022). Chlorthalidone vs. hydrochlorothiazide for hypertension–cardiovascular events. *New England Journal of Medicine*, *387*(26), 2401-2410.

Ismail, M. T., & Elbaih, A. H. (2020). Principles of intravenous fluids therapy. *EC Emerg Med Critical Care*, *4*(6), 24-46.

Israili, Z. H. (2000). Clinical pharmacokinetics of angiotensin II (AT1) receptor blockers in hypertension. *Journal of human hypertension*, *14*(1), S73-S86.

Isaac, L. (1980). Clonidine in the central nervous system: site and mechanism of hypotensive action. *Journal of cardiovascular pharmacology*, *2*, S5-20.

Iyer, P., Dirweesh, A., & Zijoo, R. (2017). *Hydralazine Induced Lupus Syndrome Presenting with Recurrent Pericardial Effusion and a Negative Antinuclear Antibody. Case Rep Rheumatol. 2017; 2017: 1–3.*

Jaber, S., Paugam, C., Futier, E., Lefrant, J. Y., Lasocki, S., Lescot, T., ... & Kipnis, E. (2018). Sodium bicarbonate therapy for patients with severe metabolic acidaemia in the intensive care unit (BICAR-ICU): a multicentre, open-label, randomised controlled, phase 3 trial. *The Lancet*, *392*(10141), 31-40.

Jackson, E.K. (2018). Drugs affecting renal excretory function. In L.L. Brunton, R. Hilal-Dandan, B.C. Knollmann (Eds.), Goodman & Gilman's The Pharmacological Basis of Therapeutics (13th Ed., pp 445-470). New York: McGraw Hill.

Jackson, K., & Moseley, K. F. (2020). Diabetes and Bone Fragility: SGLT2 Inhibitor Use in the Context of Renal and Cardiovascular Benefits. *Current osteoporosis reports*, 1-10.

James, P.A., Oparil, S., Carter, B.L., Cushman, W.C., Dennison-Himmelfarb, C., Handler, J., Lackland, D.T., . . . Ortiz, E. (2014). 2014 evidence-based guideline for the management of high blood pressure in adults. Report from the panel members appointed to the Eighth Joint National Committee (JNC8). JAMA, 311, 507-520.

Janssen Pharmaceutical Companies (2023). Canagliflozin (Invokana) Prescribing Information.

Jentzer, J. C., Anavekar, N. S., Burstein, B. J., Borlaug, B. A., & Oh, J. K. (2020). Noninvasive echocardiographic left ventricular stroke work index predicts mortality in cardiac intensive care unit patients. *Circulation: Cardiovascular Imaging*, *13*(11), e011642.

Jentzer, J. C., & Hollenberg, S. M. (2021). Vasopressor and inotrope therapy in cardiac critical care. *Journal of intensive care medicine*, *36*(8), 843-856.

Jeon, K., Song, J. U., Chung, C. R., Yang, J. H., & Suh, G. Y. (2018). Incidence of hypotension according to the discontinuation order of vasopressors in the management of septic shock: a prospective randomized trial (DOVSS). *Critical Care*, *22*, 1-12.

Jerome, R., Randhawa, J. S., Badran, S., Li, S., & Mohammadi, N. (2024). Drug-induced systemic lupus erythematosus: a rare presentation of hydralazine-induced lupus. *Cureus*, *16*(10), e72069.

Jestico, J. V., O'Brien, M. D., Teoh, R., Toseland, P. A., & Wong, H. C. (1984). Whole blood cyanide levels in patients with tobacco amblyopia. *Journal of Neurology, Neurosurgery & Psychiatry*, *47*(6), 573-578.

Jhund, P. S., McMurray, J. J., & Davie, A. P. (2000). The acute vascular effects of frusemide in heart failure. *British journal of clinical pharmacology*, *50*(1), 9.

Jia, L., Wang, P., Li, C., & Xie, J. (2023). The efficacy and safety of vasopressors for septic shock patients: A systemic review and network meta-analysis. *Shock*, *60*(6), 746-752.

Joglar, J. A., Chung, M. K., Armbruster, A. L., Benjamin, E. J., Chyou, J. Y., Cronin, E. M., ... & Van Wagoner, D. R. (2024). 2023 ACC/AHA/ACCP/HRS guideline for the diagnosis and management of atrial fibrillation: a report of the American College of Cardiology/American Heart Association Joint Committee on Clinical Practice Guidelines. *Circulation*, *149*(1), e1-e156.

Johnson & Johnson. (2013, March 29). U.S. FDA Approves INVOKANA™ (Canagliflozin) for the Treatment of Adults with Type 2 Diabetes. Retrieved on September 7, 2021from https://www.jnj.com/media-center/press-releases/us-fda-approves-invokana-canagliflozin-for-the-treatment-of-adults-with-type-2-diabetes.

Johnson & Johnson. (2018, October 30). U.S. FDA Approves INVOKANA® (canagliflozin) to Reduce the Risk of Heart Attack, Stroke or Cardiovascular Death in Adults with Type 2 Diabetes and Established Cardiovascular Disease.

Jones, D. W., Ferdinand, K. C., Taler, S. J., Johnson, H. M., Shimbo, D., ... & Williamson, J. D. (2025). 2025 AHA/ACC/AANP/AAPA/ABC/ACCP/ACPM/AGS/AMA/ASPC/NMA/PCNA/SGIM guideline for the prevention, detection, evaluation and management of high blood pressure in adults: a report of the American College of Cardiology/American Heart Association Joint Committee on Clinical Practice Guidelines. *Circulation*, *152*(11), e114-e218.

Jozwiak, M. (2022). Alternatives to norepinephrine in septic shock: which agents and when?. *Journal of Intensive Medicine*, *2*(04), 223-232.

Jozwiak, M., Geri, G., Laghlam, D., Boussion, K., Dolladille, C., & Nguyen, L. S. (2022). Vasopressors and risk of acute mesenteric ischemia: a worldwide pharmacovigilance analysis and comprehensive literature review. *Frontiers in Medicine*, *9*, 826446.

Kalmar, A. F., Allaert, S., Pletinckx, P., Maes, J. W., Heerman, J., Vos, J. J., ... & Scheeren, T. W. L. (2018). Phenylephrine increases cardiac output by raising cardiac preload in patients with anesthesia induced hypotension. *Journal of clinical monitoring and computing*, *32*, 969-976.

Kalra, S., & Gupta, Y. (2016). The insulin: glucagon ratio and the choice of glucose-lowering drugs. *Diabetes Therapy*, *7*(1), 1-9.

Kamibayashi, T., Harasawa, K., & Maze, M. (1997). Alpha-2 adrenergic agonists. *Canadian journal of anaesthesia*, *44*(Suppl 1), R13-R22.

Kaplan N. M. (1975). Antihypertensive drugs in combination: Effects of methyldopa on thiazide-induced changes in renal hemodynamics and plasma renin activity. *Archives of internal medicine*, *135*(5), 660–663.

Kaplan, K. J., Taber, M., Teagarden, J. R., Parker, M., & Davison, R. (1985). Association of Methemoglobinemia and intravenous nitroglycerin administration. *The American journal of cardiology*, *55*(1), 181-183.

Karachalios, G.N. (1986). Hypertensive emergencies treated with oral clonidine. *Eur J Clin Pharmacol* **31**, 227–229.

Katzung, B.G. (2024). Vasodilators & the Treatment of Angina Pectoris and Coronary Syndromes. In Weitz, M. & Boyle, P. (Eds.), Basic and Clinical Pharmacology (16th Ed., pp 200-218). The McGraw-Hill Companies.

Kelly, G. S., Branstetter, L. A., Moran, T. P., Hanzelka, N., & Cooper, C. D. (2023). Low-versus high-dose nitroglycerin infusion in the management of acute pulmonary edema. *The American Journal of Emergency Medicine*, *65*, 71-75.

Khajavi, M. R., Etezadi, F., Moharari, R. S., Imani, F., Meysamie, A. P., Khashayar, P., & Najafi, A. (2008). Effects of normal saline vs. lactated ringer's during renal transplantation. *Renal failure*, *30*(5), 535-539.

Khan, N., Reichel, R., Khurshid, A., Tso, K., Broussard, J., & Dass, A. (2020). Hydralazine-induced isolated lupus nephritis. *Ochsner Journal*, *20*(2), 187-192.

Khot, U. N., Novaro, G. M., Popović, Z. B., Mills, R. M., Thomas, J. D., Tuzcu, E. M., ... & Francis, G. S. (2003). Nitroprusside in critically ill patients with left ventricular dysfunction and aortic stenosis. *New England Journal of Medicine*, *348*(18), 1756-1763.

Kintscher, U., & Edelmann, F. (2023). The non-steroidal mineralocorticoid receptor antagonist finerenone and heart failure with preserved ejection fraction. *Cardiovascular Diabetology*, *22*(1), 162.

Ko, D. T., Hebert, P. R., Coffey, C. S., Curtis, J. P., Foody, J. M., Sedrakyan, A., & Krumholz, H. M. (2004). Adverse effects of β-blocker therapy for patients with heart failure: a quantitative overview of randomized trials. *Archives of internal medicine*, *164*(13), 1389-1394.

Ko, D. T., Hebert, P. R., Coffey, C. S., Sedrakyan, A., Curtis, J. P., & Krumholz, H. M. (2002). β-blocker therapy and symptoms of depression, fatigue, and sexual dysfunction. *Jama*, *288*(3), 351-357.

Kobori, H., Mori, H., Masaki, T., & Nishiyama, A. (2013). Angiotensin II blockade and renal protection. *Current pharmaceutical design*, *19*(17), 3033-3042.

Koh, K. K., Park, G. S., Song, J. H., Moon, T. H., In, H. H., Kim, J. J., ... & Kim, S. S. (1995). Interaction of intravenous heparin and organic nitrates in acute ischemic syndromes. *The American journal of cardiology*, *76*(10), 706-709.

Kotani, Y., Belletti, A., Ursoleo, J. D. A., Salvati, S., & Landoni, G. (2023). Norepinephrine dose should be reported as base equivalence in clinical research manuscripts. *Journal of Cardiothoracic and Vascular Anesthesia*, *37*(9), 1523-1524.

Krajewski, M. L., Raghunathan, K., Paluszkiewicz, S. M., Schermer, C. R., & Shaw, A. D. (2015). Meta-analysis of high-versus low-chloride content in perioperative and critical care fluid resuscitation. *Journal of British Surgery*, *102*(1), 24-36.

Kraut, J. A., & Madias, N. E. (2019). Intravenous sodium bicarbonate in treating patients with severe metabolic acidemia. *American journal of kidney diseases: the official journal of the National Kidney Foundation*, *73*(4), 572-575.

Lam, D., & Shaikh, A. (2021). Real-life prescribing of SGLT2 inhibitors: how to handle the other medications, including glucose-lowering drugs and diuretics. *Kidney360*, *2*(4), 742-746.

Lam, S. W., Sacha, G. L., Duggal, A., Reddy, A. J., & Bauer, S. R. (2021). Abrupt discontinuation versus down-titration of vasopressin in patients recovering from septic shock. *Shock*, *55*(2), 210-214.

Landry, D. W., & Oliver, J. A. (2001). The pathogenesis of vasodilatory shock. *New England Journal of Medicine*, *345*(8), 588-595.

Leavesley, H. B., Li, L., Mukhopadhyay, S., Borowitz, J. L., & Isom, G. E. (2010). Nitrite-mediated antagonism of cyanide inhibition of cytochrome c oxidase in dopamine neurons. *Toxicological Sciences*, *115*(2), 569-576.

Levin, M. A., Lin, H. M., Castillo, J. G., Adams, D. H., Reich, D. L., & Fischer, G. W. (2009). Early on–cardiopulmonary bypass hypotension and other factors associated with vasoplegic syndrome. *Circulation*, *120*(17), 1664-1671.

Lexicomp. (2023). Aliskiren.

Lexicomp. (2023). Amiloride.

Lexicomp. (2023). Amlodipine.

Lexicomp. (2026). Bumetanide.

Lexicomp. (2023). Eplerenone.

Lexicomp. (2023). Ethacrynic acid.

Lexicomp. (2023). Finerenone.

Lexicomp. (2023). Felodipine.

Lexicomp. (2023). Furosemide.

Lexicomp. (2023). Spironolactone.

Lexicomp. (2023). Torsemide.

Lexicomp. (2023). Triamterene.

Lexicon Pharmaceuticals, Inc. (2023). Sotagliflozin (Inpefa) Prescribing Information.

Li, H., Xu, T. Y., Li, Y., Chia, Y. C., Buranakitjaroen, P., Cheng, H. M., ... & Wang, J. G. (2022). Role of α1-blockers in the current management of hypertension. *The Journal of Clinical Hypertension*, *24*(9), 1180-1186.

Liamis, G., Filippatos, T. D., & Elisaf, M. S. (2016). Thiazide–associated hyponatremia in the elderly: what the clinician needs to know. *Journal of geriatric cardiology: JGC*, *13*(2), 175.

Liu, Z. M., Chen, J., Kou, Q., Lin, Q., Huang, X., Tang, Z., ... & Guan, X. D. (2018). Terlipressin versus norepinephrine as infusion in patients with septic shock: a multicentre, randomised, double-blinded trial. *Intensive care medicine*, *44*(11), 1816-1825.

Lockwood, A., Patka, J., Rabinovich, M., Wyatt, K., & Abraham, P. (2010). Sodium nitroprusside-associated cyanide toxicity in adult patients–fact or fiction? A critical review of the evidence and clinical relevance. *Open Access Journal of Clinical Trials*, 133-148.

López, A., Lorente, J. A., Steingrub, J., Bakker, J., McLuckie, A., Willatts, S., ... & Grover, R. (2004). Multiple-center, randomized, placebo-controlled, double-blind study of the nitric oxide synthase inhibitor 546C88: effect on survival in patients with septic shock. *Critical care medicine*, *32*(1), 21-30.

López-Rivera, F., Martínez, H. R. C., LaTorre, C. C., González, A. R., Vélez, J. G. R., Ferrer, V. F., ... & Monroig, H. A. G. (2019). Treatment of hypertensive cardiogenic edema with intravenous high-dose nitroglycerin in a patient presenting with signs of respiratory failure: a case report and review of the literature. *The American Journal of Case Reports*, *20*, 83.

Lotterman, S. & Sharma, S. (2023). Blood transfusion. *Stat Pearls.* [Internet].
Lu, H., Lu, H., Kosinski, C., Wojtusciszyn, A., Zanchi, A., Carron, P. N., ... & Hullin, R. (2021). SGLT2 inhibitors, what the emergency physician needs to know: a narrative review. *Journal of clinical medicine*, *10*(9), 2036.
Luis-Silva, F., Menegueti, M. G., Peres, L. M., Sepeda, C. D. R., Jordani, M. C., Mestriner, F., ... & Auxiliadora-Martins, M. (2024). Methylene blue therapy in addition to standard treatment for acute-phase septic shock: a pilot randomized controlled trial. *Frontiers in Medicine*, *11*, 1431321.
Lukacsko, P. (1982). Paradoxical bradycardia following the administration of sodium nitroprusside in the rat is abolished by indomethacin. *Cardiovascular research*, *16*(2), 95-98.
Ma, Y., Zhao, Q., Peng, H., Nalisa, D. L., Shan, P., & Jiang, H. (2023). SGLT2i in Patients with Type 1 Diabetes: Benefits, Risks, and Preventive Strategies. *Frontiers in Bioscience-Landmark*, *28*(5), 98.
Maddox, T. M., Januzzi Jr, J. L., Allen, L. A., Breathett, K., Brouse, S., Butler, J., ... & Youmans, Q. R. (2024). 2024 ACC Expert Consensus Decision Pathway for Treatment of Heart Failure With Reduced Ejection Fraction: A Report of the American College of Cardiology Solution Set Oversight Committee. *Journal of the American College of Cardiology*, *83*(15), 1444-1488.
Maddox, T. M., Januzzi Jr, J. L., Allen, L. A., Breathett, K., Butler, J., Davis, L. L., ... & Youmans, Q. R. (2021). 2021 update to the 2017 ACC expert consensus decision pathway for optimization of heart failure treatment: answers to 10 pivotal issues about heart failure with reduced ejection fraction: a report of the American College of Cardiology Solution Set Oversight Committee. *Journal of the American College of Cardiology*, *77*(6), 772-810.
Mallmann, C., Galiotto, T. M. B., de Oliveira, M. S., & Moraes, R. B. (2025). Reduction of norepinephrine versus vasopressin in the stabilization phase of septic shock: RENOVA clinical trial. *Medicina Intensiva (English Edition)*, 502147.
Manisterski, Y., Vaknin, Z., Ben-Abraham, R., Efrati, O., Lotan, D., Berkovitch, M., ... & Paret, G. (2002). Endotracheal epinephrine: a call for larger doses. *Anesthesia & Analgesia*, *95*(4), 1037-1041.
Mann, D.L. (2019). Management of heart failure patients with reduced ejection fraction. In D.P. Zipes, P. Libby, R.O. Bonow, D.L. Mann, G.F. Tomaselli (Eds.), Braunwald's Heart Disease: A Textbook of Cardiovascular Medicine (11th ed., pp. 490-522). Philadelphia: Elsevier.
Mann, J.F.E. & Flack, J.M. (2024). Choice of drug therapy in primary (essential) hypertension. In K. Law & J.P. Forman (Eds.), *UpToDate*.
Mann, J.F.E. & Hilgers, K.F. (2023). Renal effects of ACE inhibitors in hypertension. In J.P. Forman (Ed.), *UpToDate*.
Mann, J.F.E. & Hilgers, F.E. (2025). Clinical features, diagnosis, and treatment of hypertensive nephrosclerosis. In J.P. Forman (Ed.), *UpToDate*.
Mann, S. J. (2008). The silent epidemic of thiazide-induced hyponatremia. *The Journal of Clinical Hypertension*, *10*(6), 477-484.
Mann, T., Cohn, P. F., Holman, L. B., Green, L. H., Markis, J. E., & Phillips, D. A. (1978). Effect of nitroprusside on regional myocardial blood flow in coronary artery disease. Results in 25 patients and comparison with nitroglycerin. *Circulation*, *57*(4), 732-738.
Marquis-Gravel, G., Redfors, B., Leon, M. B., & Genereux, P. (2016). Medical treatment of aortic stenosis. *Circulation*, *134*(22), 1766-1784.
Marte, F., Sankar, P., Patel, P., & Cassagnol, M. (2024). Captopril. In *StatPearls [Internet]*. StatPearls Publishing.
Masarone, D., Martucci, M. L., Errigo, V., & Pacileo, G. (2021). The use of β-blockers in heart failure with reduced ejection fraction. *Journal of Cardiovascular Development and Disease*, *8*(9), 101.
Mathew, R., Di Santo, P., Jung, R. G., Marbach, J. A., Hutson, J., Simard, T., ... & Hibbert, B. (2021). Milrinone as compared with dobutamine in the treatment of cardiogenic shock. New England Journal of Medicine, 385(6), 516-525.
Matsushita, F. Y., Krebs, V. L. J., de Campos, C. V., de Vincenzi Gaiolla, P. V., & de Carvalho, W. B. (2024). Reassessing the role of milrinone in the treatment of heart failure and pulmonary hypertension in neonates and children: a systematic review and meta-analysis. *European journal of pediatrics*, *183*(2), 543-555.
Mayer, B., Brunner, F., & Schmidt, K. (1993). Inhibition of nitric oxide synthesis by methylene blue. *Biochemical pharmacology*, *45*(2), 367-374.
McComb, M. N., Chao, J. Y., & Ng, T. M. (2016). Direct vasodilators and sympatholytic agents. *Journal of cardiovascular pharmacology and therapeutics*, *21*(1), 3-19.
McIntyre, W. F., Um, K. J., Alhazzani, W., Lengyel, A. P., Hajjar, L., Gordon, A. C., ... & Belley-Côté, E. P. (2018). Association of vasopressin plus catecholamine vasopressors vs catecholamines alone with atrial fibrillation in patients with distributive shock: a systematic review and meta-analysis. *Jama*, *319*(18), 1889-1900.
McMorran, J., Crowther, D.C., Henderson, R., McMorran, S., Prince, C., Pleat, J.Yangmin, S. (2018). Acetylation of drugs. *Primary Care Notebook*. Retrieved from https://primarycarenotebook.com/pages/surgery/acetylation-of-drugs
McMurray, J. J., Packer, M., Desai, A. S., Gong, J., Lefkowitz, M. P., Rizkala, A. R., ... & Zile, M. R. (2014). Angiotensin–neprilysin inhibition versus enalapril in heart failure. *N Engl J Med*, *371*, 993-1004.
McMurray, J. J., Solomon, S. D., Inzucchi, S. E., Køber, L., Kosiborod, M. N., Martinez, F. A., ... & Langkilde, A. M. (2019). Dapagliflozin in patients with heart failure and reduced ejection fraction. *New England Journal of Medicine*, *381*(21), 1995-2008.

Melchers, M., de Smet, V., Rooijakkers, C., Huising, J., Vermeulen, W., Köktaş, B. N. N., ... & van Zanten, A. R. H. (2025). Hemodynamic effects of adjunct arginine vasopressin to norepinephrine in septic shock: insights from a prospective multicenter registry study. *Annals of Intensive Care*, *15*(1), 1-14.

Members, W. C., Ommen, S. R., Ho, C. Y., Asif, I. M., Balaji, S., Burke, M. A., ... & Waldman, C. B. (2024). 2024 AHA/ACC/AMSSM/HRS/PACES/SCMR Guideline for the Management of Hypertrophic Cardiomyopathy: A Report of the American Heart Association/American College of Cardiology Joint Committee on Clinical Practice Guidelines. *Journal of the American College of Cardiology*, *83*(23), 2324-2405.

Merck & Co., Inc. (2010). Isosorbide Mononitrate Prescribing Information.

Merck & Co., Inc. (2021). Ertugliflozin (Steglatro) Prescribing Information.

Merck Sharp & Dohme Corp (2014). Nitro-dur Transdermal Prescribing Information.

Merola, J.F. (2024). Drug induced lupus. In S.M. Case (Ed.) *UptoDate*.

Meschia, J.F., Bushnell, c., Bden-Albala, B., Braun, L.T., Bravata, D.M., Chaturvedi, S., Creager, M.A., . . . Wilson, J.A. (2014). Guidelines for the primary prevention of stroke: A statement for healthcare professionals from the American Heart Association/American Stroke Association. Stroke, 45, 3754-3832.

Messerli, F. H., Roush, G. C., & Oparil, S. (2020). Chlorthalidone and hydrochlorothiazide for treatment of patients with hypertension. *JAMA internal medicine*, *180*(8), 1133-1133.

Meyer, T. (2025). Primary pharmacologic therapy for heart failure with reduced ejection fraction. In T.F. Dardas (Ed.) UptoDate.

Mikhael, B., Steele, D. J., & Fenves, A. Z. (2022). In defense of normal saline: our perspective. *Clinical Journal of the American Society of Nephrology*, *17*(4), 588-590.

Miles, J. A., Hanumanthu, B. K., Patel, K., Chen, M., Siegel, R. M., & Kokkinidis, D. G. (2019). Torsemide versus furosemide and intermediate-term outcomes in patients with heart failure: an updated meta-analysis. *Journal of Cardiovascular Medicine*, *20*(6), 379-388.

Mirdamadi, A., Abrishamkar, R., & Kargaran, A. (2022). Comparing outcomes of clonidine and captopril in patients with hypertensive urgency: A randomized clinical trial. *ARYA atherosclerosis*, *18*(1), 1.

Miyashita, S., Kuno, T., Takagi, H., Sugiyama, T., Ando, T., Valentin, N., ... & Bangalore, S. (2020). Risk of amputation associated with sodium-glucose co-transporter 2 inhibitors: a meta-analysis of five randomized controlled trials. *Diabetes research and clinical practice*, *163*, 108136.

Moliterno, D.J., Januzzi, J.L. (2017). Evaluation and management of non-ST-segment elevation myocardial infarction. In V. Fuster, R.A. Harrington, J. Narula, Z.J. Eapen (Eds.), Hurst's The Heart (14th ed., pp. 995-1016). New York: McGraw Hill.

Molvi, S. N., Mir, S., Rana, V. S., Jabeen, F., & Malik, A. R. (2012). Role of antihypertensive therapy in mild to moderate pregnancy-induced hypertension: a prospective randomized study comparing labetalol with alpha methyldopa. *Archives of gynecology and obstetrics*, *285*, 1553-1562.

Mongardon, N., de Roux, Q., Leone, M., & Guerci, P. (2023). Norepinephrine formulation for equivalent vasopressive score. *Critical Care*, *27*(1), 62.

Morris, A. A., Page, R. L., Baumgartner, L. J., Mueller, S. W., MacLaren, R., Fish, D. N., & Kiser, T. H. (2017). Thiocyanate accumulation in critically ill patients receiving nitroprusside infusions. *Journal of Intensive Care Medicine*, *32*(9), 547-553.

Moses, R. G., Colagiuri, S., & Pollock, C. (2014). SGLT2 inhibitors: new medicines for addressing unmet needs in type 2 diabetes. *The Australasian medical journal*, *7*(10), 405.

Muluk, V., Cohn, S. & Whinney, C. (2025). Perioperative Medication Management. In H. Li (Ed.), *UpToDate*.

Münzel, T., Daiber, A., & Mülsch, A. (2005). Explaining the phenomenon of nitrate tolerance. Circulation research, 97(7), 618-628.

Murata, J., Buckley, M., Lehn, J., Agarwal, S. K., Stevenson, B., Martinez, B., & MacLaren, R. (2023). Incidence of hypotension associated with two different vasopressin discontinuation strategies in the recovery phase of septic shock. *Journal of Pharmacy Practice*, *36*(4), 830-838.

Musallam, N., Altshuler, D., Merchan, C., Zakhary, B., Aberle, C., & Papadopoulos, J. (2018). Evaluating vasopressor discontinuation strategies in patients with septic shock on concomitant norepinephrine and vasopressin infusions. *Annals of Pharmacotherapy*, *52*(8), 733-739.

Myburgh, J. A., Finfer, S., Bellomo, R., Billot, L., Cass, A., Gattas, D., ... & Webb, S. A. (2012). Hydroxyethyl starch or saline for fluid resuscitation in intensive care. *New England Journal of Medicine*, *367*(20), 1901-1911.

Myburgh, J. A., & Mythen, M. G. (2013). Resuscitation fluids. *New England Journal of Medicine*, *369*(13), 1243-1251.

Myhre, P. L., Vaduganathan, M., Claggett, B., Packer, M., Desai, A. S., Rouleau, J. L., ... & Solomon, S. D. (2019). B-type natriuretic peptide during treatment with sacubitril/valsartan: the PARADIGM-HF trial. Journal of the American College of Cardiology, 73(11), 1264-1272.

Nachawati, D., Leslie, S. W., & Patel, J. B. (2025). Alpha-Blockers. In *StatPearls [Internet]*. StatPearls Publishing.

Nagendran, M., Russell, J. A., Walley, K. R., Brett, S. J., Perkins, G. D., Hajjar, L., ... & Gordon, A. C. (2019). Vasopressin in septic shock: an individual patient data meta-analysis of randomised controlled trials. *Intensive care medicine*, *45*, 844-855.

Namigen, LLC. (2016). Sodium Nitroprusside Injection Prescribing Information.
National Kidney Foundation. (2026). ACE Inhibitors and ARBs. https://www.kidney.org/kidney-topics/ace-inhibitors-and-arbs
Neal B, Perkovic V, Mahaffey KW, de Zeeuw D, Fulcher G, Erondu N, Shaw W, Law G, Desai M, Matthews DR (2017) Canagliflozin and cardiovascular and renal events in type 2 diabetes. N Engl J Med 377:644–657
Nedel, W. L., Rech, T. H., Ribeiro, R. A., Pellegrini, J. A. S., & Moraes, R. B. (2019). Renal outcomes of vasopressin and its analogs in distributive shock: a systematic review and meta-analysis of randomized trials. *Critical Care Medicine*, *47*(1), e44-e51.
Neyra, J. A., Li, X., Canepa-Escaro, F., Adams-Huet, B., Toto, R. D., Yee, J., ... & Acute Kidney Injury in Critical Illness Study Group. (2016). Cumulative fluid balance and mortality in septic patients with or without acute kidney injury and chronic kidney disease. *Critical care medicine*, *44*(10), 1891-1900.
Nissen, S. E., & Wolski, K. (2007). Effect of rosiglitazone on the risk of myocardial infarction and death from cardiovascular causes. *New England Journal of Medicine*, *356*(24), 2457-2471.
Nottestad, S. Y., & Mascette, A. M. (1994). Nitroglycerin-induced heparin resistance: absence of interaction at clinically relevant doses. *Military medicine*, *159*(8), 569-571.
Novartis. (2015). Entresto prescribing information.
Novartis. (2023). Novartis will appeal to U.S. Court of Appeals to uphold validity of Entresto® combination patent; maintains 2023 guidance and mid-term outlook. Retrieved from https://www.novartis.com/news/media-releases/novartis-will-appeal-us-court-appeals-uphold-validity-entresto-combination-patent-maintains-2023-guidance-and-mid-term-outlook
O'Brien, S. K., Koehl, J. L., Demers, L. B., Hayes, B. D., & Barra, M. E. (2023). Safety and tolerability of 23.4% hypertonic saline administered over 2 to 5 minutes for the treatment of cerebral herniation and intracranial pressure elevation. *Neurocritical Care*, *38*(2), 312-319.
Octapharma. (2006). Albumin 5% prescribing information.
O'Gara, P.T., Kushner, F.G., Ascheim, D.D., Casey, D.E., Chung, M.K., de Lemos, J.A., Ettinger, S.M., . . . Zhao, D.X. (2013). 2013 ACCF/AHA guideline for the management of ST-elevation myocardial infarction: a report of the American College of Cardiology Foundation/American Heart Association Task Force on Practice Guidelines. Circulation. 2013;127:e362–e425.
Okuya, Y., Park, J. Y., Garg, A., & Moussa, I. (2021). Coronary artery spasm during catheter ablation caused by the intravenous infusion of isoproterenol. *Internal Medicine*, *60*(8), 1221-1224.Pham, D., Addison, D., Kayani, W., Misra, A., Jneid, H., Resar, J., ... & Alam, M. (2018). Outcomes of beta blocker use in cocaine-associated chest pain: a meta-analysis. *Emergency Medicine Journal*, *35*(9), 559-563.
Ommen, S. R., Ho, C. Y., Asif, I. M., Balaji, S., Burke, M. A., ... & Waldman, C. B. (2024). 2024 AHA/ACC/AMSSM/HRS/PACES/SCMR Guideline for the Management of Hypertrophic Cardiomyopathy: A Report of the American Heart Association/American College of Cardiology Joint Committee on Clinical Practice Guidelines. *Journal of the American College of Cardiology*, *83*(23), 2324-2405.
Omnvium Pharmaceuticals (2024). Isosorbide Mononitrate Prescribing Information.
Opie, L.H. (2013a). Beta blocking agents. In L.H Opie & B.J. Gersh (Eds.), Drugs for the Heart (8th Ed., pp 1-37). Philadelphia: Elsevier.
Opie, L.H. (2013b). Calcium channel blockers. In L.H Opie & B.J. Gersh (Eds.), Drugs for the Heart (8th Ed., pp 64-92). Philadelphia: Elsevier.
Opie, L.H. & Horowitz, J.D. (2013). Nitrates and Newer Antianginals. In L.H Opie & B.J. Gersh (Eds.), *Drugs for the Heart* (8th Ed., pp 38-63). Philadelphia: Elsevier.
Opie L.H., Krum H., Victor R. G, & Kaplan N. M. (2013). Antihypertensive therapies. In L.H. Opie& B.J. Gersh (Eds.) *Drugs for the Heart* (8th Ed., pp.224-271). W.B. Saunders.
Opie, L H., & Pfeffer, M.A. (2013). Inhibitors of the renin-angiotensin-aldosterone system. In L.H Opie & B.J. Gersh (Eds.), Drugs for the Heart (8th Ed., pp 119-168). Philadelphia: Elsevier.
Otto, C.M. (2024). Medical management of symptomatic aortic stenosis. In S.B. Yeon (Ed.), *UptoDate.*
Overgaard, C. B., & Dzavík, V. (2008). Inotropes and vasopressors: review of physiology and clinical use in cardiovascular disease. *Circulation*, *118*(10), 1047-1056.
Packer, M., Anker, S. D., Butler, J., Filippatos, G., Ferreira, J. P., Pocock, S. J., ... & EMPEROR-Reduced Trial Committees and Investigators. (2021). Effect of empagliflozin on the clinical stability of patients with heart failure and a reduced ejection fraction: the EMPEROR-Reduced trial. Circulation, 143(4), 326-336.
Packer, M., Anker, S. D., Butler, J., Filippatos, G., Pocock, S. J., Carson, P., ... & Zannad, F. (2020). Cardiovascular and renal outcomes with empagliflozin in heart failure. New England Journal of Medicine, 383(15), 1413-1424.
Packer, M., Butler, J., Zannad, F., Filippatos, G., Ferreira, J. P., Pocock, S. J., ... & Anker, S. D. (2021). Effect of empagliflozin on worsening heart failure events in patients with heart failure and a preserved ejection fraction: the EMPEROR-Preserved trial. *Circulation.*
Page, R. L., Joglar, J. A., Caldwell, M. A., Conti, J. B., Estes, M. N., Goldberger, Z. D., et al. (2016). 2015 ACC/ACC/HRS Guideline for the Management of Adult Patients with Supraventricular Tachycardia. Circulation, 133, e506-e574.

Page, R. L., O'Bryant, C. L., Cheng, D., Dow, T. J., Ky, B., Stein, C. M., ... & Lindenfeld, J. (2016). Drugs that may cause or exacerbate heart failure: a scientific statement from the American Heart Association. *Circulation*, *134*(6), e32-e69.

Palma, J., & Kaufman, H. (2025). Mechanisms, causes, and evaluation of orthostatic hypotention. In R. P. Goodeau (Ed.), *UptoDate*.

Palmer, B. F.; Clegg, D. J.. Kidney-Protective Effects of SGLT2 Inhibitors. CJASN 18(2):p 279-289, February 2023. | DOI: 10.2215/CJN.09380822

Parke-Davis Division of Pfizer (2018). Nitrostat Prescribing Information.

Parker, J. D., & Gori, T. (2001). Tolerance to organic nitrates: new ideas, new mechanisms, continued mystery. *Circulation*, *104*(19), 2263-2265.

Parker, J. O., Fung, H. L., Ruggirello, D., & Stone, J. A. (1983). Tolerance to isosorbide dinitrate: rate of development and reversal. Circulation, 68(5), 1074-1080.

Patel, M.R., Singh, M, & Gersh, B.J. (2017). ST-segment elevation myocardial infarction. In V. Fuster, R.A. Harrington, J. Narula, Z.J. Eapen (Eds.), Hurst's The Heart (14th ed., pp. 1017-1054). New York: McGraw Hill.

Patel, S., Hickman, A., Frederich, R., Johnson, S., Huyck, S., Mancuso, J. P., ... & Terra, S. G. (2020). Safety of ertugliflozin in patients with type 2 diabetes mellitus: pooled analysis of seven phase 3 randomized controlled trials. *Diabetes Therapy*, *11*(6), 1347-1367.

Perkovic V, Jardine MJ, Neal B, Bompoint S, Heerspink HJL, Charytan DM, Edwards R, Agarwal R, Bakris G, Bull S, Cannon CP, Capuano G, Chu PL, de Zeeuw D, Greene T, Levin A, Pollock C, Wheeler DC, Yavin Y, Zhang H, Zinman B, Meininger G, Brenner BM, Mahaffey KW (2019) Canagliflozin and renal outcomes in type 2 diabetes and nephropathy. N Engl J Med 380: 2295–2306.

Pfizer, Inc, (2008). Eplerenone Prescribing Information.

Pfizer, Inc. (2009). Prazosin Prescribing Information

Pfizer, Inc. (2016). Nitroglycerine in Dextrose Prescribing Information.

Pfizer, Inc. (2021). Doxazosin Prescribing Information

Pfizer, Inc. (2022a). Isosorbide Dinitrate Prescribing information.

Pfizer, Inc. (2022b). Spironolactone Prescribing Information.

Piepho, R. W. (2000). Overview of the angiotensin-converting-enzyme inhibitors. *American journal of health-system pharmacy*, *57*(suppl_1), S3-S7.

Pishdad, Reza, Paul G. Auwaerter, and Rita R. Kalyani. "Diabetes, SGLT-2 Inhibitors, and Urinary Tract Infection: a Review." *Current diabetes reports* 24, no. 5 (2024): 108-117.

Pitt, B., Anker, S. D., Böhm, M., Gheorghiade, M., Køber, L., Krum, H., ... & Filippatos, G. (2015). Rationale and design of MinerAlocorticoid Receptor antagonist Tolerability Study-Heart Failure (ARTS-HF): a randomized study of finerenone vs. eplerenone in patients who have worsening chronic heart failure with diabetes and/or chronic kidney disease. *European journal of heart failure*, *17*(2), 224-232

Plewa MC, Bryant M, King-Thiele R. Euglycemic Diabetic Ketoacidosis. In: StatPearls. StatPearls Publishing, Treasure Island (FL); 2020. PMID: 32119457.

Potura, E., Lindner, G., Biesenbach, P., Funk, G. C., Reiterer, C., Kabon, B., ... & Fleischmann, E. (2015). An acetate-buffered balanced crystalloid versus 0.9% saline in patients with end-stage renal disease undergoing cadaveric renal transplantation: a prospective randomized controlled trial. *Anesthesia & Analgesia*, *120*(1), 123-129.

Prchal, J.T. (2024). Methemoglobinemia. In J.S. Tirnauer (Ed.), *UptoDate.*

Puckrin, R., Saltiel, M. P., Reynier, P., Azoulay, L., Oriana, H. Y., & Filion, K. B. (2018). SGLT-2 inhibitors and the risk of infections: a systematic review and meta-analysis of randomized controlled trials. *Acta diabetologica*, *55*(5), 503-514.

Qasim, A., & Jain, S. K. (2020). Milrinone use in persistent pulmonary hypertension of the newborn. *Neoreviews*, *21*(3), e165-e178.

Radosevich, J. J., Patanwala, A. E., & Erstad, B. L. (2016). Norepinephrine dosing in obese and nonobese patients with septic shock. *American Journal of Critical Care*, *25*(1), 27-32.

Rangaswami, J., Bhalla, V., Blair, J. E., Chang, T. I., Costa, S., Lentine, K. L., ... & American Heart Association Council on the Kidney in Cardiovascular Disease and Council on Clinical Cardiology. (2019). Cardiorenal syndrome: classification, pathophysiology, diagnosis, and treatment strategies: a scientific statement from the American Heart Association. *Circulation*, *139*(16), e840-e878.

Rangel-Castillo, L., Gopinath, S., & Robertson, C. S. (2008). Management of intracranial hypertension. *Neurologic clinics*, *26*(2), 521-541.

Rao, S. V., O'Donoghue, M. L., Ruel, M., Rab, T., Tamis-Holland, J. E., Alexander, J. H., ... & Williams, M. S. (2025). 2025 ACC/AHA/ACEP/NAEMSP/SCAI guideline for the management of patients with acute coronary syndromes: a report of the American College of Cardiology/American Heart Association Joint Committee on Clinical Practice Guidelines. *Journal of the American College of Cardiology*, *85*(22), 2135-2237.

Rasmussen, E. R., Pottegård, A., Bygum, A., von Buchwald, C., Homøe, P., & Hallas, J. (2019). Angiotensin II receptor blockers are safe in patients with prior angioedema related to angiotensin-converting enzyme inhibitors–a nationwide registry-based cohort study. *Journal of internal medicine*, *285*(5), 553-561.

Reeder, G. S. (2022). Angiotensin converting enzyme inhibitors and receptor blockers in acute myocardial infarction: Recommendations for use. In T.F. Dardas (Ed.), *UptoDate.*

Reeder, G.S. (2023). Nitrates in the Management of Acute Coronary Syndrome. In T.F. Dardas (Ed.), *UptoDate.*

Rehnqvist, N., Olsson, G., Engvall, J., Rosenqvist, U., Nyberg, G., Åberg, A., ... & Nilsson, B. (1988). Abrupt withdrawal of isosorbide-5-mononitrate in Durules®(Imdur®) after long term treatment in patients with stable angina pectoris. *European heart journal*, *9*(12), 1339-1347.

Rindone, J. P., & Sloane, E. P. (1992). Cyanide toxicity from sodium nitroprusside: risks and management. *Annals of Pharmacotherapy*, *26*(4), 515-519.

Robben, J. H., Knoers, N. V. A. M., & Deen, P. M. T. (2004). Regulation of the vasopressin V2 receptor by vasopressin in polarized renal collecting duct cells. *Molecular biology of the cell*, *15*(12), 5693-5699.

Rochwerg, B., Alhazzani, W., Gibson, A., Ribic, C. M., Sindi, A., Heels-Ansdell, D., ... & FISSH Group (Fluids in Sepsis and Septic Shock). (2015). Fluid type and the use of renal replacement therapy in sepsis: a systematic review and network meta-analysis. *Intensive care medicine*, *41*, 1561-1571.

Rosenson, R.S., Reeder, G.S. & Kennedy, H.L. (2024). Acute myocardial infarction: role of beta blocker therapy. In T.F. Dardas (Ed.), *UptoDate.*

Rosiak, M., Grzeszczak, S., Kosior, D. A., & Postuła, M. (2014). Emerging treatments in type 2 diabetes: focus on canagliflozin. *Therapeutics and clinical risk management*, *10*, 683.

Ross, D.S. (2024). Overview of the clinical manifestations of hyperthyroidism in adults. In J.E. Mulder (Ed.), *UptoDate.*

Rossing, P., Anker, S. D., Filippatos, G., Pitt, B., Ruilope, L. M., Birkenfeld, A. L., ... & Agarwal, R. (2022a). Finerenone in patients with chronic kidney disease and type 2 diabetes by sodium–glucose cotransporter 2 inhibitor treatment: the FIDELITY analysis. *Diabetes Care*, *45*(12), 2991-2998.

Rossing, P., Caramori, M. L., Chan, J. C., Heerspink, H. J., Hurst, C., Khunti, K., ... & de Boer, I. H. (2022b). KDIGO 2022 clinical practice guideline for diabetes management in chronic kidney disease. *Kidney international*, *102*(5), S1-S127.

Rowell, S. E., Fair, K. A., Barbosa, R. R., Watters, J. M., Bulger, E. M., Holcomb, J. B., ... & PROMMTT Study Group. (2016). The impact of pre-hospital administration of lactated Ringer's solution versus normal saline in patients with traumatic brain injury. *Journal of neurotrauma*, *33*(11), 1054-1059.

Runyon, B.A. (2020). Ascites in adults with cirrhosis: Initial therapy. In M.A. Waltham (Ed.), *UptoDate.*

Ruslan, M. A., Baharuddin, K. A., Noor, N. M., Yazid, M. B., Noh, A. Y. M., & Rahman, A. (2021). Norepinephrine in septic shock: a systematic review and meta-analysis. *Western Journal of Emergency Medicine*, *22*(2), 196.

Russell, J. A. (2019). Vasopressor therapy in critically ill patients with shock. *Intensive care medicine*, *45*(11), 1503-1517.

Russell, J. A., Walley, K. R., Singer, J., Gordon, A. C., Hébert, P. C., Cooper, D. J., ... & Ayers, D. (2008). Vasopressin versus norepinephrine infusion in patients with septic shock. *New England Journal of Medicine*, *358*(9), 877-887.

Rydz, A. C., Elefritz, J. L., Conroy, M., Disney, K. A., Miller, C. J., Porter, K., & Doepker, B. A. (2022). Early initiation of vasopressin reduces organ failure and mortality in septic shock. *Shock*, *58*(4), 269-274.

Sacha, G. L., Lam, S. W., Duggal, A., Torbic, H., Reddy, A. J., & Bauer, S. R. (2018). Hypotension risk based on vasoactive agent discontinuation order in patients in the recovery phase of septic shock. *Pharmacotherapy: The Journal of Human Pharmacology and Drug Therapy*, *38*(3), 319-326.

Sacha, G. L., Lam, S. W., Wang, L., Duggal, A., Reddy, A. J., & Bauer, S. R. (2022). Association of catecholamine dose, lactate, and shock duration at vasopressin initiation with mortality in patients with septic shock. *Critical care medicine*, *50*(4), 614-623.

Sadovsky, R. (2002). Antihypertensive agents and cytochrome p450 interactions. *American Family Physician*, *65*(11), 2356.

SAFE Study Investigators. (2004). A comparison of albumin and saline for fluid resuscitation in the intensive care unit. *New England Journal of Medicine*, *350*(22), 2247-2256.

Sahoo, P., Kothari, N., Goyal, S., Sharma, A., & Bhatia, P. K. (2022). Comparison of norepinephrine and terlipressin vs norepinephrine alone for management of septic shock: a randomized control study. *Indian journal of critical care medicine: peer-reviewed, official publication of Indian Society of Critical Care Medicine*, *26*(6), 669.

Samuel, E., & Lee, J. (2017). Sodium-Glucose Cotransporter 2 Inhibitors: An Overview. *US Pharm*, *42*(10), 42-46.

Saunders, E., & Gavin III, J. R. (2003). Blockade of the renin-angiotensin system in African Americans with hypertension and cardiovascular disease. *The Journal of Clinical Hypertension*, *5*(1), 12-17.

Savage Laboratories (2021). NITRO-BID Nitroglycerine Ointment Prescribing Information

Sawan, Z. H., Soliman, H. M., Mostafa, A. E. A., & Kamel, R. A. (2023). A Review of Nitroglycerin: Present and Future. *The Egyptian Journal of Hospital Medicine*, *91*(1), 4972-4974.

Schulz, L. T., Elder, E. J., Jones, K. J., Vijayan, A., Johnson, B. D., Medow, J. E., & Vermeulen, L. (2010). Stability of sodium nitroprusside and sodium thiosulfate 1: 10 intravenous admixture. *Hospital pharmacy*, *45*(10), 779-784.

Schulz, V., Bonn, R., & Kindler, J. (1979). Kinetics of elimination of thiocyanate in 7 healthy subjects and in 8 subjects with renal failure. *Klinische Wochenschrift*, *57*(5), 243-247.

Schwartz, R. H., Hernandez, S., Noor, N., Topfer, J., Farrell, K., Singh, N., ... & Kaye, A. D. (2022). A comprehensive review of the use of alpha 2 agonists in spinal anesthetics. *Pain physician*, *25*(2), E193.

Scott, J.H., Menouar, M.A., Dunn, R.J. (2023). Physiology, Aldosterone. In: StatPearls [Internet]. Treasure Island (FL): StatPearls Publishing.

Sedhai, Y. R., Shrestha, D. B., Budhathoki, P., Memon, W., Acharya, R., Gaire, S., ... & Kashiouris, M. G. (2022). Vasopressin versus norepinephrine as the first-line vasopressor in septic shock: A systematic review and meta-analysis. *Journal of Clinical and Translational Research*, *8*(3), 185.

Self, W. H., Semler, M. W., Wanderer, J. P., Wang, L., Byrne, D. W., Collins, S. P., ... & Rice, T. W. (2018). Balanced crystalloids versus saline in noncritically ill adults. *New England Journal of Medicine*, *378*(9), 819-828.

Semler, M. W., Self, W. H., Wanderer, J. P., Ehrenfeld, J. M., Wang, L., Byrne, D. W., ... & Rice, T. W. (2018). Balanced crystalloids versus saline in critically ill adults. *New England Journal of Medicine*, *378*(9), 829-839.

Senewiratne, N.L., Woodall, A., Can, A.S. (2024). Sodium Bicarbonate. StatPearls.

Shah, K. B., Inoue, Y., & Mehra, M. R. (2006). Amyloidosis and the heart: a comprehensive review. *Archives of internal medicine*, *166*(17), 1805-1813.

Shah, N. (2025). Ascites in adults with cirrhosis: Initial therapy. In C. Meyer (Ed.), *UptoDate.*

Shastri, P., Burmeister, C., Tomcho, J., Patel, M., Elzanaty, A., Bhuta, S., ... & Beran, A. (2021). Continuous infusion versus intermittent bolus furosemide for acute decompensated heart failure: a systematic review and meta-analysis. *Journal of the American College of Cardiology*, *77*(18_Supplement_1), 616-616.

Shaw, A. D., Bagshaw, S. M., Goldstein, S. L., Scherer, L. A., Duan, M., Schermer, C. R., & Kellum, J. A. (2012). Major complications, mortality, and resource utilization after open abdominal surgery: 0.9% saline compared to Plasma-Lyte. *Annals of surgery*, *255*(5), 821-829.

Sica, D.A. (2004a). Diuretic-Related Side Effects: Development and Treatment. *Medscape.*

Sica, D.A. (2004b). Minoxidil: an underused vasodilator for resistant or severe hypertension. *The Journal of Clinical Hypertension*, *6*(5), 283-287.

Sica, D. A. (2007). Centrally acting antihypertensive agents: an update. *The Journal of Clinical Hypertension*, *9*(5), 399-405.

Sica, D. A. (2015). Centrally acting antihypertensive agents in the treatment of hypertension. In *Pathophysiology and pharmacotherapy of cardiovascular disease* (pp. 853-868). Cham: Springer International Publishing.

Sica, D. A., & Gehr, T. W. (2001). Direct vasodilators and their role in hypertension management: minoxidil. *The Journal of Clinical Hypertension*, *3*(2), 110-114.

Sica, D. A., & Grubbs, R. (2005). Transdermal clonidine: therapeutic considerations. *Journal of clinical hypertension (Greenwich, Conn.)*, *7*(9), 558–562.

Sidhu, G. & Puckett, Y. (2023). Bumetanide. In: StatPearls [Internet]. Treasure Island (FL): StatPearls Publishing.

Silverthorn, D. U. (2016). Isosmotic is not always isotonic: the five-minute version. *Advances in Physiology Education*, *40*(4), 499-500.

Singh, B., Cusick, A. S., Goyal, A., & Patel, P. (2025). ACE inhibitors. In *StatPearls [Internet]*. StatPearls Publishing.

Solomon, S. D., McMurray, J. J., Claggett, B., de Boer, R. A., DeMets, D., Hernandez, A. F., ... & Langkilde, A. M. (2022). Dapagliflozin in heart failure with mildly reduced or preserved ejection fraction. *New England Journal of Medicine*, *387*(12), 1089-1098.

Solomon, S. D., McMurray, J. J., Vaduganathan, M., Claggett, B., Jhund, P. S., Desai, A. S., ... & Viswanathan, P. (2024). Finerenone in heart failure with mildly reduced or preserved ejection fraction. *New England Journal of Medicine*, *391*(16), 1475-1485.

Song, X., Liu, X., Evans, K. D., Frank, R. D., Barreto, E. F., Dong, Y., ... & Kashani, K. B. (2021). The order of vasopressor discontinuation and incidence of hypotension: a retrospective cohort analysis. *Scientific Reports*, *11*(1), 16680.

Spitalewitz S, Porush JG, Oguagha C. Use of oral clonidine for rapid titration of blood pressure in severe hypertension. Chest. 1983 Feb;83(2 Suppl):404-7. doi: 10.1378/chest.83.2_supplement.404. PMID: 6822138.

Sridhar, V. S., Tuttle, K. R., & Cherney, D. Z. (2020). We can finally stop worrying about SGLT2 inhibitors and acute kidney injury. *American journal of kidney diseases: the official journal of the National Kidney Foundation*, *76*(4), 454-456.

Srivastava, U., Sarkar, M. E., Kumar, A., Gupta, A., Agarwal, A., Singh, T. K., ... & Dwivedi, Y. (2014). Comparison of clonidine and dexmedetomidine for short-term sedation of intensive care unit patients. *Indian journal of critical care medicine: peer-reviewed, official publication of Indian Society of Critical Care Medicine*, *18*(7), 431.

Sterns, R.H. (2023a). Diuretic indued hyponatremia. In J.P. Forman (Ed.), *UptoDate.*

Sterns, R.H. (2023b). Causes of hypotonic hyponatremia in adults. In J.P. Forman (Ed.), *UpToDate*.

Sterns, R.H. (2023c). Treatment of hyponatremia: Syndrome of inappropriate diuretic hormone secretion (SIADH) and rest osmostat. In J.P. Forman (Ed.), *UpToDate*.

Sterns, R.H. (2024). Overview of the treatment of hyponatremia in adults. In J.P. Forman (Ed.), *UpToDate*.

Strandvik, G. F. (2009). Hypertonic saline in critical care: a review of the literature and guidelines for use in hypotensive states and raised intracranial pressure. *Anaesthesia*, *64*(9), 990-1003.

Sunwoo, Y. E., Nguyen, P. T. T., Chien, C. M., Ryu, J. Y., Shon, J., & Shin, J. G. (2019). Effect of rifampin on enantioselective disposition and anti-hypertensive effect of benidipine. *British Journal of Clinical Pharmacology*, *85*(4), 737-745.

Suwa, S., Sumiyoshi, M., Mineda, Y., Ohta, H., Kojima, S., & Nakata, Y. (2004). Vasovagal response induced by a low dose of isoproterenol infusion before tilting-up. *Circulation Journal*, *68*(9), 876-877.
Svensson, C. K. (2022). Attenuation of response to repeated drug administration: A proposal for differentiating tachyphylaxis and tolerance. The Journal of Pharmacology and Experimental Therapeutics, 381(1), 22-32.
Taylor, A., Jones, T., Forehand, C. C., Smith, S. E., Dykes, H., & Newsome, A. S. (2022). Vasopressor discontinuation order in septic shock with reduced left ventricular function. *Journal of pharmacy practice*, *35*(6), 879-885.
Taylor, A. L., Ziesche, S., Yancy, C., Carson, P., D'Agostino Jr, R., Ferdinand, K., ... & Cohn, J. N. (2004). Combination of isosorbide dinitrate and hydralazine in blacks with heart failure. *New England Journal of Medicine*, *351*(20), 2049-2057.
Tang, H. L., Li, D. D., Zhang, J. J., Hsu, Y. H., Wang, T. S., Zhai, S. D., & Song, Y. Q. (2016). Lack of evidence for a harmful effect of sodium-glucose co-transporter 2 (SGLT2) inhibitors on fracture risk among type 2 diabetes patients: a network and cumulative meta-analysis of randomized controlled trials. *Diabetes, Obesity and Metabolism*, *18*(12), 1199-1206.
Theracos Bio, LLC. (2023). Bexagliflozin (Brenzavvy) Prescribing Information.
Timlin, H., Wu, M., Crespo-Bosque, M., Geetha, D., Ingolia, A., Haque, U., ... & Grader-Beck, T. (2019). Clinical characteristics of hydralazine-induced lupus. *cureus*, *11*(6).
Tinawi, M. (2021). New trends in the utilization of intravenous fluids. *Cureus*, *13*(4).
Toporek, A. H., Semler, M. W., Self, W. H., Bernard, G. R., Wang, L., Siew, E. D., ... & Casey, J. D. (2021). Balanced crystalloids versus saline in critically ill adults with hyperkalemia or acute kidney injury: secondary analysis of a clinical trial. *American journal of respiratory and critical care medicine*, *203*(10), 1322-1325.
Townsend, R.R. (2022). Major side effects of angiotensin-converting enzyme inhibitors and angiotensin II receptor blockers. In J.P. Forman (Ed.), *UpToDate*.
TruPharma, LLC. (2024). Clonidine Extended Release Prescribing Information.
UptoDate®,Lexidrug™ (2026). Aliskiren.
UptoDate®,Lexidrug™ (2024). Albumin.
UptoDate®,Lexidrug™ (2026). Amiloride.
UptoDate®,Lexidrug™ (2026). Amlodipine.
UptoDate®,Lexidrug™ (2024). Bexagliflozin.
UptoDate®,Lexidrug™ (2026). Bumetanide.
UptoDate®,Lexidrug™ (2024). Canagliflozin.
UptoDate®,Lexidrug™ (2026). Candesartan.
UptoDate®,Lexidrug™ (2026). Carvedilol.
UptoDate®,Lexidrug™ (2026). Chlorothiazide.
UptoDate®,Lexidrug™ (2026). Chlorthalidone.
UptoDate®,Lexidrug™ (2024). Clevidipine.
UptoDate®,Lexidrug™ (2025). Clonidine.
UptoDate®,Lexidrug™ (2026). Conivaptan.
UptoDate®,Lexidrug™ (2024). Dapagliflozin.
UptoDate®,Lexidrug™ (2024). Dextran.
UptoDate®,Lexidrug™ (2026). Diltiazem.
UptoDate®,Lexidrug™ (2024). Dobutamine.
UptoDate®,Lexidrug™ (2024). Dopamine.
UptoDate®,Lexidrug™ (2025). Doxazosin.
UptoDate®,Lexidrug™ (2024). Empagliflozin.
UptoDate®,Lexidrug™ (2026). Enalapril.
UptoDate®,Lexidrug™ (2024). Epinephrine.
UptoDate®,Lexidrug™ (2026). Eplerenone.
UptoDate®,Lexidrug™ (2024). Ertugliflozin.
UptoDate®,Lexidrug™ (2026). Felodipine.
UptoDate®,Lexidrug™ (2026). Finerenone.
UptoDate®,Lexidrug™ (2026). Furosemide.
UptoDate®,Lexidrug™ (2025). Guanfacine.
UptoDate®,Lexidrug™ (2025). Hydralazine.
UptoDate®,Lexidrug™ (2026). Hydrochlorothiazide.
UptoDate®,Lexidrug™ (2026). Irbesartan.
UptoDate®,Lexidrug™ (2024). Isoproterenol.
UptoDate®,Lexidrug™ (2025). Isosorbide Dinitrate.
UptoDate®,Lexidrug™ (2025). Isosorbide Mononitrate.
UptoDate®,Lexidrug™ (2026). Lisinopril.
UptoDate®,Lexidrug™ (2026). Losartan.
UptoDate®,Lexidrug™ (2025). Methyldopa.

UptoDate®,Lexidrug™ (2026). Metoprolol.
UptoDate®,Lexidrug™ (2025). Milrinone.
UptoDate®,Lexidrug™ (2025). Minoxidil.
UptoDate®,Lexidrug™ (2024). Nicardipine.
UptoDate®,Lexidrug™ (2024) Nitroglycerine.
UptoDate®, Lexidrug™ (2024) Nitroprusside.
UptoDate®,Lexidrug™ (2024). Norepinephrine.
UptoDate®,Lexidrug™ (2024). Phenylephrine.
UptoDate®,Lexidrug™ (2025). Prazosin.
UptoDate®,Lexidrug™ (2026). Ramipril.
UptoDate®,Lexidrug™ (2026). Sacubitril and valsartan.
UptoDate®,Lexidrug™ (2026). Sodium chloride preparations.
UptoDate®,Lexidrug™ (2024). Sotagliflozin.
UptoDate®,Lexidrug™ (2026). Spironolactone.
UptoDate®,Lexidrug™ (2025). Terazosin.
UptoDate®,Lexidrug™ (2026). Tolvaptan.
UptoDate®,Lexidrug™ (2026). Torsemide.
UptoDate®,Lexidrug™ (2026). Triamterene.
UptoDate®,Lexidrug™ (2026). Valsartan.
UptoDate®,Lexidrug™ (2026). Verapamil.

Vadiei, N., Daley, M. J., Murthy, M. S., & Shuman, C. S. (2017). Impact of norepinephrine weight-based dosing compared with non–weight-based dosing in achieving time to goal mean arterial pressure in obese patients with septic shock. *Annals of Pharmacotherapy*, *51*(3), 194-202.

Valeant Pharmaceuticals North America LLC (2015) Isosorbide Dinitrate Prescribing information.

Vanholder, R., Carpentier, J., Schurgers, M., & Clement, D. L. (1977). Rebound phenomenon during gradual withdrawal of clonidine. *British Medical Journal*, *1*(6069), 1138.

Vargas Pelaez, A. F., Gao, Z., Ahmad, T. A., Leuenberger, U. A., Proctor, D. N., Maman, S. R., & Muller, M. D. (2016). Effect of adrenergic agonists on coronary blood flow: a laboratory study in healthy volunteers. *Physiological reports*, *4*(10), e12806.

Varon, J. & Elliott, W. J. (2025). Management of severe hypertension (hypertensive urgencies) in adults. In J.P. Forman (ED), *UptoDate.*

Verresen, L., Fink, E., Lemke, H. D., & Vanrenterghem, Y. (1994). Bradykinin is a mediator of anaphylactoid reactions during hemodialysis with AN69 membranes. *Kidney international*, *45*(5), 1497-1503.

Vincent, J. L., & De Backer, D. (2013). Circulatory shock. *New England Journal of Medicine*, *369*(18), 1726-1734.

Wang, J. G., Belley-Coté, E., Burry, L., Duffett, M., Karachi, T., Perri, D., ... & Rochwerg, B. (2017). Clonidine for sedation in the critically ill: a systematic review and meta-analysis. *Critical Care*, *21*(1), 75.

Wang, K. M., & Isom, R. T. (2020). SGLT2 inhibitor–induced euglycemic diabetic ketoacidosis: A case report. *Kidney Medicine*, *2*(2), 218-221.

Wang, M. T., Su, C. Y., Chan, A. L., Lian, P. W., Leu, H. B., & Hsu, Y. J. (2010). Risk of digoxin intoxication in heart failure patients exposed to digoxin–diuretic interactions: a population-based study. *British journal of clinical pharmacology*, *70*(2), 258-267.

Wang, Y. H., Huang, L. C., Tsai, S. H. L., Chen, Y. J., Wu, C. L., & Kang, Y. N. (2022). Risk of intraoperative floppy iris syndrome among selective alpha-1 blockers—A consistency model of 6,488 cases. *Frontiers in Medicine*, *9*, 941130.

Watts, N. B., Bilezikian, J. P., Usiskin, K., Edwards, R., Desai, M., Law, G., & Meininger, G. (2016). Effects of canagliflozin on fracture risk in patients with type 2 diabetes mellitus. *The Journal of Clinical Endocrinology*, *101*(1), 157-166.

Weinstein, J., Girard, L. P., Lepage, S., McKelvie, R. S., & Tennankore, K. (2021). Prevention and management of hyperkalemia in patients treated with renin–angiotensin–aldosterone system inhibitors. *Cmaj*, *193*(48), E1836-E1841.

Welsh, T. J., & Mitchell, A. (2023). Centrally acting antihypertensives and alpha-blockers in people at risk of falls: therapeutic dilemmas—a clinical review. *European geriatric medicine*, *14*(4), 675-682.

Westfall, T. C., Macarthur, H. & Westfall, D.P. (2018). Adrenergic Agonists and Antagonists. In L.L. Brunton, R. Hilal-Dandan, B.C. Knollmann (Eds.), Goodman & Gilman's The Pharmacological Basis of Therapeutics (13th Ed., pp 191-224). New York: McGraw Hill.

Whelton, P. K., Carey, R. M., Aronow, W. S., Casey, D. E., Collins, K. J., Dennison Himmelfarb, C., ... & Wright, J. T. (2018). 2017 ACC/AHA/AAPA/ABC/ACPM/AGS/APhA/ASH/ASPC/NMA/PCNA guideline for the prevention, detection, evaluation, and management of high blood pressure in adults: a report of the American College of Cardiology/American Heart Association Task Force on Clinical Practice Guidelines. *Journal of the American College of Cardiology*, *71*(19), e127-e248.

White, W.B. (2024) Treatment of hypertension in patients with diabetes mellitus. In: Nathan, D.M. (Ed), *UpToDate.*

Wilkes, MM, & Navickis, RJ. (2001). Patient survival after human albumin administration: a meta-analysis of randomized, controlled trials. *Ann Intern Med*, *135*(3), 149.

Williams, B., Mancia, G., Spiering, W., Rosei, E.A., Azizi, M,. Burnier, M., Clement, D.L., . . . Desormais, I. (2018). 2018 ESC/ESH guidelines for the management of arterial hypertension. European Heart Journal, 39, 3021-3104.

Wiviott, S. D., Raz, I., Bonaca, M. P., Mosenzon, O., Kato, E. T., Cahn, A., ... & Sabatine, M. S. (2019). Dapagliflozin and cardiovascular outcomes in type 2 diabetes. *New England Journal of Medicine*, *380*(4), 347-357.

Wrenn, K. (1990). The hazards of defibrillation through nitroglycerin patches. *Annals of emergency medicine*, *19*(11), 1327-1328.

Xu, Q. Y., Jin, Y. H., Fu, L., & Li, Y. Y. (2025). Application of norepinephrine in the treatment of septic shock: A meta-analysis. *Irish Journal of Medical Science (1971-)*, *194*(1), 361-369.

Yancy, C. W., Jessup, M., Bozkurt, B., Butler, J., Casey, D. E., Drazner, M. H., ... & Wilkoff, B. L. (2013). 2013 ACCF/AHA guideline for the management of heart failure: executive summary: a report of the American College of Cardiology Foundation/American Heart Association Task Force on practice guidelines. *Journal of the American College of Cardiology*, *62*(16), 1495-1539.

Yao, R. Q., Xia, D. M., Wang, L. X., Wu, G. S., Zhu, Y. B., Zhao, H. Q., ... & Yao, Y. M. (2020). Clinical efficiency of vasopressin or its analogs in comparison with catecholamines alone on patients with septic shock: a systematic review and meta-analysis. *Frontiers in pharmacology*, *11*, 563.

Yasaei, R, & Saadabadi, A.(2023). Clonidine. [Updated 2023 Jul 17]. In: StatPearls [Internet]. Treasure Island (FL): StatPearls Publishing.

Yokogawa, N., & Vivino, F. B. (2009). Hydralazine-induced autoimmune disease: comparison to idiopathic lupus and ANCA-positive vasculitis. *Modern rheumatology*, *19*(3), 338-347.

Yuan, Z., DeFalco, F. J., Ryan, P. B., Schuemie, M. J., Stang, P. E., Berlin, J. A., ... & Rosenthal, N. (2018). Risk of lower extremity amputations in people with type 2 diabetes mellitus treated with sodium-glucose co-transporter-2 inhibitors in the USA: a retrospective cohort study. *Diabetes, Obesity and Metabolism*, *20*(3), 582-589.

Zampieri, F. G., Machado, F. R., Biondi, R. S., Freitas, F. G., Veiga, V. C., Figueiredo, R. C., ... & Pfingsten, L. E. (2021). Effect of intravenous fluid treatment with a balanced solution vs 0.9% saline solution on mortality in critically ill patients: the BaSICS randomized clinical trial. *Jama*, *326*(9), 818-829.

Zarychanski, R., Abou-Setta, A. M., Turgeon, A. F., Houston, B. L., McIntyre, L., Marshall, J. C., & Fergusson, D. A. (2013). Association of hydroxyethyl starch administration with mortality and acute kidney injury in critically ill patients requiring volume resuscitation: a systematic review and meta-analysis. *Jama*, *309*(7), 678-688.

Zhang, F., Wang, W., & Hou, X. (2021). Effectiveness and safety of ertugliflozin for type 2 diabetes: a meta-analysis data from randomized controlled trials. *Journal of Diabetes Investigation*.

Zhang, Y., He, D., Zhang, W., Xing, Y., Guo, Y., Wang, F., ... & Lin, S. (2020). ACE inhibitor benefit to kidney and cardiovascular outcomes for patients with non-dialysis chronic kidney disease stages 3–5: a network meta-analysis of randomised clinical trials. *Drugs*, *80*(8), 797-811.

Ziaeian, B., Fonarow, G. C., & Heidenreich, P. A. (2017). Clinical effectiveness of hydralazine–isosorbide dinitrate in African-American patients with heart failure. *JACC: Heart Failure*, *5*(9), 632-639.

Zinman, B., Wanner, C., Lachin, J. M., Fitchett, D., Bluhmki, E., Hantel, S., ... & Inzucchi, S. E. (2015). Empagliflozin, cardiovascular outcomes, and mortality in type 2 diabetes. *New England Journal of Medicine*, *373*(22), 2117-2128.

Zisman, A. L. (2024). Thiazides for nephrolithiasis prevention: written in stone? *American Journal of Kidney Diseases*, *84*(2), 241-243.

Zuraw, B. (2022). An overview of angioedema: clinical features, diagnosis, and management. In S. Sarbjit (Ed.), *UptoDate*.

Note: FDA = U.S. Food and Drug Administration.

Index

A

D

E

F

G

H

I

L

M

S

T

V

W